Multimodality Treatments in Metastatic Gastric Cancer

Multimodality Treatments in Metastatic Gastric Cancer

Editor

Angelica Petrillo

MDPI • Basel • Beijing • Wuhan • Barcelona • Belgrade • Manchester • Tokyo • Cluj • Tianjin

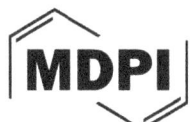

Editor
Angelica Petrillo
Medical Oncology Unit
Ospedale del Mare
Naples
Italy

Editorial Office
MDPI
St. Alban-Anlage 66
4052 Basel, Switzerland

This is a reprint of articles from the Special Issue published online in the open access journal *Journal of Clinical Medicine* (ISSN 2077-0383) (available at: https://www.mdpi.com/journal/jcm/special_issues/Gastric_Treatments).

For citation purposes, cite each article independently as indicated on the article page online and as indicated below:

LastName, A.A.; LastName, B.B.; LastName, C.C. Article Title. *Journal Name* **Year**, *Volume Number*, Page Range.

ISBN 978-3-0365-2592-1 (Hbk)
ISBN 978-3-0365-2593-8 (PDF)

Cover image courtesy of Sandro Iovanella

© 2021 by the authors. Articles in this book are Open Access and distributed under the Creative Commons Attribution (CC BY) license, which allows users to download, copy and build upon published articles, as long as the author and publisher are properly credited, which ensures maximum dissemination and a wider impact of our publications.

The book as a whole is distributed by MDPI under the terms and conditions of the Creative Commons license CC BY-NC-ND.

Contents

About the Editor vii

Angelica Petrillo
Multimodality Treatment in Metastatic Gastric Cancer: Working Together to Tailor the Continuum of Care
Reprinted from: *J. Clin. Med.* **2021**, *10*, 5492, doi:10.3390/jcm10235492 1

Gianpaolo Marte, Andrea Tufo, Francesca Steccanella, Ester Marra, Piera Federico, Angelica Petrillo and Pietro Maida
Efficacy of Surgery for the Treatment of Gastric Cancer Liver Metastases: A Systematic Review of the Literature and Meta-Analysis of Prognostic Factors
Reprinted from: *J. Clin. Med.* **2021**, *10*, 1141, doi:10.3390/jcm10051141 5

Angelica Petrillo, Emilio Francesco Giunta, Annalisa Pappalardo, Davide Bosso, Laura Attademo, Cinzia Cardalesi, Anna Diana, Antonietta Fabbrocini, Teresa Fabozzi, Pasqualina Giordano, Margaret Ottaviano, Mario Rosanova, Antonia Silvestri, Piera Federico and Bruno Daniele
Bone Metastases from Gastric Cancer: What We Know and How to Deal with Them
Reprinted from: *J. Clin. Med.* **2021**, *10*, 1777, doi:10.3390/jcm10081777 29

Valentina Gambardella, Tania Fleitas, Noelia Tarazona, Federica Papaccio, Marisol Huerta, Susana Roselló, Francisco Gimeno-Valiente, Desamparados Roda and Andrés Cervantes
Precision Medicine to Treat Advanced Gastroesophageal Adenocarcinoma: A Work in Progress
Reprinted from: *J. Clin. Med.* **2020**, *9*, 3049, doi:10.3390/jcm9093049 55

Michele Ghidini, Angelica Petrillo, Andrea Botticelli, Dario Trapani, Alessandro Parisi, Anna La Salvia, Elham Sajjadi, Roberto Piciotti, Nicola Fusco and Shelize Khakoo
How to Best Exploit Immunotherapeutics in Advanced Gastric Cancer: Between Biomarkers and Novel Cell-Based Approaches
Reprinted from: *J. Clin. Med.* **2021**, *10*, 1412, doi:10.3390/ jcm10071412 71

Csongor György Lengyel, Sadaqat Hussain, Dario Trapani, Khalid El Bairi, Sara Cecilia Altuna, Andreas Seeber, Andrew Odhiambo, Baker Shalal Habeeb and Fahmi Seid
The Emerging Role of Liquid Biopsy in Gastric Cancer
Reprinted from: *J. Clin. Med.* **2021**, *10*, 2108, doi:10.3390/jcm10102108 95

Irene Y. Chong, Naureen Starling, Alistair Rust, John Alexander, Lauren Aronson, Marta Llorca-Cardenosa, Ritika Chauhan, Asif Chaudry, Sacheen Kumar, Kerry Fenwick, Ioannis Assiotis, Nik Matthews, Ruwaida Begum, Andrew Wotherspoon, Monica Terlizzo, David Watkins, Ian Chau, Christopher J. Lord, Syed Haider, Sheela Rao and David Cunningham
The Mutational Concordance of Fixed Formalin Paraffin Embedded and Fresh Frozen Gastro-Oesophageal Tumours Using Whole Exome Sequencing
Reprinted from: *J. Clin. Med.* **2021**, *10*, 215, doi:10.3390/jcm10020215 111

**Margherita Rimini, Annarita Pecchi, Francesco Prampolini, Chiara Bussei,
Massimiliano Salati, Daniela Forni, Francesca Martelli, Filippo Valoriani, Fabio Canino,
Alessandro Bocconi, Fabio Gelsomino, Linda Reverberi, Stefania Benatti, Federico Piacentini,
Renata Menozzi, Massimo Dominici, Gabriele Luppi and Andrea Spallanzani**
The Prognostic Role of Early Skeletal Muscle Mass Depletion in Multimodality Management of Patients with Advanced Gastric Cancer Treated with First Line Chemotherapy: A Pilot Experience from Modena Cancer Center
Reprinted from: *J. Clin. Med.* **2021**, *10*, 1705, doi:10.3390/jcm10081705 . . . . **123**

**Silvia Catanese, Giacomo Aringhieri, Caterina Vivaldi, Francesca Salani, Saverio Vitali,
Irene Pecora, Valentina Massa, Monica Lencioni, Enrico Vasile, Rachele Tintori,
Francesco Balducci, Alfredo Falcone, Carla Cappelli and Lorenzo Fornaro**
Role of Baseline Computed-Tomography-Evaluated Body Composition in Predicting Outcome and Toxicity from First-Line Therapy in Advanced Gastric Cancer Patients
Reprinted from: *J. Clin. Med.* **2021**, *10*, 1079, doi:10.3390/jcm10051079 . . . . **139**

About the Editor

Angelica Petrillo, MD. Bio: Dr Angelica Petrillo graduated in 2012 from the University of study of Campania "L. Vanvitelli" with the best grade, laude, special mention and recommendation for publication. Then, she graduated in 2018 as Medical Oncology specialist at the University of study of Campania "L. Vanvitelli" with the best grade cum laude. During her career, Dr Petrillo has attended international institutes of research in the field of gastrointestinal tumours, such as the Medical Oncology Unit of Hospital Clinico Universitario of Valencia (Spain), under the guide of Prof. A. Cervantes and the gastrointestinal Unit of the Addenbrooke's Hospital-Cambridge University NHS Foundation Trust (UK), under the supervision of Dr E. Smyth. She is the recipient of many prizes and grants: prize as best students of University of study of Campania "L.Vanvitelli" in 2009, grant to attend a clinical research unit in Italy in 2011 (Medical Oncology Unit of Policlinico S.Orsola-Malpighi, Bologna), prize for the best oral abstract presentation during the XX GOIM Congress in 2018, grant as fellow into the ESMO Clinical Unit Fellowship program. Currently, Dr Petrillo is a consultant in Medical Oncology at the Medical Oncology Unit of Ospedale del Mare in Naples (Italy). She is specialized in the treatment of gastrointestinal cancers and she is in charge of the Gastric cancer multidisciplinary team at the hospital. Dr. Petrillo is the principal investigator and sub-investigator in many phase II and III national and international clinical trials in the field of gastrointestinal cancers, presenter at national and international congresses and author in various national and international publications and abstracts. Dr Petrillo is a peer reviewer for several international papers. She is a member of various medical associations, such as ESMO, AIOM, EORTC GI group, ASCO, Women4Oncology. Additionally, she is attending the ESMO Leader Generation program course; she is the representative for AIOM young oncologists in her region and one of the administrator of the international ONCOLLEGE community, with the aim to enhance access to the best education possibilities in oncology through an evidence-based and value-driven approach, especially for colleagues from low and middle-income countries.

Journal of Clinical Medicine

Editorial

Multimodality Treatment in Metastatic Gastric Cancer: Working Together to Tailor the Continuum of Care

Angelica Petrillo

Medical Oncology Unit, Ospedale del Mare, 80147 Naples, Italy; angelic.petrillo@gmail.com

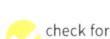

Citation: Petrillo, A. Multimodality Treatment in Metastatic Gastric Cancer: Working Together to Tailor the Continuum of Care. *J. Clin. Med.* 2021, *10*, 5492. https://doi.org/10.3390/jcm10235492

Academic Editor: Emmanuel Andrès

Received: 15 November 2021
Accepted: 22 November 2021
Published: 24 November 2021

Publisher's Note: MDPI stays neutral with regard to jurisdictional claims in published maps and institutional affiliations.

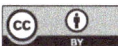

Copyright: © 2021 by the author. Licensee MDPI, Basel, Switzerland. This article is an open access article distributed under the terms and conditions of the Creative Commons Attribution (CC BY) license (https://creativecommons.org/licenses/by/4.0/).

Gastric cancer (GC) represents one of the most frequent and lethal tumors worldwide today, finding itself in fifth place in terms of incidence and third in terms of mortality [1]. Surgery remains the only curative treatment for localized tumors, but only 20% of patients are suitable for surgery due to the lack of specific symptoms and the late diagnosis, especially in Western countries [2]. Additionally, even in patients who receive curative treatment, the rates of locoregional relapse and distant metastases remain high [3]. Palliative chemotherapy is the principal treatment in cases of metastatic disease; however, the prognosis of patients receiving chemotherapy is still poor. In this context, one of the most important conceptual achievements of the last few decades in the field of metastatic GC is represented by the "continuum of care", meaning the possibility to treat patients with multiple subsequent lines of therapy in order to obtain longer survival. In fact, almost 40% of patients receiving first-line treatment for metastatic disease maintain a good performance status after progression; they are able to receive a second and even a third line of treatment. Additionally, there is an unmet need for a better understanding of genetic alterations and prognostic and predictive factors in metastatic GC that could be useful when choosing the best-tailored therapy for each patient [4].

Therefore, a multidisciplinary evaluation is crucial in order to individualize treatment for patients with metastatic GC—according to the concept of precision medicine—and to define the right sequence of treatment from the diagnosis—according to the concept of "continuum of care". Taking all these facts into account, the aim of this Special Issue was to focus on the results and problems of multimodality treatment in metastatic GC, the search for prognostic and predictive factors, and the evaluation of novel strategies for individualized treatment.

In this regard, the management of patients with oligometastatic GC is challenging. In particular, the treatment for patients with only liver metastases is changing and the latest advances in the research in this field suggest a potential role for multimodality treatment, including curative surgery. In this Special Issue, Marte, G. et al. [5] provided a systematic review and metanalysis of 40 studies with the aim of evaluating the efficacy of hepatectomy for metastatic GC with liver metastases. The authors showed that an approach consisting of the resection of the primary tumor alongside liver metastases by hepatectomy is feasible in this population and provides benefits in terms of long-term survival. However, the clear definition of oligometastatic disease and the role of multimodality treatment for these patients are still a matter of debate; clinical trials are ongoing in this setting. Additionally, a strict selection of patients that could benefit from curative surgery is mandatory and requires a multidisciplinary evaluation.

In the field of metastatic GC today, it is still unclear how the metastatic sites may affect the prognosis and little evidence exists regarding the impact of rare metastatic locations (e.g., lung, bone and brain). Therefore, a narrative review regarding the role of bone metastases in GC and their potential implication in treatment choice was also included in this Special Issue [6].

A nutritional assessment is crucial in the multidisciplinary evaluation of metastatic GC patients. However, few data about the link between nutritional status and survival are available in this field and the role of sarcopenia in metastatic GC is controversial today. In this Special Issue, Rimini, M. et al. [7] evaluated the prognostic role of tissue modifications (assessed using computed tomography) during treatment in 40 metastatic GC patients and the benefit of a scheduled nutritional assessment in this setting. Interestingly, the authors showed that an early skeletal muscle mass depletion >10% in the first months of treatment significantly influenced the overall survival ($p = 0.0023$). Additionally, Catanese, S. et al. [8] investigated the role of baseline computed-tomography-evaluated body composition in predicting the outcome and toxicity of first-line therapy in 78 advanced GC patients. In this paper, even if sarcopenia failed to show an association with the outcomes, skeletal muscle mass depletion was linked to the development of high-grade neutropenia ($p = 0.048$) and mucositis ($p = 0.054$). On the other hand, the fat distribution (visceral versus subcutaneous) exhibits a robust impact on survival.

However, although GC has been considered as a single entity for a long time, nowadays it is acknowledged that it represents a heterogeneous disease, deserving to be treated according to the own peculiarities of each subtype. Based on this background, several molecular classifications have been developed over the last few decades in an attempt to select molecular alterations, which might act as a driver for each subtype [4].

In this context, the application of sequencing has led to the identification of aberrant druggable pathways and somatic mutations within therapeutically relevant genes in GC. However, since the majority of those evaluations use formalin-fixed paraffin-embedded (FFPE) samples, an assessment of the concordance between comprehensive exome-wide sequencing data from archival FFPE samples would be beneficial in order to find some potential biomarker in GC. In this regard, Chong, I.Y. et al. [9] reported in this Special Issue the analysis of whole-exome sequencing data from 16 matched fresh-frozen and FFPE gastro-esophageal tumors (N = 32) with the aim of defining the mutational concordance. The authors found a high median mutational concordance (97%) between fresh-frozen and FFPE gastro-esophageal tumor-derived exomes, suggesting that comprehensive genomic data can be generated from the exome sequencing of selected DNA samples extracted from archival FFPE samples.

The molecular peculiarities of GC subtypes can influence the treatment choice in the metastatic setting. Based on that, Gambardella, V. et al. [10] provided a comprehensive overview of the role of precision medicine in metastatic GC. In particular, the authors described the novel pathways implicated in GC and the state of the art of target therapies in those tumors, according to molecular classifications and alterations. Even if the road toward a personalized approach requires further studies, this paper underlined the importance of molecular selection to use tailored treatments for metastatic GC.

In this scenario, the development of immunotherapy could also represent a promising strategy in a selected population affected by metastatic GC. In this Special Issue, Ghidini, M. et al. [11] conducted an update of the predictive biomarkers of response to immunotherapy in GC. Additionally, the authors provided an overview regarding the translational meaning of those findings in the practice, alongside descriptions of the landmark and ongoing clinical trials in this field.

Lastly, one of the most important frontiers in the GC scenario is represented by the development and use of liquid biopsy, both in localized and metastatic disease. In this Special Issue, Lengyel, C.G. et al. [12] summarized the state of the art and future application of liquid biopsy in GC, showing that, although preliminary results are promising, more research is required to obtain better insights into the molecular mechanisms, as well as to validate and standardize the methods for liquid biopsy.

In conclusion, the papers collected in this Special Issue highlight that the treatment of metastatic GC is challenging. A careful and comprehensive evaluation of these patients by a multidisciplinary team in dedicated and high-volume centers is crucial in order to improve the outcomes. The multidisciplinary evaluation should include a nutritional assessment, since sarcopenia and fat distributions might affect the prognosis and the rate of drug toxicities, as well as the evaluation of metastases' distribution and the definition of oligometastatic disease, which is at the forefront of metastatic GC research today. In this context, the role of surgery as part of a multimodal strategy for metastatic disease is improving. We should consider that GC is a very heterogeneous disease; therefore, we should attempt to treat each patient according to the tumor and patient characteristics, which lead to the choice of a unique and personalized treatment journey, based on the milestone concepts of precision medicine and a continuum of care.

However, the journey to discover the molecular mechanisms that control GC behavior has just started and further investigation is still required. Thus, working together as a multidisciplinary team including different professional figures, such as oncologists, nutritionists, surgeons, pathologists, radiotherapists, gastroenterologists, etc., is the only way to achieve proper patient care in the complex and evolving landscape of metastatic GC.

Conflicts of Interest: The author received personal fees from Eli-Lilly, Servier, Merck and MSD. No fees are connected with the submitted paper.

References

1. Sung, H.; Ferlay, J.; Siegel, R.L.; Laversanne, M.; Soerjomataram, I.; Jemal, A.; Bray, F. Global cancer statistics 2020: GLOBOCAN estimates of incidence and mortality worldwide for 36 cancers in 185 countries. *CA Cancer J. Clin.* **2021**, *71*, 209–249. [CrossRef] [PubMed]
2. De Vita, F.D.; Tirino, G.; Pompella, L.; Petrillo, A. Gastric Cancer: Advanced/Metastatic Disease. In *Practical Medical Oncology Textbook*; Russo, A., Peeters, M., Incorvaia, L., Rolfo, C., Eds.; Springer: Cham, Switzerland, 2021; pp. 587–604.
3. Petrillo, A.; Smyth, E.C. Multimodality treatment for localized gastric cancer: State of the art and new insights. *Curr. Opin. Oncol.* **2020**, *32*, 347–355. [CrossRef] [PubMed]
4. Petrillo, A.; Smyth, E.C. Biomarkers for Precision Treatment in Gastric Cancer. *Visc. Med.* **2020**, *36*, 364–372. [CrossRef] [PubMed]
5. Marte, G.; Tufo, A.; Steccanella, F.; Marra, E.; Federico, P.; Petrillo, A.; Maida, P. Efficacy of Surgery for the Treatment of Gastric Cancer Liver Metastases: A Systematic Review of the Literature and Meta-Analysis of Prognostic Factors. *J. Clin. Med.* **2021**, *10*, 1141. [CrossRef] [PubMed]
6. Petrillo, A.; Giunta, E.F.; Pappalardo, A.; Bosso, D.; Attademo, L.; Cardalesi, C.; Diana, A.; Fabbrocini, A.; Fabozzi, T.; Giordano, P.; et al. Bone Metastases from Gastric Cancer: What We Know and How to Deal with Them. *J. Clin. Med.* **2021**, *10*, 1777. [CrossRef] [PubMed]
7. Rimini, M.; Pecchi, A.; Prampolini, F.; Bussei, C.; Salati, M.; Forni, D.; Martelli, F.; Valoriani, F.; Canino, F.; Bocconi, A.; et al. The Prognostic Role of Early Skeletal Muscle Mass Depletion in Multimodality Management of Patients with Advanced Gastric Cancer Treated with First Line Chemotherapy: A Pilot Experience from Modena Cancer Center. *J. Clin. Med.* **2021**, *10*, 1705. [CrossRef] [PubMed]
8. Catanese, S.; Aringhieri, G.; Vivaldi, C.; Salani, F.; Vitali, S.; Pecora, I.; Massa, V.; Lencioni, M.; Vasile, E.; Tintori, R.; et al. Role of Baseline Computed-Tomography-Evaluated Body Composition in Predicting Outcome and Toxicity from First-Line Therapy in Advanced Gastric Cancer Patients. *J. Clin. Med.* **2021**, *10*, 1079. [CrossRef] [PubMed]
9. Chong, I.Y.; Starling, N.; Rust, A.; Alexander, J.; Aronson, L.; Llorca-Cardenosa, M.; Chauhan, R.; Chaudry, A.; Kumar, S.; Fenwick, K.; et al. The Mutational Concordance of Fixed Formalin Paraffin Embedded and Fresh Frozen Gastro-Oesophageal Tumours Using Whole Exome Sequencing. *J. Clin. Med.* **2021**, *10*, 215. [CrossRef] [PubMed]
10. Gambardella, V.; Fleitas, T.; Tarazona, N.; Papaccio, F.; Huerta, M.; Roselló, S.; Gimeno-Valiente, F.; Roda, D.; Cervantes, A. Precision Medicine to Treat Advanced Gastroesophageal Adenocarcinoma: A Work in Progress. *J. Clin. Med.* **2020**, *9*, 3049. [CrossRef] [PubMed]
11. Ghidini, M.; Petrillo, A.; Botticelli, A.; Trapani, D.; Parisi, A.; La Salvia, A.; Sajjadi, E.; Piciotti, R.; Fusco, N.; Khakoo, S. How to Best Exploit Immunotherapeutics in Advanced Gastric Cancer: Between Biomarkers and Novel Cell-Based Approaches. *J. Clin. Med.* **2021**, *10*, 1412. [CrossRef]
12. Lengyel, C.G.; Hussain, S.; Trapani, D.; El Bairi, K.; Altuna, S.C.; Seeber, A.; Odhiambo, A.; Habeeb, B.S.; Seid, F. The Emerging Role of Liquid Biopsy in Gastric Cancer. *J. Clin. Med.* **2021**, *10*, 2108. [CrossRef] [PubMed]

Review

Efficacy of Surgery for the Treatment of Gastric Cancer Liver Metastases: A Systematic Review of the Literature and Meta-Analysis of Prognostic Factors

Gianpaolo Marte [1,*], Andrea Tufo [1], Francesca Steccanella [1], Ester Marra [1], Piera Federico [2], Angelica Petrillo [2] and Pietro Maida [1]

1. Department of General Surgery, Ospedale del Mare, 80147 Naples, Italy; tufo.andrea@gmail.com (A.T.); fra.steccanella@gmail.com (F.S.); estermarra9@gmail.com (E.M.); p.maida@libero.it (P.M.)
2. Medical Oncology Unit, Ospedale del Mare, 80147 Naples, Italy; pierafederico@yahoo.it (P.F.); angelic.petrillo@gmail.com (A.P.)
* Correspondence: gianpaolo.marte@gmail.com; Tel.: +39-08118775110

Abstract: Background: In the last 10 years, the management of patients with gastric cancer liver metastases (GCLM) has changed from chemotherapy alone, towards a multidisciplinary treatment with liver surgery playing a leading role. The aim of this systematic review and meta-analysis is to assess the efficacy of hepatectomy for GCLM and to analyze the impact of related prognostic factors on long-term outcomes. Methods: The databases PubMed (Medline), EMBASE, and Google Scholar were searched for relevant articles from January 2010 to September 2020. We included prospective and retrospective studies that reported the outcomes after hepatectomy for GCLM. A systematic review of the literature and meta-analysis of prognostic factors was performed. Results: We included 40 studies, including 1573 participants who underwent hepatic resection for GCLM. Post-operative morbidity and 30-day mortality rates were 24.7% and 1.6%, respectively. One-year, 3-years, and 5-years overall survival (OS) were 72%, 37%, and 26%, respectively. The 1-year, 3-years, and 5-years disease-free survival (DFS) were 44%, 24%, and 22%, respectively. Well-moderately differentiated tumors, pT1–2 and pN0–1 adenocarcinoma, R0 resection, the presence of solitary metastasis, unilobar metastases, metachronous metastasis, and chemotherapy were all strongly positively associated to better OS and DFS. Conclusion: In the present study, we demonstrated that hepatectomy for GCLM is feasible and provides benefits in terms of long-term survival. Identification of patient subgroups that could benefit from surgical treatment is mandatory in a multidisciplinary setting.

Keywords: gastric cancer; liver metastasis; conversion surgery; hepatectomy; stage iv gastric cancer

1. Introduction

Gastric cancer (GC) is the fourth most common cancer worldwide and the second among cancer deaths [1]. Distant metastases are found in 30–35% of patients at their first clinical observation and they spread commonly to the liver (48% of metastatic cancer patients), peritoneum (32%), lung (15%), and bone (12%). Patients with stage IV GC have a median survival of 3 months, which is worst among those with bone and liver metastases (2 months) [2]. According to current guidelines, systemic chemotherapy is recommended as a single modality treatment for stage IV GC [3]. However, despite the development of new molecular targeting agents, the prognosis remains unsatisfactory, with a reported median overall survival (OS) of 13.8 months [4,5].

The role of surgical resection of GC metastases has always been debated. However, in the last 10 years, many studies showed encouraging results. Recently, Yoshida et al. proposed a new classification of stage IV GC, dividing the stage IV in four categories which results in different treatment approaches (Figure 1) [6]. Gastric cancer liver metastases (GCLM) without peritoneal carcinomatosis belong to categories 1 and 2; in those patients, the authors suggest using the so-called "conversion therapy", which consists of intensive chemotherapy followed by adjuvant surgery if radical resection is achievable. In addition, the last revision of the Japanese Gastric Cancer guidelines stated that hepatectomy can be considered for a subset of patients such as cases with solitary liver metastasis [7]. This approach is also endorsed by the Italian Group on Gastric Cancer Research [8].

		Stage IV Gastric Cancer	
Macroscopic Peritoneal Dissemination (-)	Category 1	Potentially resectable metastasis	Resectable one liver metastasis or few para-aortic lymph node (16a2,b1) or CY1
	Category 2	Marginally resectable metastasis	Liver mets > 1 or tumor size > 5 cm, close to vein or distant mets (lung, Virchow) or para-aortic lymph node (16a1,b1)
Macroscopic Peritoneal Dissemination (+)	Category 3	Incurable and unresectable metastasis (except for local palliation needs)	Other organ (-)
	Category 4	Non-curable metastasis	Other organ (+)

Figure 1. Yoshida categories for stage IV gastric cancer (GC).

However, GC patients often present with metastases in multiple sites and only 0.4–1% of patients have liver metastases amenable to radical resection [7]. Most recent reports in the literature showed promising results after adopting aggressive multidisciplinary management, including surgery, to treat patients with GCLM [9].

In our study, we performed a systematic review of the literature of the last decade to evaluate the OS and disease-free survival (DFS) after hepatectomy for GCLM, and a meta-analysis of the prognostic factors, in order to clarify which patients would benefit more from surgical treatment.

2. Materials and Methods

A systematic review protocol was registered at the International Prospective Register of Systematic Reviews (PROSPERO): database registration number CRD42021218350 [10]. This study is reported in compliance with the Transparent Reporting of Systematic Reviews and Meta-analyses (PRISMA) statement [11].

2.1. Criteria for Considering Studies for This Review

2.1.1. Type of Studies

We included prospective and retrospective studies reporting survival outcomes after hepatectomy for GCLM. We have selected only studies involving humans and available as full text in English published in the last decade. We excluded case reports, animal and other experimental, as well as purely imaging studies.

2.1.2. Type of Participants

We included studies where all participants who had hepatectomy for GCLM were eligible for upfront radical resection (R0) of both primary tumor and metastasis in the liver. In order to avoid selection bias, studies including participants with metastatic sites other than the liver were excluded.

2.1.3. Type of Interventions and Outcomes

We included only studies in which there were reported short-term outcomes (postoperative morbidity and 30-day mortality) and long-term outcomes (1-, 3-, 5-years OS and DFS) after hepatectomy for GCLM. We investigated the impact of the prognostic factors collected from the studies on OS and DFS.

2.2. Search Methods for Identification of Studies

2.2.1. Electronic Searches

Two independent reviewers (G.M. and F.S.) performed a systematic search of the literature, from January 2010 to September 2020. The authors did not consider previous articles as the management of gastric liver metastases has changed significantly over the last decade.

We searched the PubMed (Medline), Cochrane, EMBASE, and Google Scholar databases using MeSH and free text words (tw) for GC and liver metastases.

We performed the search using different combinations of the following keywords: "gastric AND cancer AND hepatectomy", "gastric AND cancer AND metastases" "gastric AND cancer AND metastasectomy", "stomach AND cancer AND hepatectomy", "stomach AND cancer AND metastasectomy". The same search was then repeated changing the word "cancer" with "carcinoma", "cancer" with "neoplasm", "metastases with "metastasis", and "hepatectomy" with "liver resection".

2.2.2. Searching Other Resources

We also checked the references of the selected studies in order to find further relevant trials.

2.3. Data Collection and Analysis

Two authors (G.M. and F.S.) independently selected studies and two authors (G.M. and A.T.) extracted data from those trials in a pre-piloted data extraction form created using Microsoft Excel (Microsoft, Redmond, WA, USA).

Study Selection

Study selection was performed by first screening the titles and abstracts in order to exclude the studies that were clearly not eligible. Then, using the predefined inclusion and exclusion criteria, the full texts of the studies were screened. Figure 2 illustrates the flow-chart diagram of the study selection.

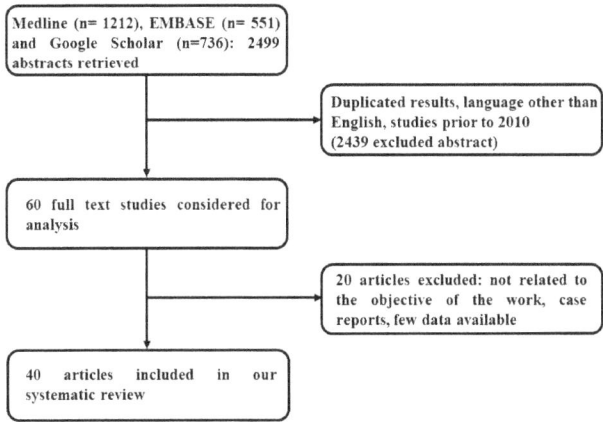

Figure 2. Flow-chart diagram of the study selection.

Then, some papers were excluded after discussion between the two reviewers (G.M. and F.S.), because they were not strictly linked to the topic of the review.

Ethical approval and informed consent were not needed for this paper as per local rules at our institution.

2.4. Literature Search

2.4.1. Data Extraction and Management

Two independent reviewers performed data collection (G.M. and A.T.) and included the following data:

1. Year of publication.
2. Country of recruitment.
3. Study interval (year(s) in which the trial was conducted).
4. Inclusion and exclusion criteria.
5. Population details, such as age, sex, characteristics of the primary tumor, and liver metastases.
6. Outcomes (mentioned in 'Type of interventions and outcomes').
7. Details of the prognostic factor(s).

The reviewer extract survival data from tables, directly from the text whenever possible or by manual interpolation in case of data available only in graphs. The clarification of unclear or missing information was done by direct contact with the authors of each study. We solved any differences in opinion through discussion.

2.4.2. Assessment of Risk of Bias in Included Studies

Due to the nature of this systematic review, the study quality or risk of bias was assessed by the Oxford Centre for Evidence-Based Medicine (CEBM) classification only for descriptive purposes [12].

2.4.3. Data Synthesis

One, three, and five-year OS and DFS were calculated as the proportion of patients alive and free from the tumor at 1, 3, and 5 years and the total of patients included in the study. Median Survival Time (MST) was also calculated. StatsDirect Software (StatsDirect Ltd., Birkenhead, UK) was used to calculate the meta-analysis of proportion [13].

Hazard ratio (HR) with corresponding 95% confidence intervals (95% CIs) were calculated to assess the impact on OS and DFS of the liver metastases related prognostic factors using the inverse variance method with Review Manager 5.4 (Cochrane Collaboration) [14].

The HR and its variance were obtained from the study or calculated according to the data presentation: annual mortality rates, survival curves, number of deaths, or percentage freedom from death [15].

A random-effects model was used to perform a meta-analysis due to the clinical heterogeneity among studies. Funnel plots were used to graphically represent publication bias and in order to find asymmetry and any outliers. Heterogeneity across the studies was assessed using the Cochran Q test and/or the I^2 statistic to measure the degree of variation not attributable to chance alone. This was graded as low ($I^2 < 25\%$), moderate ($I^2 = 25\%$ to 75%), or high ($I^2 > 75\%$) [16].

A significant *p* value < 0.05 was considered in order to assess statistically significant differences in each analysis. Forest plots showed the results of the current meta-analysis. Calculations were performed by A.T. and verified by G.M.

2.4.4. Subgroup Analysis

We performed a subgroup analysis of the OS and DFS based on ethnicity. One, three, and five-year OS and DFS were calculated as the proportion of patients alive and free from tumor at 1, 3, and 5 years and the total patients included in the study. StatsDirect Software was used to calculate the meta-analysis of proportion [17].

3. Results

We identified 2499 references through electronic searches of Medline (n = 1212), EMBASE (n = 551), and Google Scholar (n = 736). We excluded 2439 duplicates and clearly irrelevant references through reading the abstracts. The remaining 60 records were retrieved as full text for further assessment. Then, we discharged the other 4 references (for further details, see the section "Characteristic of excluded studies" below). At least, 40 studies were included in the study and were finally analyzed.

3.1. Characteristics of the Included Studies

The 40 included studies [8,18–57] included 1573 participants who underwent hepatic resection for GCLM. All studies were reported in English. All studies were retrospective analyses. No prospective studies or randomized trials were found (Tables 1 and 2). The majority of the studies were conducted in Asia (33 studies: 82.5%), whereas only 7 trials included data from Western countries (17.5%).

The median age of the whole population was 64 years old (range 30–89), the majority of whom were men (1050 participants, 66.8%). Two hundred eighty-five participants (30.3%) had pT1–2 and 656 (69.7%) pT3–4 gastric adenocarcinoma in 26 studies reporting this data. Four hundred twenty participants (37%) had pN0–1 and 714 (63%) pN2–3 gastric adenocarcinoma in 25 studies reporting this data. Lymphatic invasion was present in 230 patients (48%) included in 10 studies, whereas 216 patients (53.7%) included in 7 studies had a venous invasion. Nine studies reported the size of the primary tumor: 94 participants (37.3%) had primary tumor <5 cm and 158 (62.3%) >5 cm (median 5.2 cm). The tumor was poorly differentiated in 236 patients (16.4%), whereas it was well or moderately differentiated in 1201 (83.6%) participants in 19 studies reporting this data. Six hundred twelve participants (63.4%) underwent surgical resection for solitary hepatic metastasis and 354 (36.6%) were treated for multiple hepatic metastases in 27 studies reporting this data. Three hundred fifteen participants (78.5%) underwent surgical resection for unilobar hepatic metastases and 86 (21.5%) were treated for bilobar hepatic metastases in 13 studies reporting this data. Eight hundred seventy-six participants (62.3%) underwent surgical resection for synchronous liver metastases and 529 (37.7%) were treated for metachronous hepatic metastases in 33 studies reporting this data.

The median time between gastrectomy and the onset of hepatic metastases was 12.5 months (range 7–135) in 12 studies reporting this data.

The median size of the hepatic metastases was 28 mm (range 17–160 mm) and 52 participants (57.7%) had liver tumor >3 cm and 38 <3cm (42.3%) in 18 studies reporting this data. Seven hundred ninety-nine participants (77%) underwent minor hepatectomy and 239 (23%) major hepatectomy in 18 studies reporting this data. A total of 757 participants (86.3%) underwent R0 hepatic resection, 72 (8.2%) had R1 resection, and 48 (5.5%) R2 in 12 studies reporting this data.

One hundred fifty-one participants (12.3%) underwent neoadjuvant whereas 610 (48.6%) underwent adjuvant chemotherapy in 30 studies reporting this data.

Table 1. Patient characteristics according to the primary tumor.

Author Year	Country	Study Design	Study Interval	N. Patients	Median Age	Female/Male	pT1-2/pT3-4	pN0-1/pN2-3	Lymphatic Invasion	Venous Invasion	Primary Tumor Median Size (cm)	Histology Well-Moderate/Poor Differentiated
Choi 2010 [57]	Korea	Retro	1986–2007	14	65	NR	NR	NR	NR	NR	NR	NR
Makino 2010 [58]	Japan	Retro	1992–2007	16	NR	3/13	NR/8	NR/13	12	14	NR	8/8
Tsujimoto 2010 [19]	Japan	Retro	1980–2007	17	66	1/16	12/5	12/5	8	9	5.7	NR
Dittmar 2012 [4]	Germany	Retro	1995–2009	10	57	NR	NR	NR	11	NR	NR	NR
Garancini 2012 [41]	Italy	Retro	1998–2007	21	64	7/14	NR/8	19/11	NR	13	NR	8/13
Liu J. 2012 [51]	China	Retro	1995–2010	35	NR	8/29	19/16	12/23	10	NR	NR	0/25
Miki 2012 [52]	Japan	Retro	1995–2009	25	72	2/23	8/17	14/11	NR	NR	NR	NR
Schildberg 2012 [53]	Germany	Retro	1972–2008	31	65	11/20	NR	NR	NR	NR	NR	NR
Takemura 2012 [54]	Japan	Retro	1993–2011	64	65	49/15	NR/49	22/42	NR	NR	NR	42/22
Wang Y.N. 2012 [55]	China	Retro	2003–2008	30	60	3/27	4/26	10/20	NR	NR	3.7	NR
Baek 2013 [56]	Korea	Retro	1998–2009	12	61	1/11	3/9	9/3	7	2	NR	9/1
Chen 2013 [20]	China	Retro	2007–2012	20	54	8/12	6/14	12/8	NR	NR	NR	16/4
Qiu 2013 [1]	China	Retro	1998–2009	25	NR	3/22	17/8	4/21	NR	NR	NR	9/16
Vigano 2013 [2]	Italy	Retro	1997–2008	14	61.5	NR	NR	NR	NR	NR	NR	NR
Aizawa 2014 [7]	Japan	Retro	1997–2010	74	66	18/56	NR	NR	NR	NR	NR	NR
Komeda 2014 [24]	Japan	Retro	2000–2012	24	69.5	3/21	17/7	10/14	NR	NR	NR	23/16
Wang W. 2014 [25]	China	Retro	1996–2008	39	64	13/26	8/31	23/16	NR	NR	NR	NR
Guner 2015 [26]	Korea	Retro	1998–2013	68	61	12/56	17/52	32/36	35	36	NR	NR
Kinoshita 2015 [27]	Japan	Retro	1990–2010	256	64	49/207	74	54/204	105	129	NR	173/NR
Li Z. 2015 [28]	China	Retro	2008–2011	13	NR	NR	NR	NR	NR	NR	NR	NR
Liu Q. 2015 [29]	China	Retro	1990–2009	35	56	13/22	6/29	4/31	20	NR	NR	15/20
Ohkura 2015 [61]	Japan	Retro	1985–2014	13	63	0/13	NR	NR	NR	NR	NR	NR
Shinohara 2015 [32]	Japan	Retro	1995–2010	18	NR	NR	NR	NR	NR	NR	NR	NR
Markar 2016 [3]	UK	Retro	1997–2012	78	65	51/7	NR	NR	NR	NR	NR	NR
Oguro 2016 [44]	Japan	Retro	2002–2012	26	69.5	3/23	8/18	NR/8	NR	NR	NR	18/8
Tatsubayashi 2016 [45]	Japan	Retro	2004–2014	28	72	5/23	8/20	3/25	NR	NR	5.6	22/6
Tiberio 2016 [5]	Italy	Retro	1990–2013	105	68	34/71	38/46	36/40	NR	NR	NR	NR
Fukami 2017 [36]	Japan	Retro	2001–2012	14	66	3/11	2/12	NR/11	NR	NR	NR	11/3
Lee J.W. 2017 [37]	Korea	Retro	2000–2014	7	59.2	2/5	NR	NR	NR	NR	NR	NR
Li J. 2017 [8]	China	Retro	2006–2016	30	NR	NR	NR	NR	NR	NR	NR	NR
Li S.C. 2017 [9]	Taiwan	Retro	1996–2012	34	62	11/23	NR	NR	NR	NR	NR	NR
Ryu 2017 [46]	Japan	Retro	1997–2005	14	NR	NR	NR	NR	NR	NR	NR	NR
Song 2017 [42]	China	Retro	2001–2012	96	63	24/72	47/59	28/68	NR	NR	NR	62/34
Ministrini 2018 [43]	Italy	Retro	1990–2017	144	68	50/94	23/93	48/68	NR	NR	NR	13/22
Nishi 2018 [44]	Japan	Retro	2001–2013	10	71.7	1/9	8/2	NR	NR	NR	NR	NR
Shirasu 2018 [45]	Japan	Retro	2004–2015	9	74	1/8	NR	NR	NR	NR	NR	11/3
Gao 2019 [5]	China	Retro	1975–2013	54	57	11/43	29/25	18/36	NR	NR	NR	9/NR
Nonaka 2019 [51]	Japan	Retro	2016	10	68	1/9	3/7	7/3	8	NR	NR	NR
Kawahara 2020 [48]	Japan	Retro	2006–2016	20	73.5	7/13	NR/4	8/12	14	13	NR	14/3
Tang 2020 [49]	China	Retro	2008–2018	20	61	4/16	2/18	10/10	NR	NR	NR	0/12

Abbreviations: retro: retrospective; NR: not reported.

Table 2. Patient Characteristics according to liver metastases.

Author Year	Synchronous/Metachronous	Solitary/Multiple	Unilobar/Bilobar	Median Size Liver Metastases (mm)	Minor/Major Hepatectomy	R0/R1/R2 Liver Resection Margin	Neoadjuvant/Adjuvant Chemotherapy
Choi 2010 [ ]	0/14	9/5	NR	NR	NR	NR	NR
Makino 2010 [ ]	9/7	9/7	11/5	NR	14/2	NR	5/9
Tsujimoto 2010 [ ]	9/8	13/4	NR	48	NR	NR	0/14
Dittmar 2012 [ ]	12/9	NR	NR	26	8/2	NR	0/NR
Garancini 2012 [ ]	12/9	12/9	16/5	30	17/4	19/2/0	NR
Liu J 2012 [ ]	NR	NR	NR	NR	NR	NR	NR
Miki 2012 [ ]	16/9	18/7	20/5	20	NR	NR	0/10
Schildberg 2012 [ ]	17/14	NR	NR	NR	21/10	23/3/5	2/9
Takemura 2012 [ ]	32/32	37/27	NR	NR	50/14	55/9/0	18/26
Wang Y.N. 2012 [ ]	30/0	22/8	27/3	31	23/7	NR	0/30
Baek 2013 [ ]	3/9	10/1	NR	NR	9/3	11/1/0	NR/6
Chen 2013 [ ]	20/0	8/12	11/9	41	6/14	NR	20/20
Qiu 2013 [ ]	25/0	19/6	21/4	20	NR	NR	4/14
Vigano 2013 [ ]	9/5	9/5	NR	NR	NR	NR	8/0
Aizawa 2014 [ ]	74/0	NR	NR	NR	NR	53/0/21	NR
Komeda 2014 [ ]	1/23	17/	NR	28	NR	NR	11/15
Wang W. 2014 [ ]	39/0	31/8	34/5	27	NR	NR	0/39
Guner 2015 [ ]	26/42	45/23	60/8	30	47/21	NR	0/66
Kinoshita 2015 [ ]	106/150	168/88	NR	NR	183/73	230/26/0	45/84
Li Z. 2015 [ ]	13/0	NR	NR	NR	NR	NR	13/NR
Liu Q. 2015 [ ]	35/0	27/8	30/5	NR	29/6	30/5/0	0/35
Ohkura 2015 [ ]	9/4	4/9	NR	NR	NR	NR	0/12
Shinohara 2015 [ ]	NR	NR	NR	NR	NR	NR	NR
Markar 2016 [ ]	78/0	16/10	NR	37	66/12	NR	NR
Oguro 2016 [ ]	6/20	20/8	NR	24.5	27/1	NR	3/12
Tatsubayashi 2016 [ ]	15/13	9/5	NR	NR	94/11	89/7/9	0/29
Tiberio 2016 [ ]	74/31	5/2	NR	28	NR	NR	NR/14
Fukami 2017 [ ]	1/13	NR	6/1	NR	NR	NR	0/6
Lee J.W. 2017 [ ]	NR	NR	NR	NR	30/0/0	30/0/0	NR
Li J. 2017 [ ]	0/34	NR	NR	NR	NR	NR	NR
Li S.C. 2017 [ ]	NR	NR	NR	42	7/7	NR	NR
Ryu 2017 [ ]	59/37	42/54	57/29	NR	61/35	91/5/0	0/58
Song 2017 [ ]	112/32	NR	NR	NR	132/12	117/14/13	20/32
Ministrini 2018 [ ]	6/4	6/4	NR	23.5	5/5	NR	2/6
Nishi 2018 [ ]	6/3	0/9	5/4	25	NR	9/0/0	NR/3
Shirasu 2018 [ ]	NR	38/16	NR	NR	NR	NR	0/24
Gao 2019 [ ]	4/6	7/3	NR	NR	NR	NR	0/0
Nonaka 2019 [ ]	11/9	11/9	NR	25	NR	NR	0/20
Tang 2020 [ ]	19/1	NR	17/3	29	NR	NR	0/17

Abbreviations: NR: not reported.

3.2. Characteristics of the Excluded Studies, Risk of Bias, and Applicability Concerns

Three studies were excluded because authors included also patients with peritoneal metastasis [58–60].

Data from one study were excluded from all the analyses because the authors did not specify if the patients underwent liver resection or other treatments (Radiofrequency ablation (RFA), Microwave ablation, others) [60]. Data from 4 studies were included from the analysis of the short-term outcomes (morbidity and mortality) but excluded from the analysis of the OS, DFS, and the analysis of the prognostic factors because the authors did not specify if the patients underwent liver resection or other treatments [33,39,41,42].

All the studies included in the analysis had a type 2b quality of evidence, according to the Oxford Centre for Evidence-Based Medicine scoring system.

3.3. Discrimination Results

3.3.1. Morbidity and Mortality

Surgical resection of GCLM was performed with 24.7% of morbidity from the 19 studies reporting this data (250/1011) and 1.6% of 30-day mortality from the 30 studies reporting this data (22/1338). Short- and long-term outcomes are shown in Table 3.

3.3.2. Survival Data

After a median follow-up of 26 months (range 8–77), the 1-year, 3-year, and 5-year OS were 72% (range 66–77%), 37% (range 31–43%), and 26% (range 21–30%), respectively (Figure 3).

The 1-year, 3-year and 5-year DFS were 44% (range 40–48%), 24% (range 19–29%), and 22% (range 15–31%), respectively (Figure 4).

Subgroup meta-analyses based on ethnicity were performed (Figures 5 and 6). Eastern studies showed better 1-year (75% vs. 59%), (HR 0.38, 0.29–0.49, $p < 0.00001$, I^2 78.9%), 3-year (39% vs. 28%) (HR 0.44, 0.32–0.60, $p < 0.00001$, I^2 72.3%), and 5 year (27% vs. 19%) (HR 0.36, 0.21–0.60, $p = 0.0001$, I^2 66.2%) OS. The results of the DFS for Eastern and Western studies at 1 year (42% vs. 28%) (HR 1.26, 0.85–1.86, $p = 0.25$, I^2 4.8%) and 3 years (25% vs. 21%) (HR 0.69, 0.43–1.11, $p = 0.13$, I^2 46.2%) were similar, while the 5-year DFS was better in the Eastern studies (25% vs. 10%) (HR 0.29, 0.15–0.54, $p = 0.0001$, I^2 77.9%).

The analysis of the funnel plots showed the presence of a slight asymmetry. However, even if the presence of a small study bias cannot be excluded at all, the data suggest that it seems unlikely.

Heterogeneity was significant, so the variability cannot be related only to ethnicity.

3.3.3. Analysis of Prognostic Factors

The results of the meta-analysis of prognostic factors are shown in Tables 4 and 5.

Table 3. Short- and long-term outcomes after hepatectomy.

Author Year	Post-Operative Morbidity (%)	Post-Operative 30-Day Mortality (%)	Overall Survival				Disease-Free Survival			
			1 Year (%)	3 Years (%)	5 Years (%)	MST (Months)	1 Year (%)	3 Years (%)	5 Years (%)	MST (Months)
Choi 2010 [57]	NR	NR	67	38.3	NR	NR	28.5	NR	NR	NR
Makino 2010 [58]	NR	0	82.3	46.4	37.1	31.2	NR	NR	NR	NR
Tsujimoto 2010 [59]	NR	NR	75	37.5	31.5	34	NR	NR	NR	NR
Dittmar 2012 [60]	NR	0	NR	NR	NR	NR	NR	NR	NR	NR
Garancini 2012 [41]	19	0	68	31	19	11	51	25	14	NR
Liu J. 2012 [51]	NR	NR	58.1	21.7	NR	15	NR	NR	NR	5
Miki 2012 [62]	NR	NR	73.9	42.8	36.7	33.4	NR	NR	NR	NR
Schildberg 2012 [53]	29	6	NR	NR	13	NR	42	27	NR	9
Takemura 2012 [54]	27	0	84	50	37	34	NR	NR	NR	NR
Wang Y.N. 2012 [65]	13	0	43.3	16.7	16.7	11	NR	NR	NR	NR
Baek 2013 [66]	NR	0	65	NR	39	31	NR	NR	NR	NR
Chen 2013 [20]	NR	0	NR	NR	15	22.3	NR	NR	NR	NR
Qiu 2013 [21]	NR	0	96	70.4	29.4	38	56	22.3	11.1	18
Vigano 2013 [22]	40	0	95	63.2	33.2	52.3	NR	NR	NR	NR
Aizawa 2014 [23]	NR	0	NR	NR	17	13	NR	NR	NR	NR
Komeda 2014 [24]	NR	0	78.3	40.1	40.1	22.3	NR	NR	NR	NR
Wang W 2014 [25]	8	0	56.4	17.9	10.3	14	30.8	10.3	7.7	8
Guner 2015 [26]	28	1	79.1	40.6	30	24	49.3	30.4	26	NR
Kinoshita 2015 [27]	11	2	77.3	41.9	31.1	31.1	43.6	32.4	30.1	9.4
Li Z. 2015 [28]	NR	0	NR	NR	NR	16.3	NR	NR	NR	NR
Liu Q. 2015 [29]	6	0	NR	NR	14.3	33	NR	NR	NR	NR
Ohkura 2015 [31]	NR	0	NR	NR	NR	NR	NR	NR	NR	NR
Shinohara 2015 [32]	NR	0	NR	NR	38.5	NR	NR	NR	NR	NR
Markar 2016 [33]	NR	10	64.1	NR	13.9	20.1	NR	NR	NR	16.8
Oguro 2016 [34]	NR	NR	NR	NR	32	49	NR	NR	29	NR
Tatsubayashi 2016 [35]	4	0	NR	20.3	13.1	14.6	48	20.2	8.6	10
Tiberio 2016 [8]	13	1	58.2	42.9	42.9	27.9	NR	NR	NR	NR
Fukami 2017 [36]	21	0	71.4	NR	68.6	67.5	NR	NR	80	74.1
Lee J.W. 2017 [37]	29	NR	NR	NR	NR	NR	–	–	NR	–
Li J. 2017 [38]	NR	0	–	36.9	24.5	26.16	NR	NR	NR	NR
Li S.C. 2017 [39]	NR	NR	73.5	51.3	51.3	NR	NR	NR	NR	NR
Ryu 2017 [40]	NR	0	84.6	47.6	21.7	34	NR	NR	NR	NR
Song 2017 [42]	55	0	87.5	19.4	11.6	12	NR	NR	NR	NR
Ministrini 2018 [43]	22	2	49.5	17.8	NR	21.5	20	NR	NR	4.7
Nishi 2018 [44]	10	0	88.9							

Table 3. Cont.

Author Year	Post-Operative Morbidity (%)	Post-Operative 30-Day Mortality (%)	Overall Survival				Disease-Free Survival			
			1 Year (%)	3 Years (%)	5 Years (%)	MST (Months)	1 Year (%)	3 Years (%)	5 Years (%)	MST (Months)
SHIRASU 2018 [47]	44	0	NR	NR	NR	24.8	NR	NR	NR	7.9
Gao 2019 [50]	NR	NR	77.8	37	25.9	29.3	NR	NR	NR	NR
Nonaka 2019 [51]	NR	NR	78	33.3	22.2	30	44.4	22.2	22.2	NR
Kawahara 2020 [48]	0	0	80	55.5	31.7	42	35	24	18	10.5
Tang 2020 [49]	25	15	NR	23.5	NR	20	NR	23.5	NR	NR

Abbreviations: MST: median survival time; NR: not reported.

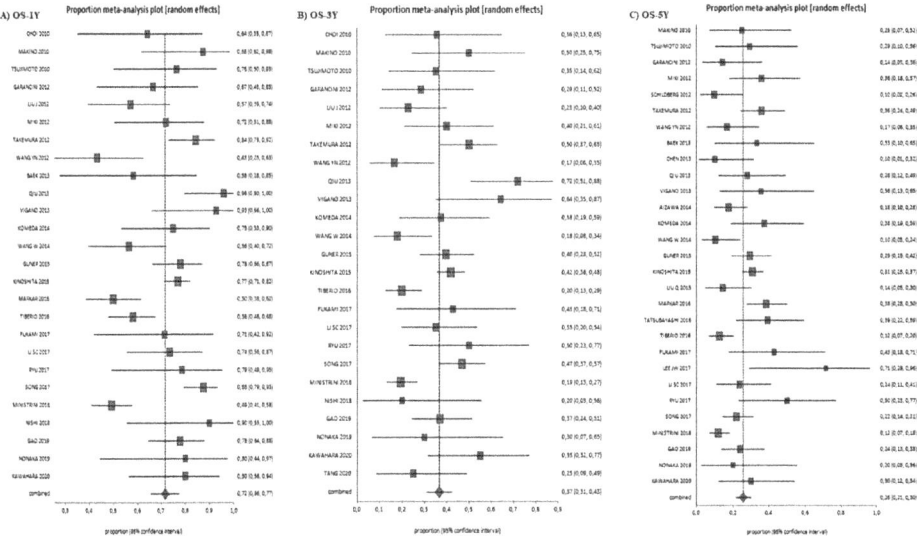

Figure 3. Overall survival results. (**A**): 1-year OS, (**B**): 3-years OS, (**C**): 5-year OS.

Nevertheless, we could not include all the studies due to missing data. The analysis demonstrated that the primary cancer factors associated with higher OS were well-moderately differentiated tumors, pT1–2 and pN0–1 adenocarcinoma. Chemotherapy was also a strong prognostic factor as well as R0 resections. Considering the burden of the disease, the presence of solitary metastasis, unilobar and metachronous metastases were all strongly positively associated with OS. On the contrary, older age, sex, size of primary tumor or metastasis, and the presence of lymphatic or venous invasion by the primary tumor were not significantly associated with OS.

The factors associated with a higher DFS were pT1–pT2 primary cancers, the absence of lymphatic invasion by the primary tumors, metachronous liver metastases, solitary metastasis, and the size of liver metastasis <3 cm. However, for the analysis of the prognostic factors related to DFS, less than 5 studies reported the results for each outcome.

The majority of the analyses had mild or low levels of heterogeneity, suggesting that the impact of those prognostic factors on OS and DFS is quite similar despite the well-known differences in the studies.

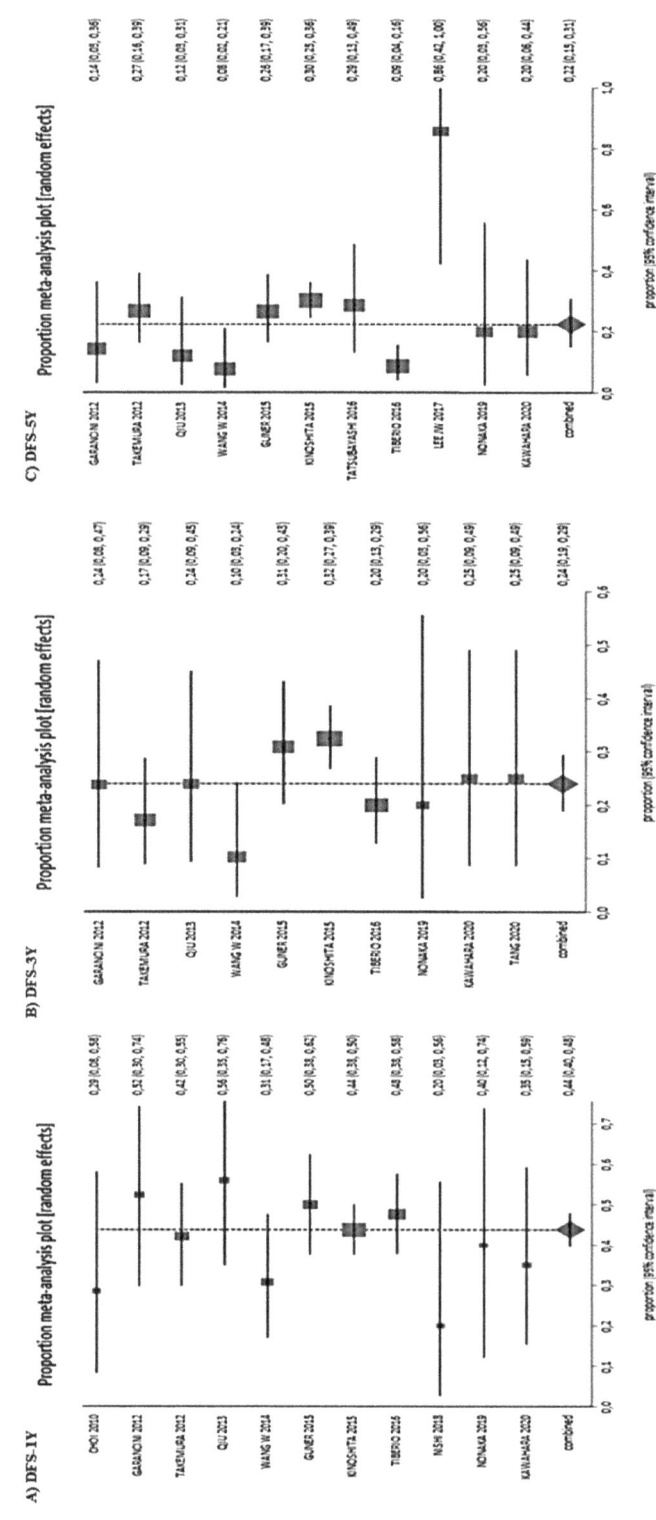

Figure 4. Disease-free survival results. (**A**): 1-year DFS, (**B**): 3-year-DFS, (**C**): 5-year DFS.

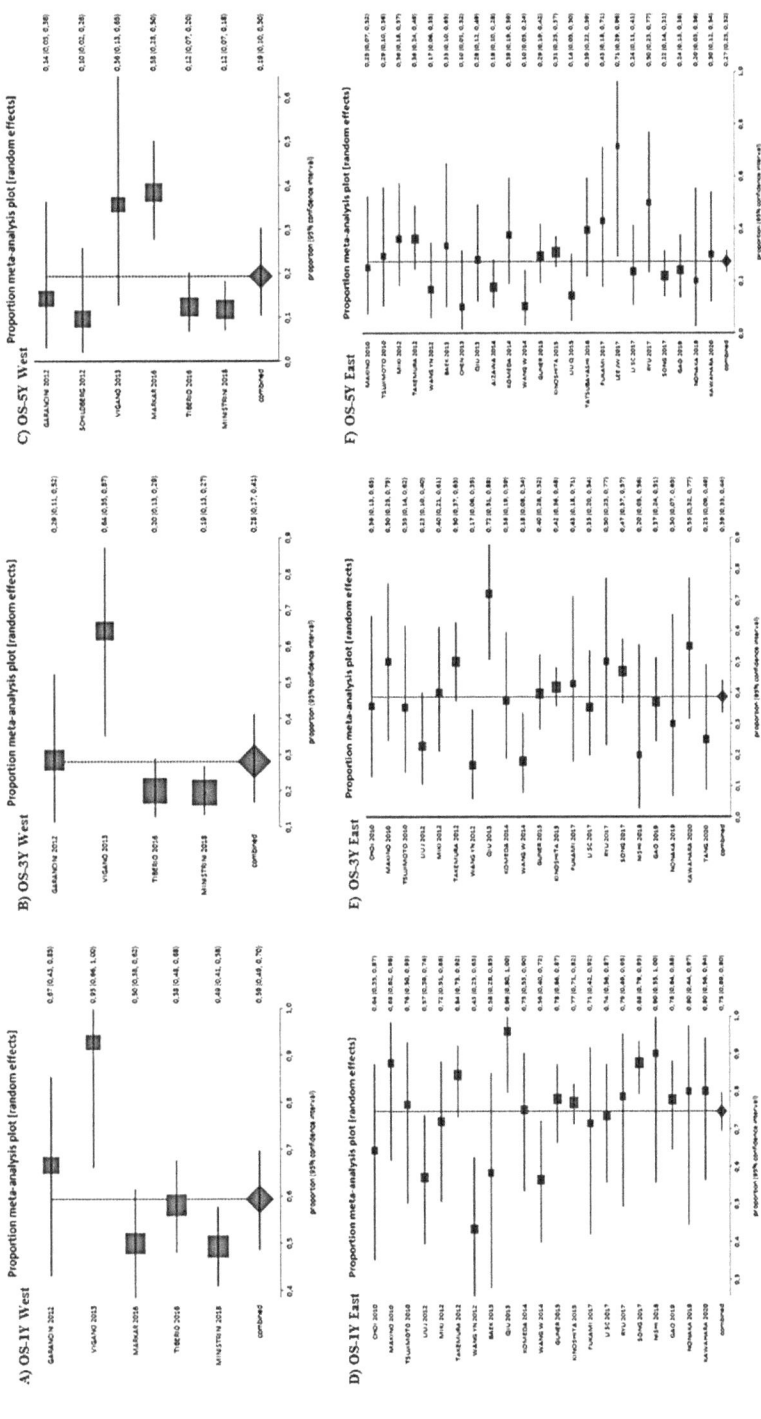

Figure 5. Overall survival according to subgroup analysis (Asian versus Western countries). (**A**): 1-year OS West, (**B**): 3-year OS West, (**C**): 5-year OS West, (**D**): 1-year OS East, (**E**): 3-year OS East, (**F**): 5-year OS East.

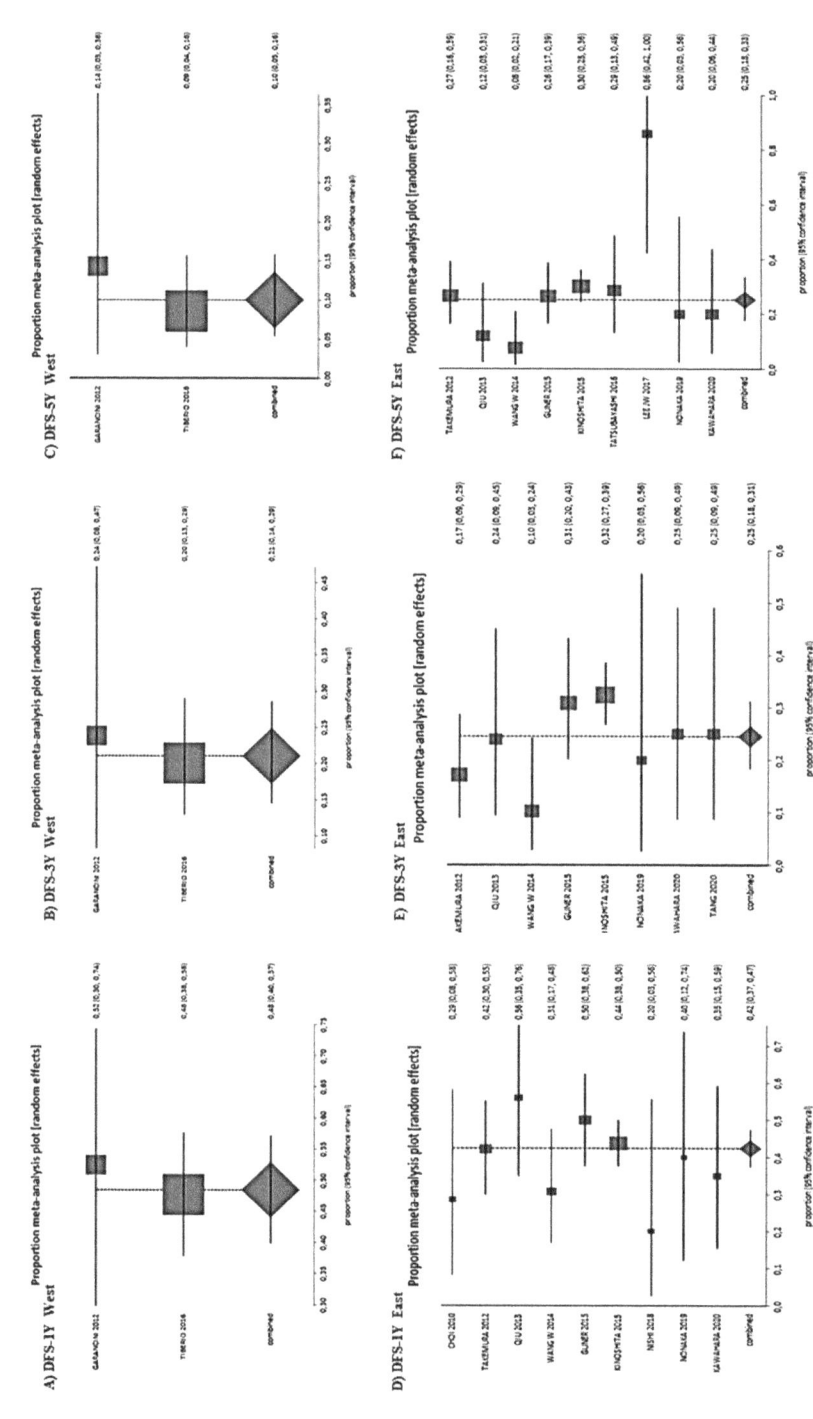

Figure 6. Disease-free survival according to subgroup analysis (Asian versus Western countries). (**A**): 1-year DFS West, (**B**): 3-year DFS West, (**C**): 5-year DFS West, (**D**): 1-year DFS East, (**E**): 3-year DFS East, (**F**): 5-year DFS East.

Table 4. Analysis of prognostic factors related to overall survival.

Prognostic Factor	N. of Studies	Participants	HR (95% CI)	p	I²
Male sex	16	788	0.86 (0.68–1.09)	0.21	0%
Age >65	19	896	0.86 (0.49–1.51)	0.60	94%
Synchronous liver metastases	14	730	1.62 (1.17–2.25)	0.004	62%
Multiple liver metastases	17	788	1.66 (1.44–1.91)	<0.00001	4%
Bilobar liver metastases	9	495	1.96 (1.34–2.87)	0.0005	69%
>3 cm liver metastases	19	803	2.39 (1.14–5.04)	0.02	98%
R + liver resection margin	6	400	4.15 (2.37–7.26)	<0.00001	33%
Chemotherapy before/after liver resection	11	781	1.49 (1.11–1.99)	0.008	73%
Primary tumor Size >5 cm	7	179	1.50 (0.99–2.26)	0.06	14%
pT3–4	21	1084	1.77 (1.31–2.41)	0.0002	51%
pN2–3	16	750	1.54 (1.28–1.85)	<0.00001	11%
Lymphatic invasion present	9	467	1.28 (0.96–1.70)	0.09	72%
Venous invasion present	7	364	1.23 (0.93–1.62)	0.15	0%
Primary tumor poorly differentiated	17	796	1.34 (1.10–1.63)	0.004	14%

Table 5. Analysis of prognostic factors related to disease-free survival.

Prognostic Factor	N. of Studies	Participants	HR (95% CI)	p	I²
Male sex	3	291	0.94 (0.65–1.36)	0.76	0%
Age >65	4	301	0.96 (0.70–1.31)	0.80	39%
Synchronous liver metastases	4	302	1.50 (1.21–1.86)	0.0002	0%
Multiple liver metastases	4	301	2.34 (1.67–3.29)	<0.00001	0%
Bilobar liver metastases	1	25	3.39 (1.09–10.56)	0.04	-
>3 cm liver metastases	4	301	1.51 (1.10–2.07)	0.01	0%
Chemotherapy before/after liver resection	3	291	0.77 (0.56–1.06)	0.11	0%
Primary tumor Size >5 cm	1	10	3.22 (0.71–14.57)	0.13	-
pT3–4	4	301	1.43 (1.06–1.94)	0.02	0%
pN2–3	3	292	1.35 (0.93–1.97)	0.11	35%
Lymphatic invasion present	3	291	1.46 (1.02–2.08)	0.04	43%
Venous invasion present	2	266	1.25 (0.92–1.70)	0.16	0%
Primary tumor poorly differentiated	4	317	1.27 (0.80–2.01)	0.31	46%

4. Discussion

This systematic review and meta-analysis demonstrate that surgical resection of GCLM, in the absence of peritoneal disease, is a safe procedure, with a 1.6% risk of mortality. It can achieve a 5-year OS of 26%. Those results are in line with the results of recent studies. Long et al., in a meta-analysis [61] of 39 studies, showed a 5-year OS rate of 27%. Similarly, Liao et al. [62], in a comparative analysis of 8 retrospective studies between hepatectomy and chemotherapy only, showed better OS in the surgical group with an odds ratio of 0.17 and 0.15 at 1 and 2 years. Up to now, no other meta-analysis has investigated DFS and prognostic factors related to DFS. We found that liver resection was associated with 5-year DFS of 22%.

Those positive results were particularly highlighted in the Asian studies. Historically, GC survival has always been substantially different in Asian and Western countries. However, results from recent systematic review and meta-analysis are discordant. While Gavriilidis et al. [63] showed no significant difference between Eastern and Western countries in terms of OS, Markar et al. [64] reported a better survival rate for the Eastern studies compared to Western. Furthermore, the results on this topic should be interpreted carefully due to differences between populations in terms of characteristics related to primary cancer, population screening, and dietary habits [65].

In clinical practice, patient selection is crucial in order to achieve acceptable mortality and morbidity. However, in addition to the importance of precision medicine, the role of a careful evaluation of each patient by multidisciplinary teams is improving. In fact, a multidisciplinary approach could increase the proportion of patients' candidates to curative treatment also in the metastatic setting. In this context, tools to perform a better selection of candidates for hepatectomy, such as the assessment of patients' performance status, hepatic invasiveness, and the feasibility of obtaining R0 resection, play a central role. Although there are still discordant results in the literature, we believe that radical resection of primary tumor and metastases is vital to achieve good outcomes.

Beom et al. demonstrated in a retrospective study the central role of conversion surgery following chemotherapy for 101 patients with metastatic GC [66]. In the trial, 65 patients (64.4%) had a major response and 11 patients (10.9%) received metastasectomy. Fifty-seven patients (56.4%) had a complete macroscopic resection, with a median survival of 26 months. The importance of R0 resection clearly emerged also in the study of Morgagni et al. [67], in which 11/54 metastatic GC underwent R0 resection. The authors concluded that conversion surgery in metastatic GC could be beneficial only if R0 resection could be achieved. We showed the same results in our analysis, with R1 resection strongly associated with poor OS and DFS. On the other hand, Cheon et al. [68] observed a similar survival rate after R0 or R1 resection, in contrast with our findings. However, the fact that a higher percentage of patients in the Korean series (88% vs. 27.6% in our series) received chemotherapy could be responsible for the differences in the outcomes, due to the positive impact of active treatment on survival. In general, in the case of synchronous disease, achieving an R0 resection both for primary tumor and for the hepatic metastases is recommend. Median survival exceeds 16 months after radical resections and drops to 6 months in case of R1 resections [8]. In our meta-analysis, R0 resection was found strongly associated with a better outcome, in terms of both OS and DFS. In addition to radical resection, other factors have been demonstrated to have a huge impact on prognosis.

In the study of Kinoshita et al. [35], a significant association with poor OS was found in the case of lymphatic and serosal invasion, when the liver metastases were more than 3, the maximum liver metastasis diameter was > 5 cm, or when there was high baseline CEA and CA19.9. Tiberio et al. [8], in an Italian cohort of 105 patients, showed that T-stage, R0 resection, and use of adjuvant chemotherapy were prognostic factors. Montangini et al. [69] showed that T and N staging, lymphovascular invasion of the primary tumor, and the burden of liver disease (i.e., number and diameter of the metastases) were strongly linked with survival. In particular, patients with involvement of the serosa or lymph nodes as well as with lymphovascular invasion had a poor prognosis. Otherwise, ≤3 liver metastases, tumor maximum diameter <5 cm, metachronous presentation, and R0 resections were linked to a better prognosis.

Other authors showed that some clinical and pathologic parameters, such as nodal status and histologic grade of the primary tumor, could impact the prognosis [48]. In this context, the lymph node ratio (number of metastatic lymph nodes on the number of the lymph nodes removed by surgery) is recognized to be an important factor linked to a poor prognosis among patients with GCLM who received combined surgical resection [70,71]. In fact, high lymph node ratio was significantly related to the more advanced pN stage, larger primary tumor dimension, microvascular invasion, and neoadjuvant chemotherapy.

In case of peritoneal involvement from GC, the survival is extremely poor. In those patients, hepatic resection does not add any benefit to survival [72,73]. For this reason, we excluded from the analysis the studies that included patients with peritoneal metastases.

Previous studies [22,56,74] have shown that the presence of multiple or synchronous liver metastases [74] were significant negative prognostic factors. However, in a recent meta-analysis, Cui et al. [75] showed that only the presence of synchronous GCLM was a negative prognostic factor, but they concluded that synchronous or multiple liver metastases should not be considered absolute contraindications for surgery.

Better survival could be obtained in presence of multiple scattered metastases in both lobes if R0 resection can be obtained [8]. In our study, the size of primary tumor and liver metastases were not unfavorable prognostic factors, as well as the presence of lymphatic or venous invasion by the primary tumor. However, we found that the best candidate for aggressive treatment is the patient with a well-moderately differentiated, pT1–2 and pN0–1 primary tumor and solitary, unilobar, and metachronous metastasis. Of course, R0 resection is vital in all cases.

Thus, three main treatment options have been identified for resectable GCLM: chemotherapy, upfront surgery, and preoperative chemotherapy followed by surgery [76]. In Western countries, there is no difference in the treatment strategy in case of synchronous or metachronous GCLM, whereas in Japan, upfront surgery is the preferred treatment option for the synchronous disease. According to international guidelines [5,77], a multimodality approach based on preoperative chemotherapy followed by surgery is considered the best treatment for both synchronous and metachronous resectable GCLM.

Although the REGATTA trial [77] is often cited in support of those guidelines, nowadays many oncologists still do not take the surgical approach into consideration in stage IV GC based on those results. In this phase 3 trial, 175 patients with GC and a single metastatic site confined to liver, peritoneum, or para-aortic lymph nodes were randomized to receive chemotherapy alone or gastrectomy followed by chemotherapy. The study failed to show an improvement in the survival of the experimental arm; additionally, it showed a detrimental effect of gastrectomy in this setting (median OS: 14.3 versus 16.6 months in the chemotherapy arm). However, those results should be interpreted with caution since two main concerns, at least, emerged: first, patients in the REGATTA trial did not receive neoadjuvant chemotherapy; second, the trial was designed to assess only the role of primary tumor site resection (gastrectomy with D1 lymphadenectomy) without any resection of metastatic lesions. That said, it is clear that the surgical treatment in the trial cannot be considered curative but only palliative. Additionally, in the trial, only 9% of the metastatic GC patients had a liver limited disease. Therefore, for all these reasons, the REGATTA trial should not be considered as strong evidence to discharge a multimodality strategy for patients with GCLM.

We believe that for surgeons a new era started since FLOT regimen (5FU, Folinic acid, Oxaliplatin, Docetaxel) was widely approved as the standard of care for advanced GC [78]. The neoadjuvant strategy was widely accepted for >T1N+, and oligometastatic GC has been increasingly recognized as a distinct clinical entity. It is characterized by limited metastatic spread and benefits from a multimodality strategy including chemotherapy and surgery [79]. Despite some limitations due to a non-randomized trial and a relatively small sample size, the phase 2 AIO/FLOT3 [58] showed an increased OS in oligometastatic GC patients treated with neoadjuvant chemotherapy (FLOT schedule) followed surgery. The trial underlined the concept that a more aggressive treatment strategy including preoperative chemotherapy and surgical resection of metastases might have better results in terms of survival in this setting.

Still, open questions are unsolved on which sub-population could really benefit from this strategy. In this regard, the results of the ongoing phase 3 RENAISSANCE/AIO-FLOT5 trial (NCT02578368) [80] are awaited.

In general, our study showed some interesting results that support the new surgical trend of approaching GCLM. However, the importance of neoadjuvant chemotherapy and the number of cycles of adjuvant chemotherapy should be taken into account. In our study, poor data were found for neoadjuvant CT to draw any firm conclusion, although, in our forest plot analysis regarding chemotherapy, including adjuvant and neoadjuvant, HR was 1.49 ($p = 0.008$). If we analyze separately, adjuvant chemotherapy had HR 1.5 ($p = 0.01$) instead of neoadjuvant CT with HR 1.39 ($p = 0.34$), therefore not significant (Figure 7, supplementary Figures S1–S25).

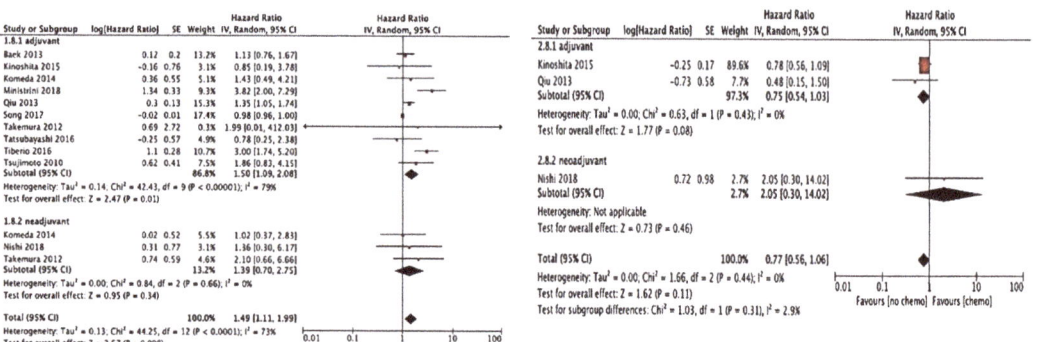

Figure 7. Forest plot showing the impact of chemotherapy on overall survival (OS) and disease-free survival (DFS). (**A**): Forest plot Chemotherapy related to OS (**B**): Forest plot Chemotherapy related to DFS.

Systemic chemotherapy remains the mainstay for the treatment of metastatic GC and progression during chemotherapy is probably the most relevant contraindication for any surgical approach.

In a study focusing on GCLM responder to induction chemotherapy, an R0 resection rate of 100% was obtained in all patients who underwent radical gastric resection plus liver metastasectomy after Docetaxel-Cisplatin-5-FU (DCF) chemotherapy [81]. Kinoshita et al. [82] reported a case series of 18 patients with liver metastases from GC and treated with DCF. In this experience, the majority of patients underwent conversion gastrectomy after chemotherapy (11 patients; 5 patients received also liver metastasectomy), showing an improvement in MST and 3-years OS rate if compared to patients who did not receive surgery (MST: 18.9 vs. 15.6 months; 3-year OS rate: 40.4% vs. 27.5%)

Another retrospective case series including 29 patients with GCLM reported that six patients underwent conversion surgery after DCF chemotherapy (complete response in two patients), two patients received partial hepatectomies with a complete pathological response and two were treated with radiofrequency ablation (RFA) [83]. Additionally, Yamaguchi et al. [84] showed a conversion rate of 21.5% in patients with GCLM liver treated with chemotherapy and subsequent metastasectomy. Same results regarding the good impact of surgery on the survival of those patients were reported in different analyses [66].

Regarding morbidity, most of the studies included in our analysis did not specify if the complications were major or minor. The 30-day morbidity and mortality were 24.7% and 1.6%, respectively, in our study.

Low mortality rate and a limited morbidity rate are not requisites to push patients with GCLM towards a surgical strategy, but certainly these data, in agreement with our results in terms of OS and DFS, reinforce the importance of future randomized prospective studies, needed to validate this strategy and recognize subgroups of patients who can really benefit from it.

Like previous works available in the literature, our study has some limitations. First, all the studies included in the analysis are retrospective and characterized by heterogeneous patient groups. Then, the results may have been affected by selection, institutional and national bias, underpowered sample size, and smaller oncological burden.

5. Conclusions

Japanese guidelines have begun to change attitudes towards GCLM, reporting surgical resection as recommended for cases with small number of metastases with no other incurable factor even though with a weak level of evidence [7,85]. Our findings suggest the possibility of expanding surgical indications for patients with GCLM if R0 can be achieved, always in a multidisciplinary setting.

Resection of GCLM is feasible, and a benefit in terms of long-term survival emerged despite the current guidelines. Identification of patient subgroups that would benefit from surgery is mandatory and in a multidisciplinary setting, we should take into consideration the stage of primary cancer, mainly with regard to serosal infiltration and lymph node ratio, and the characteristics of the liver metastases. The presence of solitary or unilobar metastases are positive prognostic factors, whereas size does not matter if GCLM are resectable and R0 could be achieved. Pre- and postoperative chemotherapy plays a key role in the treatment of these patients, even though the role of neoadjuvant CT should be better investigated. The ongoing FLOT 5 trial and a prospective register in the coming years will specify these findings and probably will change the current guidelines. A European registry from which a randomized controlled trial could be developed is necessary in the near future.

Supplementary Materials: The following are available online at https://www.mdpi.com/2077-0383/10/3/1141/s1, Figure S1: Forest plot of age related to OS; Figure S2: Forest of plot histology related to OS; Figure S3: Forest plot of lymphatic invasion related to OS; Figure S4: Forest plot of pN related to OS; Figure S5: Forest plot of pT related to OS; Figure S6: Forest plot of R0 related to OS; Figure S7: Forest plot of size liver mets related to OS; Figure S8: Forest plot of size primary tumor related to OS; Figure S9: Forest plot of solitary vs. multiple mets related to OS; Figure S10: Forest plot of synchronous vs. metachronous related to OS; Figure S11: Forest plot of unilobar vs. bilobar related to OS; Figure S12: Forest plot of venous invasion related to OS; Figure S13: Forest plot of sex related to OS; Figure S14: Forest plot of age related to DFS; Figure S15: Forest plot of histology related to DFS; Figure S16: Forest plot of lymphatic invasion related to DFS; Figure S17: Forest plot of pN related to DFS; Figure S18: Forest plot of pT related to DFS; Figure S19: Forest plot of size liver mets related to DFS; Figure S20: Forest plot of size primary tumor related to DFS; Figure S21: Forest plot of solitary vs. multiple mets related to DFS; Figure S22: Forest plot of synchronous vs. metachronous related to DFS; Figure S23: Forest plot of unilobar vs. bilobar related to DFS; Figure S24: Forest plot of venous invasion related to DFS. Figure S25: Forest plot of sex related to DFS.

Author Contributions: G.M. and F.S. contributed to the initial literature search for the content of the manuscript, filling the database, and design of the manuscript. A.T. and E.M. contributed significantly to the drafting of the manuscript, providing materials, and reviewing the English language. A.T. independently analyzed all the data and extracted the results. P.F., A.P., and P.M. gave a critical review of the content and were involved in the design of the manuscript. All authors contributed to the final manuscript drafting. All authors have read and agreed to the published version of the manuscript.

Funding: This research received no external funding.

Institutional Review Board Statement: Ethics approval was not required due to the retrospective nature of the analysis and quality of the article design.

Informed Consent Statement: The study was conducted according to the guidelines of the Declaration of Helsinki, and approved by Ethics Committee of our Hospital.

Conflicts of Interest: A.P. reported fees from Eli-Lilly, MSD, and Servier outside the submitted work. The other authors have no conflict of interest.

References

1. Ferlay, J.; Shin, H.-R.; Bray, F.; Forman, D.; Mathers, C.; Parkin, D.M. Estimates of worldwide burden of cancer in 2008: GLOBOCAN 2008. *Int. J. Cancer* **2010**, *127*, 2893–2917. [CrossRef] [PubMed]
2. Riihimäki, M.; Hemminki, A.; Sundquist, K.; Sundquist, J.; Hemminki, K. Metastatic spread in patients with gastric cancer. *Oncotarget* **2016**, *7*, 52307–52316. [CrossRef]
3. Ajani, J.A.; D'Amico, T.A.; Almhanna, K.; Bentrem, D.J.; Chao, J.; Das, P.; Denlinger, C.S.; Fanta, P.; Farjah, F.; Fuchs, C.S.; et al. Gastric Cancer, Version 3.2016; Clinical Practice Guidelines in Oncology. *J. Natl. Compr. Cancer Netw.* **2016**, *14*, 1286–1312. [CrossRef] [PubMed]

4. Bang, Y.-J.; Van Cutsem, E.; Feyereislova, A.; Chung, H.C.; Shen, L.; Sawaki, A.; Lordick, F.; Ohtsu, A.; Omuro, Y.; Satoh, T.; et al. Trastuzumab in combination with chemotherapy versus chemotherapy alone for treatment of HER2-positive advanced gastric or gastro-oesophageal junction cancer (ToGA): A phase 3, open-label, randomised controlled trial. *Lancet* **2010**, *376*, 687–697. [CrossRef]
5. Smyth, E.C.; Verheij, M.; Allum, W.; Cunningham, D.; Cervantes, A.; Arnold, D. Gastric cancer: ESMO Clinical Practice Guidelines for diagnosis, treatment and follow-up. *Ann. Oncol.* **2016**, *27*, v38–v49. [CrossRef]
6. Yoshida, K.; Yamaguchi, K.; Okumura, N.; Tanahashi, T.; Kodera, Y. Is conversion therapy possible in stage IV gastric cancer: The proposal of new biological categories of classification. *Gastric Cancer* **2015**, *19*, 329–338. [CrossRef]
7. Kodera, Y.; Fujitani, K.; Fukushima, N.; Ito, S.; Muro, K.; Ohashi, N.; Yoshikawa, T.; Kobayashi, D.; Tanaka, C.; Fujiwara, M. Surgical resection of hepatic metastasis from gastric cancer: A review and new recommendation in the Japanese gastric cancer treatment guidelines. *Gastric Cancer* **2013**, *17*, 206–212. [CrossRef]
8. Tiberio, G.; Ministrini, S.; Gardini, A.; Marrelli, D.; Marchet, A.; Cipollari, C.; Graziosi, L.; Pedrazzani, C.; Baiocchi, G.; La Barba, G.; et al. Factors influencing survival after hepatectomy for metastases from gastric cancer. *Eur. J. Surg. Oncol.* **2016**, *42*, 1229–1235. [CrossRef] [PubMed]
9. Gadde, R.; Tamariz, L.; Hanna, M.; Avisar, E.; Livingstone, A.; Franceschi, D.; Yakoub, D. Metastatic gastric cancer (MGC) patients: Can we improve survival by metastasectomy? A systematic review and meta-analysis. *J. Surg. Oncol.* **2015**, *112*, 38–45. [CrossRef]
10. Booth, A.; Clarke, M.; Dooley, G.; Ghersi, D.; Moher, D.; Petticrew, M.; Stewart, L. The nuts and bolts of PROSPERO: An international prospective register of systematic reviews. *Syst. Rev.* **2012**, *1*, 2. [CrossRef]
11. Moher, D.; Liberati, A.; Tetzlaff, J.; Altman, D.G. For the PRISMA Group Preferred reporting items for systematic reviews and meta-analyses: The PRISMA statement. *BMJ* **2009**, *339*, b2535. [CrossRef]
12. University of Oxford. *OCEBM Levels of Evidence Working Group, "The Oxford Levels of Evidence 1"*; University of Oxford: Oxford, UK, 2009.
13. Freemantle, N. CD: StatsDirect—Statistical Software for Medical Research in the 21st Century. *BMJ* **2000**, *321*, 1536. [CrossRef]
14. The Cochrane Collaboration. *Review Manager (RevMan) [Computer Program]*, version 5.3; Nordic Cochrane Centre: Copenhagen, Denmark, 2014.
15. Parmar, M.K.B.; Torri, V.; Stewart, L. Extracting Summary Statistics to Perform Meta-Analyses of the Published Literature for Survival Endpoints. *Stat. Med.* **1998**, *17*, 2815–2834. [CrossRef]
16. Higgins, J.P.T.; Thompson, S.G. Quantifying heterogeneity in a meta-analysis. *Stat. Med.* **2002**, *21*, 1539–1558. [CrossRef]
17. StatsDirect. StatsDirect Statistical Software. 2008. Available online: www.statsdirect.com (accessed on 26 November 2020).
18. Makino, H.; Kunisaki, C.; Izumisawa, Y.; Tokuhisa, M.; Oshima, T.; Nagano, Y.; Fujii, S.; Kimura, J.; Takagawa, R.; Kosaka, T.; et al. Indication for hepatic resection in the treatment of liver metastasis from gastric cancer. *Anticancer Res.* **2010**, *30*, 2367–2376. [PubMed]
19. TsujimotoTakashi, H.; Ichikura, T.; Ono, S.; Sugasawa, H.; Hiraki, S.; Sakamoto, N.; Yaguchi, Y.; Hatsuse, K.; Yamamoto, J.; Hase, K. Outcomes for patients following hepatic resection of metastatic tumors from gastric cancer. *Hepatol. Int.* **2010**, *4*, 406–413. [CrossRef] [PubMed]
20. Chen, L.; Song, M.-Q.; Lin, H.-Z.; Hao, L.-H.; Jiang, X.-J.; Li, Z.-Y.; Chen, Y.-X. Chemotherapy and resection for gastric cancer with synchronous liver metastases. *World J. Gastroenterol.* **2013**, *19*, 2097–2103. [CrossRef] [PubMed]
21. Qiu, J.-L.; Deng, M.-G.; Li, W.; Zou, R.-H.; Li, B.-K.; Zheng, Y.; Lao, X.-M.; Zhou, K.; Yuan, Y.-F. Hepatic resection for synchronous hepatic metastasis from gastric cancer. *Eur. J. Surg. Oncol.* **2013**, *39*, 694–700. [CrossRef] [PubMed]
22. Viganò, L.; Vellone, M.; Ferrero, A.; Giuliante, F.; Nuzzo, G.; Capussotti, L. Liver resection for gastric cancer metastases. *Hepato Gastroenterol.* **2013**, *60*, 557–562.
23. Aizawa, M.; Nashimoto, A.; Yabusaki, H.; Nakagawa, S.; Matsuki, A. Clinical benefit of surgical management for gastric cancer with synchronous liver metastasis. *Hepato Gastroenterol.* **2014**, *61*, 1439–1445. [CrossRef]
24. Komeda, K.; Hayashi, M.; Kubo, S.; Nagano, H.; Nakai, T.; Kaibori, M.; Wada, H.; Takemura, S.; Kinoshita, M.; Koga, C.; et al. High Survival in Patients Operated for Small Isolated Liver Metastases from Gastric Cancer: A Multi-institutional Study. *World J. Surg.* **2014**, *38*, 2692–2697. [CrossRef]
25. Wang, W.; Liang, H.; Zhang, H.; Wang, X.; Xue, Q.; Zhang, R. Prognostic significance of radical surgical treatment for gastric cancer patients with synchronous liver metastases. *Med. Oncol.* **2014**, *31*, 258. [CrossRef] [PubMed]
26. Guner, A.; Son, T.; Cho, I.; Kwon, I.G.; An, J.Y.; Kim, H.-I.; Cheong, J.-H.; Noh, S.H.; Hyung, W.J. Liver-directed treatments for liver metastasis from gastric adenocarcinoma: Comparison between liver resection and radiofrequency ablation. *Gastric Cancer* **2016**, *19*, 951–960. [CrossRef] [PubMed]
27. Kinoshita, T.; Saiura, A.; Esaki, M.; Sakamoto, H.; Yamanaka, T. Multicentre analysis of long-term outcome after surgical resection for gastric cancer liver metastases. *BJS* **2014**, *102*, 102–107. [CrossRef] [PubMed]
28. Li, Z.; Fan, B.; Shan, F.; Tang, L.; Bu, Z.; Wu, A.; Zhang, L.; Wu, X.; Zong, X.; Li, S.; et al. Gastrectomy in comprehensive treatment of advanced gastric cancer with synchronous liver metastasis: A prospectively comparative study. *World J. Surg. Oncol.* **2015**, *13*, 212. [CrossRef]
29. Liu, Q.; Bi, J.-J.; Tian, Y.-T.; Feng, Q.; Zheng, Z.-X.; Wang, Z. Outcome after Simultaneous Resection of Gastric Primary Tumour and Synchronous Liver Metastases: Survival Analysis of a Single-center Experience in China. *Asian Pac. J. Cancer Prev.* **2015**, *16*, 1665–1669. [CrossRef]

30. Dittmar, Y.; Altendorf-Hofmann, A.; Rauchfuss, F.; Götz, M.; Scheuerlein, H.; Jandt, K.; Settmacher, U. Resection of liver metastases is beneficial in patients with gastric cancer: Report on 15 cases and review of literature. *Gastric Cancer* **2011**, *15*, 131–136. [CrossRef]
31. Ohkura, Y.; Shinohara, H.; Haruta, S.; Ueno, M.; Hashimoto, M.; Sakai, Y.; Udagawa, H. Hepatectomy Offers Superior Survival Compared with Non-surgical Treatment for ≤3 Metastatic Tumors with Diameters. *World J. Surg.* **2015**, *39*, 2757–2763. [CrossRef]
32. Shinohara, T.; Maeda, Y.; Hamada, T.; Futakawa, N. Survival Benefit of Surgical Treatment for Liver Metastases from Gastric Cancer. *J. Gastrointest. Surg.* **2015**, *19*, 1043–1051. [CrossRef] [PubMed]
33. Markar, S.R.; MacKenzie, H.; Mikhail, S.; Mughal, M.; Preston, S.R.; Maynard, N.D.; Faiz, O.; Hanna, G.B. Surgical resection of hepatic metastases from gastric cancer: Outcomes from national series in England. *Gastric Cancer* **2017**, *20*, 379–386. [CrossRef]
34. Oguro, S.; Imamura, H.; Yoshimoto, J.; Ishizaki, Y.; Kawasaki, S. Liver metastases from gastric cancer represent systemic disease in comparison with those from colorectal cancer. *J. Hepato Biliary Pancreat. Sci.* **2016**, *23*, 324–332. [CrossRef] [PubMed]
35. Tatsubayashi, T.; Tanizawa, Y.; Miki, Y.; Tokunaga, M.; Bando, E.; Kawamura, T.; Sugiura, T.; Kinugasa, Y.; Uesaka, K.; Terashima, M. Treatment outcomes of hepatectomy for liver metastases of gastric cancer diagnosed using contrast-enhanced magnetic resonance imaging. *Gastric Cancer* **2017**, *20*, 387–393. [CrossRef] [PubMed]
36. Fukami, Y.; Kaneoka, Y.; Maeda, A.; Takayama, Y.; Takahashi, T.; Uji, M.; Kumada, T. Adjuvant hepatic artery infusion chemotherapy after hemihepatectomy for gastric cancer liver metastases. *Int. J. Surg.* **2017**, *46*, 79–84. [CrossRef] [PubMed]
37. Lee, J.W.; Choi, M.H.; Lee, Y.J.; Ali, B.; Yoo, H.M.; Song, K.Y.; Park, C.H. Radiofrequency ablation for liver metastases in patients with gastric cancer as an alternative to hepatic resection. *BMC Cancer* **2017**, *17*, 1–8. [CrossRef] [PubMed]
38. Li, J.; Xi, H.; Cui, J.; Zhang, K.; Gao, Y.; Liang, W.; Cai, A.; Wei, B.; Chen, L. Minimally invasive surgery as a treatment option for gastric cancer with liver metastasis: A comparison with open surgery. *Surg. Endosc.* **2017**, *32*, 1422–1433. [CrossRef] [PubMed]
39. Li, S.C.; Lee, C.H.; Hung, C.L.; Wu, J.C.; Chen, J.H. Surgical resection of metachronous hepatic metastases from gastric cancer improves long-term survival: A population-based study. *PLoS ONE* **2017**, *12*, e0182255. [CrossRef]
40. Ryu, T.; Takami, Y.; Wada, Y.; Tateishi, M.; Matsushima, H.; Yoshitomi, M.; Saitsu, H. Oncological outcomes after hepatic resection and/or surgical microwave ablation for liver metastasis from gastric cancer. *Asian J. Surg.* **2019**, *42*, 100–105. [CrossRef]
41. Garancini, M.; Uggeri, F.; Degrate, L.; Nespoli, L.; Gianotti, L.; Nespoli, A.; Uggeri, F.; Romano, F. Surgical treatment of liver metastases of gastric cancer: Is local treatment in a systemic disease worthwhile? *HPB* **2012**, *14*, 209–215. [CrossRef] [PubMed]
42. Song, A.; Zhang, X.; Yu, F.; Li, D.; Shao, W.; Zhou, Y. Surgical resection for hepatic metastasis from gastric cancer: A multi-institution study. *Oncotarget* **2017**, *8*, 71147–71153. [CrossRef]
43. Ministrini, S.; Solaini, L.; Cipollari, C.; Sofia, S.; Marino, E.; D'Ignazio, A.; Bencivenga, M.; Tiberio, G.A.M. Surgical treatment of hepatic metastases from gastric cancer. *Updates Surg.* **2018**, *70*, 273–278. [CrossRef] [PubMed]
44. Nishi, M.; Shimada, M.; Yoshikawa, K.; Higashijima, J.; Tokunaga, T.; Kashihara, H.; Takasu, C.; Ishikawa, D.; Wada, Y.; Eto, S. Results of Hepatic Resection for Liver Metastasis of Gastric Cancer—A single center experience. *J. Med. Investig.* **2018**, *65*, 27–31. [CrossRef]
45. Shirasu, H.; Tsushima, T.; Kawahira, M.; Kawai, S.; Kawakami, T.; Kito, Y.; Yoshida, Y.; Hamauchi, S.; Todaka, A.; Yokota, T.; et al. Role of hepatectomy in gastric cancer with multiple liver-limited metastases. *Gastric Cancer* **2017**, *21*, 338–344. [CrossRef] [PubMed]
46. Gao, J.; Wang, Y.; Li, F.; Zhu, Z.; Han, B.; Wang, R.; Xie, R.; Xue, Y. Prognostic Nutritional Index and Neutrophil-to-Lymphocyte Ratio Are Respectively Associated with Prognosis of Gastric Cancer with Liver Metatasis Undergoing and without Hepatectomy. *BioMed Res. Int.* **2019**, *2019*, 4213623–4213627. [CrossRef] [PubMed]
47. Nonaka, Y.; Hiramatsu, K.; Kato, T.; Shibata, Y.; Yoshihara, M.; Aoba, T.; Kamiya, T. Evaluation of Hepatic Resection in Liver Metastasis of Gastric Cancer. *Indian J. Surg. Oncol.* **2019**, *10*, 204–209. [CrossRef] [PubMed]
48. Kawahara, K.; Makino, H.; Kametaka, H.; Hoshino, I.; Fukada, T.; Seike, K.; Kawasaki, Y.; Otsuka, M. Outcomes of surgical resection for gastric cancer liver metastases: A retrospective analysis. *World J. Surg. Oncol.* **2020**, *18*, 1–8. [CrossRef] [PubMed]
49. Tang, K.; Zhang, B.; Dong, L.; Wang, L.; Tang, Z. Radiofrequency ablation versus traditional liver resection and chemotherapy for liver metastases from gastric cancer. *J. Int. Med. Res.* **2020**, *48*, 300060520940509. [CrossRef] [PubMed]
50. Ceniceros, L.; Chopitea, A.; Pardo, F.; Rotellar, F.; Arbea, L.; Sangro, B.; Benito, A.; Rodríguez, J.; Sola, J.J.; Subtil, J.C.; et al. Intensified neoadjuvant multimodal approach in synchronous liver metastases from gastric cancer: A single institutional experience. *Clin. Transl. Oncol.* **2017**, *20*, 658–665. [CrossRef]
51. Liu, J.; Li, J.-H.; Zhai, R.-J.; Wei, B.; Shao, M.-Z.; Chen, L. Predictive factors improving survival after gastric and hepatic surgical treatment in gastric cancer patients with synchronous liver metastases. *Chin. Med. J.* **2012**, *125*, 165–171.
52. Miki, Y.; Fujitani, K.; Hirao, M.; Kurokawa, Y.; Mano, M.; Tsujie, M.; Miyamoto, A.; Nakamori, S.; Tsujinaka, T. Significance of surgical treatment of liver metastases from gastric cancer. *Anticancer Res.* **2012**, *32*, 665–670.
53. Schildberg, C.W.; Croner, R.; Merkel, S.; Schellerer, V.; Müller, V.; Yedibela, S.; Hohenberger, W.; Peros, G.; Perrakis, A. Outcome of Operative Therapy of Hepatic Metastatic Stomach Carcinoma: A Retrospective Analysis. *World J. Surg.* **2012**, *36*, 872–878. [CrossRef] [PubMed]
54. Takemura, N.; Saiura, A.; Koga, R.; Arita, J.; Yoshioka, R.; Ono, Y.; Hiki, N.; Sano, T.; Yamamoto, J.; Kokudo, N.; et al. Long-term outcomes after surgical resection for gastric cancer liver metastasis: An analysis of 64 macroscopically complete resections. *Langenbeck Arch. Surg.* **2012**, *397*, 951–957. [CrossRef] [PubMed]

55. Wang, Y.-N.; Shen, K.-T.; Ling, J.-Q.; Gao, X.-D.; Hou, Y.-Y.; Wang, X.-F.; Qin, J.; Sun, Y.-H.; Qin, X.-Y. Prognostic analysis of combined curative resection of the stomach and liver lesions in 30 gastric cancer patients with synchronous liver metastases. *BMC Surg.* 2012, *12*, 20. [CrossRef] [PubMed]
56. Baek, H.-U.; Kim, S.B.; Cho, E.-H.; Jin, S.-H.; Yu, H.J.; Lee, J.-I.; Bang, H.-Y.; Lim, C.-S. Hepatic Resection for Hepatic Metastases from Gastric Adenocarcinoma. *J. Gastric Cancer* 2013, *13*, 86–92. [CrossRef] [PubMed]
57. Choi, S.B.; Song, J.; Kang, C.M.; Hyung, W.J.; Kim, K.S.; Choi, J.S.; Lee, W.J.; Noh, S.H.; Kim, C.B. Surgical outcome of metachronous hepatic metastases secondary to gastric cancer. *Hepato Gastroenterol.* 2010, *57*, 29–34.
58. Al-Batran, S.-E.; Homann, N.; Pauligk, C.; Illerhaus, G.; Martens, U.M.; Stoehlmacher, J.; Schmalenberg, H.; Luley, K.B.; Prasnikar, N.; Egger, M.; et al. Effect of Neoadjuvant Chemotherapy Followed by Surgical Resection on Survival in Patients With Limited Metastatic Gastric or Gastroesophageal Junction Cancer. *JAMA Oncol.* 2017, *3*, 1237–1244. [CrossRef] [PubMed]
59. Kokkola, A.; Louhimo, J.; Puolakkainen, P. Does non-curative gastrectomy improve survival in patients with metastatic gastric cancer? *J. Surg. Oncol.* 2012, *106*, 193–196. [CrossRef] [PubMed]
60. Oki, E.; Kyushu Study Group of Clinical Cancer; Tokunaga, S.; Emi, Y.; Kusumoto, T.; Yamamoto, M.; Fukuzawa, K.; Takahashi, I.; Ishigami, S.; Tsuji, A.; et al. Surgical treatment of liver metastasis of gastric cancer: A retrospective multicenter cohort study (KSCC1302). *Gastric Cancer* 2016, *19*, 968–976. [CrossRef]
61. Long, D.; Yu, P.-C.; Huang, W.; Luo, Y.-L.; Zhang, S. Systematic review of partial hepatic resection to treat hepatic metastases in patients with gastric cancer. *Medicine* 2016, *95*, e5235. [CrossRef]
62. Liao, Y.-Y.; Peng, N.-F.; Long, D.; Yu, P.-C.; Zhang, S.; Zhong, J.-H.; Li, L.-Q. Hepatectomy for liver metastases from gastric cancer: A systematic review. *BMC Surg.* 2017, *17*, 1–7. [CrossRef]
63. Gavriilidis, P.; Roberts, K.J.; De'Angelis, N.; Sutcliffe, R.P. Gastrectomy Alone or in Combination with Hepatic Resection in the Management of Liver Metastases from Gastric Cancer: A Systematic Review Using an Updated and Cumulative Meta-Analysis. *J. Clin. Med. Res.* 2019, *11*, 600–608. [CrossRef] [PubMed]
64. Markar, S.R.; Mikhail, S.; Malietzis, G.; Athanasiou, T.; Mariette, C.; Sasako, M.; Hanna, G.B. Influence of Surgical Resection of Hepatic Metastases from Gastric Adenocarcinoma on Long-term Survival. *Ann. Surg.* 2016, *263*, 1092–1101. [CrossRef]
65. Griniatsos, J.; Trafalis, D. Differences in gastric cancer surgery outcome between East and West: Differences in surgery or different diseases? *J. Buon* 2018, *23*, 1210–1215.
66. Beom, S.-H.; Choi, Y.Y.; Baek, S.-E.; Li, S.-X.; Lim, J.S.; Son, T.; Kim, H.-I.; Cheong, J.-H.; Hyung, W.J.; Choi, S.H.; et al. Multidisciplinary treatment for patients with stage IV gastric cancer: The role of conversion surgery following chemotherapy. *BMC Cancer* 2018, *18*, 1116. [CrossRef] [PubMed]
67. Morgagni, P.; Solaini, L.; Framarini, M.; Vittimberga, G.; Gardini, A.; Tringali, D.; Valgiusti, M.; Monti, M.; Ercolani, G. Conversion surgery for gastric cancer: A cohort study from a western center. *Int. J. Surg.* 2018, *53*, 360–365. [CrossRef] [PubMed]
68. Cheon, S.H.; Rha, S.Y.; Jeung, H.-C.; Im, C.-K.; Kim, S.H.; Kim, H.R.; Ahn, J.B.; Roh, J.K.; Noh, S.H.; Chung, H.C. Survival benefit of combined curative resection of the stomach (D2 resection) and liver in gastric cancer patients with liver metastases. *Ann. Oncol.* 2008, *19*, 1146–1153. [CrossRef] [PubMed]
69. Montagnani, F.; Crivelli, F.; Aprile, G.; Vivaldi, C.; Pecora, I.; De Vivo, R.; Clerico, M.A.; Fornaro, L. Long-term survival after liver metastasectomy in gastric cancer: Systematic review and meta-analysis of prognostic factors. *Cancer Treat. Rev.* 2018, *69*, 11–20. [CrossRef] [PubMed]
70. Kurokawa, Y.; Shibata, T.; Sasako, M.; Sano, T.; Tsuburaya, A.; Iwasaki, Y.; Fukuda, H. Validity of response assessment criteria in neoadjuvant chemotherapy for gastric cancer (JCOG0507-A). *Gastric Cancer* 2013, *17*, 514–521. [CrossRef]
71. Li, M.-X.; Jin, Z.-X.; Zhou, J.-G.; Ying, J.-M.; Liang, Z.-Y.; Mao, X.-X.; Bi, X.-Y.; Zhao, J.-J.; Li, Z.-Y.; Huang, Z.; et al. Prognostic Value of Lymph Node Ratio in Patients Receiving Combined Surgical Resection for Gastric Cancer Liver Metastasis. *Medicine* 2016, *95*, e3395. [CrossRef]
72. Schmidt, B.; Look-Hong, N.; Maduekwe, U.N.; Chang, K.; Hong, T.S.; Kwak, E.L.; Lauwers, G.Y.; Rattner, D.W.; Mullen, J.T.; Yoon, S.S. Noncurative Gastrectomy for Gastric Adenocarcinoma Should only be Performed in Highly Selected Patients. *Ann. Surg. Oncol.* 2013, *20*, 3512–3518. [CrossRef]
73. Ambiru, S.; Miyazaki, M.; Ito, H.; Nakagawa, K.; Shimizu, H.; Yoshidome, H.; Shimizu, Y.; Nakajima, N. Benefits and limits of hepatic resection for gastric metastases. *Am. J. Surg.* 2001, *181*, 279–283. [CrossRef]
74. Sakamoto, Y.; Sano, T.; Shimada, K.; Esaki, M.; Saka, M.; Fukagawa, T.; Katai, H.; Kosuge, T.; Sasako, M. Favorable indications for hepatectomy in patients with liver metastasis from gastric cancer. *J. Surg. Oncol.* 2007, *95*, 534–539. [CrossRef] [PubMed]
75. Cui, J.-K.; Liu, M.; Shang, X.-K. Hepatectomy for Liver Metastasis of Gastric Cancer: A Meta-Analysis. *Surg. Innov.* 2019, *26*, 692–697. [CrossRef] [PubMed]
76. Kataoka, K.; Kinoshita, T.; Moehler, M.; Mauer, M.; Shitara, K.; Wagner, A.D.; Schrauwen, S.; Yoshikawa, T.; Roviello, F.; Tokunaga, M.; et al. Current management of liver metastases from gastric cancer: What is common practice? New challenge of EORTC and JCOG. *Gastric Cancer* 2017, *20*, 904–912. [CrossRef] [PubMed]
77. Fujitani, K.; Yang, H.-K.; Mizusawa, J.; Kim, Y.-W.; Terashima, M.; Han-Kwang, Y.; Iwasaki, Y.; Hyung, W.J.; Takagane, A.; Park, D.J.; et al. Gastrectomy plus chemotherapy versus chemotherapy alone for advanced gastric cancer with a single non-curable factor (REGATTA): A phase 3, randomised controlled trial. *Lancet Oncol.* 2016, *17*, 309–318. [CrossRef]

78. Al-Batran, S.-E.; Hartmann, J.T.; Hofheinz, R.; Homann, N.; Rethwisch, V.; Probst, S.; Stoehlmacher, J.; Clemens, M.R.; Mahlberg, R.; Fritz, M.; et al. Biweekly fluorouracil, leucovorin, oxaliplatin, and docetaxel (FLOT) for patients with metastatic adenocarcinoma of the stomach or esophagogastric junction: A phase II trial of the Arbeitsgemeinschaft Internistische Onkologie. *Ann. Oncol.* **2008**, *19*, 1882–1887. [CrossRef]
79. Salati, M.; Valeri, N.; Spallanzani, A.; Braconi, C.; Cascinu, S. Oligometastatic gastric cancer: An emerging clinical entity with distinct therapeutic implications. *Eur. J. Surg. Oncol.* **2019**, *45*, 1479–1482. [CrossRef]
80. Al-Batran, S.-E.; Goetze, T.O.; Mueller, D.W.; Vogel, A.; Winkler, M.; Lorenzen, S.; Novotny, A.; Pauligk, C.; Homann, N.; Jungbluth, T.; et al. The RENAISSANCE (AIO-FLOT5) trial: Effect of chemotherapy alone vs. chemotherapy followed by surgical resection on survival and quality of life in patients with limited-metastatic adenocarcinoma of the stomach or esophagogastric junction—A phase III trial of the German AIO/CAO-V/CAOGI. *BMC Cancer* **2017**, *17*, 1–7. [CrossRef]
81. Han, D.-S.; Suh, Y.-S.; Kong, S.-H.; Lee, H.-J.; Im, S.-A.; Bang, Y.-J.; Kim, W.-H.; Yang, H.-K. Outcomes of surgery aiming at curative resection in good responder to induction chemotherapy for gastric cancer with distant metastases. *J. Surg. Oncol.* **2012**, *107*, 511–516. [CrossRef]
82. Kinoshita, J.; Fushida, S.; Tsukada, T.; Oyama, K.; Okamoto, K.; Makino, I.; Nakamura, K.; Miyashita, T.; Tajima, H.; Takamura, H.; et al. Efficacy of conversion gastrectomy following docetaxel, cisplatin, and S-1 therapy in potentially resectable stage IV gastric cancer. *Eur. J. Surg. Oncol.* **2015**, *41*, 1354–1360. [CrossRef] [PubMed]
83. Sato, Y.; Ohnuma, H.; Nobuoka, T.; Hirakawa, M.; Sagawa, T.; Fujikawa, K.; Takahashi, Y.; Shinya, M.; Katsuki, S.; Takahashi, M.; et al. Conversion therapy for inoperable advanced gastric cancer patients by docetaxel, cisplatin, and S-1 (DCS) chemotherapy: A multi-institutional retrospective study. *Gastric Cancer* **2017**, *20*, 517–526. [CrossRef] [PubMed]
84. Yamaguchi, K.; Yoshida, K.; Tanahashi, T.; Takahashi, T.; Matsuhashi, N.; Tanaka, Y.; Tanabe, K.; Ohdan, H. The long-term survival of stage IV gastric cancer patients with conversion therapy. *Gastric Cancer* **2017**, *21*, 315–323. [CrossRef] [PubMed]
85. Ma, G. Japanese Gastric Cancer Treatment Guidelines 2018, 5th edition. *Gastric Cancer* **2020**, *24*, 1–21. [CrossRef]

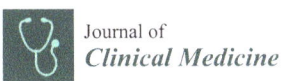

Review

Bone Metastases from Gastric Cancer: What We Know and How to Deal with Them

Angelica Petrillo [1,2,*], Emilio Francesco Giunta [1,2], Annalisa Pappalardo [1,2], Davide Bosso [1], Laura Attademo [1], Cinzia Cardalesi [1], Anna Diana [1,2], Antonietta Fabbrocini [1], Teresa Fabozzi [1], Pasqualina Giordano [1], Margaret Ottaviano [1,3,4], Mario Rosanova [1], Antonia Silvestri [1], Piera Federico [1] and Bruno Daniele [1]

1. Medical Oncology Unit, Ospedale del Mare, 80147 Naples, Italy; emiliofrancescogiunta@gmail.com (E.F.G.); annalisa.pappalardo88@gmail.com (A.P.); davidebosso84@gmail.com (D.B.); laura.attademo@gmail.com (L.A.); cinzia.cardalesi@gmail.com (C.C.); annadiana88@gmail.com (A.D.); antonietta.fabbrocini@gmail.com (A.F.); fabozzit79@gmail.com (T.F.); giopas@email.it (P.G.); margaretottaviano@gmail.com (M.O.); rosanovamario@hotmail.com (M.R.); antonia.silv@libero.it (A.S.); pierafederico@yahoo.it (P.F.); b.daniele@libero.it (B.D.)
2. Department of Precision Medicine, School of Medicine, University of Study of Campania "L. Vanvitelli", 80131 Naples, Italy
3. Department of Clinical Medicine and Surgery, University of Naples "Federico II", 80131 Naples, Italy
4. CRCTR Rare Tumors Reference Center of Campania Region, 80131 Naples, Italy
* Correspondence: angelic.petrillo@gmail.com

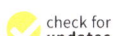

Abstract: Gastric cancer (GC) is the third cause of cancer-related death worldwide; the prognosis is poor especially in the case of metastatic disease. Liver, lymph nodes, peritoneum, and lung are the most frequent sites of metastases from GC; however, bone metastases from GC have been reported in the literature. Nevertheless, it is unclear how the metastatic sites may affect the prognosis. In particular, knowledge about the impact of bone metastases on GC patients' outcome is scant, and this may be related to the rarity of bone lesions and/or their underestimation at the time of diagnosis. In fact, there is still a lack of specific recommendation for their detection at the diagnosis. Then, the majority of the evidences in this field came from retrospective analysis on very heterogeneous study populations. In this context, the aim of this narrative review is to delineate an overview about the evidences existing about bone metastases in GC patients, focusing on their incidence and biology, the prognostic role of bone involvement, and their possible implication in the treatment choice.

Keywords: metastatic gastric cancer; target therapy; bone flare; stage IV; treatment; RANK-L

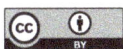

1. Introduction

Gastric cancer (GC) is the third cause of cancer-related death worldwide [1]. In particular, even today, survival is dismal, and only 5.5% of patients diagnosed with metastatic GC are alive at 5 years [2]. Although over the last decades the research in GC has focused on the role of novel and targeted treatments, chemotherapy based on a doublet with platin and fluorouracil remains the standard of care for the first-line therapy in case of metastatic disease without overexpression of human epithelial growth factor 2 receptor (HER2) [3]. To date, trastuzumab is the unique target agent approved for first-line treatment of HER2-positive metastatic GC in addition to the doublet chemotherapy backbone, due to the fact that all the other targeted agents failed to improve survival outcomes in this setting [4,5]. Recently, the immune checkpoint inhibitors have shown promising results in the treatment of first-line metastatic GC [6–8]. However, data are preliminary, and the final results of the trials are awaited in order to clarify their role in the first-line treatment of metastatic GC. Therefore, these agents have not been approved by the regulatory authorities yet, and their use is not a standard of care at the time of writing.

In the last decades, one of the most important conceptual achievements in this field is represented by the "continuum of care", meaning the possibility to treat patients with multiple subsequent lines of therapy in order to obtain longer survivals. In fact, almost 40% of patients receiving a first-line treatment for metastatic disease maintains a good performance status after progression; they are able to receive a second and even a third line of treatment [9,10]. In the second line, a treatment with paclitaxel and ramucirumab is the standard of care in case of patients with good performance status (PS 0–1 according to the Eastern Cooperative Oncology Group (ECOG) scale); otherwise, ramucirumab as monotherapy is the preferred choice in case of patients with ECOG PS 2 [3]. Then, up to date, triflurifine/tipiracil is the unique agent to have shown a benefit as third line treatment in patients with metastatic GC and good PS, representing the standard choice in this field after the approval of local authorities [3]. Thus, moving from the experience in colorectal cancer patients [11], the definition of the right sequence of treatment from the diagnosis is becoming crucial in GC as well [12].

Over the last decades, a better understanding of molecular patterns of metastatic GC led to validated molecular classifications [13,14], indicating that GC is no longer a single entity, while it includes many subgroups with their own peculiarities and different behavior. However, so far, these molecular classifications have not been applied diffusely in the everyday clinical practice. Additionally, there is still a lack of validated prognostic and predictive biomarkers in GC able to guide the choice of a tailored treatment for each patient [15]. Therefore, the treatment algorithm for metastatic GC is often painted according to the patient's (age, PS, comorbidities, and nutritional assessment) or tumor's (tumor burden, symptomatic disease, metastatic sites) characteristics. Thus, a multidisciplinary evaluation of each patient is crucial in the treatment decision process.

In this context, it is unclear how the sites of metastases may affect the prognosis. In fact, if the presence of peritoneal disease or of multiple metastatic sites is considered a well-known worse prognostic factor [16], the knowledge about the role of bone metastases or other visceral sites, such as lung, is scant. This could be related to the rarity of bone involvement in GC, representing the fifth metastatic site after liver, peritoneum, lymph nodes, and—according to the series—lung. Additionally, they are often underestimated at the diagnosis due to the lack of specific recommendation for their detection. Thus, bone metastases have been typically searched for only in case of appearance of new symptoms (e.g., pain), and a consistent fraction of them have been recognized only post-mortem during autopsy in case of non-symptomatic disease [17].

Based on this background, the aim of this narrative review is to describe the evidence existing about bone metastases in GC patients, focusing on their incidence and biology, their prognostic role, and possible implication in the treatment choice.

2. The Biological Basis of Bone Involvement in Metastatic Gastric Cancer

From a biological point of view, bones are a unique and favored site for metastases from several types of cancer, and complex mechanisms are responsible for the development of bone metastasis [18,19]. The cells mostly responsible for bone metabolism are osteoblasts, osteoclasts and osteocytes. In general, osteoblasts produce a bone matrix, called osteoid, which consists of proteins, mainly type I collagen (95%), and they synthesize hydroxyapatite crystals, mineralizing the bone matrix; at the end of their synthetic processes, some osteoblasts are "trapped" into their own matrix and become osteocytes [20]. Osteoblasts, which derived from mesenchymal stem cells, are primarily responsible for bone formation; however, they are also involved in bone destruction [21]. In fact, these cells could be stimulated in both physiological and pathological conditions through the excretion of parathormone (PTH) or, in pathological conditions only, through its related peptide-PTHrP- to overproduce the Receptor Activator of Nuclear factor-κB Ligand (RANK-L) [22]. RANK-L—a member of the RANKL/RANK/osteoprotegerin (OPG) pathway and belonging to tumor necrosis factor (TNF) superfamily—exists both as a transmembrane protein and as a soluble form; it interacts with RANK on the surface of osteoclasts, resulting in their activation via transcription factors [23,24]. Preclinical studies have shown that RANK-L is able to promote the migration of breast cancer cells [25] but also of GC cells. Interestingly, in GC it could interact with epidermal growth factor receptor (EGFR) [26]. Osteoblasts are also able to reduce osteoclastogenic activity by expressing OPG, which is a decoy receptor for RANKL that prevents RANK signaling activation [27].

Osteoclasts are multinucleated cells deriving from the monocyte/macrophage lineage, which is responsible for bone resorption by creating sealed zones. In these zones, they can dissolve bone minerals and degrade extracellular matrix (ECM) bone proteins through the secretion of H+, Cl- and enzymes such as cathepsin K and matrix metalloproteinases (MMPs) [28]. During this process, growth factors—namely bone morphogenetic proteins (BMPs) and fibroblast growth factors—are released from the bone matrix; this release causes the attraction of osteoblasts and the start of a new cycle inside the Bone Remodeling Compartment [29,30]. In adulthood, in physiological conditions, bone remodeling reaches equilibrium between formation and resorption. Nevertheless, the quantity of bone loss is not entirely replaced over the years, causing an unrelenting decline in bone mass with aging [31,32].

Several steps are required for bone metastases development: first of all, cells from the primary tumor should reach bones through systemic circulation; then, they enter the bone microenvironment, especially in areas of the skeleton characterized by high vascularization, such as bones with red marrow [33]. The hypothesis of vascular niches in the bone microenvironment, which promotes the skeletal localization of tumor cells through their extravasation and docking, is supported by the discovery of biological and molecular mechanisms, such as cytokines, adhesion molecules, and skeletal endothelial cells properties [34]. Additionally, the dormancy of disseminated tumor cells, followed by their reactivation and proliferation, is a poorly understood process involved in bone metastases development [35].

Although during metastatic dissemination, the circulating tumor cells could localize in bone marrow virtually in all types of solid tumors [36], differences in the incidence of bone metastases across distinct primary tumor sites have suggested the implication of specific and histotype-related mechanisms. In fact, there are several mechanisms—that are not entirely understood—that could lead to a distinct pattern of metastatization, also according to the heterogeneity of primary tumor. In this context, an analysis on 910 samples from 100 patients affected by renal cancer showed that monoclonal tumors tend to provide a more rapid metastatization to multiple sites. Otherwise, heterogeneous tumors had late progression as single metastatic lesions [19]. Nevertheless, bone metastases from gastrointestinal cancers are quite uncommon [33].

Regarding GC, it is still not very clear how the tumor cells colonize the bone microenvironment. Since bone metastases are the results of hematogenous spreading of cancer cells, preferential ways among venous systems, potentially used by GC cells to reach the skeleton, have not been identified [37]. Angiogenesis, which is involved in gastric carcinogenesis and tumor progression, could play a primary role in bone metastasis growth [38]. Among the actors of tumoral angiogenesis, mast cells positive to tryptase (MCPT) have demonstrated to be positively associated with neovascularization in bone metastases from GC, identifying them as a new potential anti-tumor target [39].

PTHrP has been found to be expressed in several epithelial cancers, including gastric adenocarcinoma [40], where it was found to be overexpressed in moderately and poorly differentiated tumors as well as in metastatic sites [41,42]. However, no association with an increased risk of bone metastases has been reported in gastric adenocarcinomas overproducing PTHrP [42].

RANKL expression in resected GC has been associated to high risk of distant metastases and poor prognosis [43]. However, to date no correlation between RANKL expression and bone metastases development risk has been found in those tumors.

Finally, BMP4 has been described to be overexpressed in GC [44]. In an in vivo model of prostate cancer, BMP4 favors tumor growth in bone by tumor-induced osteogenesis [45]. In GC cells, BMP4 could be responsible for the development of metastasis by enhancing epithelial–mesenchymal transition (EMT) [46]. However, despite of these evidences, the role of BMP4 role in bone metastases from GC should be further elucidated.

3. Clinical Overview on Bone Metastases from Gastric Cancer

The skeleton has been considered a typical metastatic site in some kind of tumors, such as breast or prostate cancer [47,48]. However, bone involvement is considered unusual in GC. In fact, the little evidence that exists in the literature has shown that bone metastases occur in metastatic GC patients in a range between 0.9% and 13.4%, according to the study population [17,49–62]. However, it is important to note that these data mostly come from retrospective analysis and case series. Therefore, no prospective evaluation regarding the characteristics and distribution of bone metastasis in GC exists to date.

In general, the most important issues to consider in the knowledge of bone metastases in GC patients are the time of onset (at diagnosis—synchronous, or at the time of progression—metachronous), the type of metastases (osteolytic, osteoblastic, or mixed), their distribution (axial versus appendicular skeleton), the prognostic implications of metastatic bone involvement and correlation with other patients' and tumor's clinicopathological characteristics.

3.1. Incidence, Onset, Type and Distribution

Moving from the first historical report by Yoshikawa et al. in 1983 [17], showing 33 GC patients with bone metastases, the research has focused on this topic especially over the last decade. Table 1 summarizes the most significant data reported in the literature regarding the descriptive evaluation of bone metastases in GC, including time of onset, type, and distribution. Of note, the articles that were not available in English were not considered in this review.

Among the available studies, a retrospective Italian analysis, which collected the data from 2000 metastatic GC patients treated at 22 centers over 12 years (from 1998 to 2011), is one of the largest multicenter experiences in this context [55]. The trial showed a bone involvement in 10% of metastatic GC patients (208 patients); of them, 28% were diagnosed with bone metastasis (synchronous disease), whereas 62% had a bone progression of disease (metachronous disease). The majority of patients were young (<61 years old: 52.9%), male (66%), showing an ECOG PS 1 (43.9%); the most frequent disease characteristics were the following: intestinal subtype according to Lauren classification (38.9%) [63], grade 3 (81.3%), N2 involvement according to TNM stage (41.5%), and concurrent visceral metastasis (86.3%). It is important to underline that 27% of patients had an ECOG PS 2–3 at the diagnosis of bone involvement; additionally, 33% of patients had a diffuse tumor subtype according to Lauren classification [63]. Regarding the type and distribution of the lesions, the majority of patients included in the study population had multiple bone metastasis, especially in the long bones (52%); those lesions were mostly osteolytic (52% versus 25% mixed lesions and 23% osteoblastic ones).

Table 1. Clinical overview about bone metastases characteristics in gastric cancer patients.

Author and year *	Study Design, Timeline, Country	N Patients Analyzed	N Patient with Bone Metastasis (%)	Onset	Type	Distribution	Main Patients' Characteristics	Main Tumor's Characteristics	Outcomes
Yoshikawa et al., 1983 [17]	Retrospective Monoinstitutional 1970–1979 Japan	1945	23 (1.2%)	NR	NR	Thoracic vertebrae: 69.6%; Lumbar vertebrae: 69.6%; Pelvic bones: 26.1%; Ribs: 21.7%	Young (age <60: 78.3%); male: 56.5%	NR	NR
Park et al., 2011 [59]	Retrospective Monoinstitutional 1998–2008 Korea	8633	203 (2.4%)	Synchronous: 62%; Metachronous: 38%	NR	NR	Median age: 51 years; multiple metastatic sites (bone and visceral): 84.7%; multiple bone metastasis: 88.7%; ECOG PS 0–2: 82%	Poorly differentiated: 72%	mOS: 3.4 months
Park et al., 2013 [64]	Retrospective Monoinstitutional 1989–2008 Korea	1683	30 (1.8%)	Metachronous: 100%	NR	Vertebrae: 93.3%; pelvic bones: 40%; ribs: 33.3%	young (median age 53.1 years old) male: 63.3%	Undifferentiated: 73% N3: 43.3%	mOS after bone recurrence: 6 months
Silvestri N et al., 2013 [55]	Retrospective Multicenter 1998–2011 Italy	2000	208 (10%)	Synchronous: 28%; Metachronous: 62%	Osteolytic: 52%; mixed: 25%; osteoblastic: 23%	Long bones: 52%; Hip: 38%; Spine: 20%	young (median age 61 years old): 52.9%; male: 66%; ECOG PS 0–1: 43.9%; multiple metastatic sites (bone and visceral): 86.3%; multiple bone metastasis: 68.6%	Intestinal: 38.9%; G3: 81.3%; N2: 41.5%.	mOS: 14 months; mOS from the diagnosis: 6 months; mOS SRE versus no SRE: 3 versus 5 months
Nakamura et al., 2014 [60]	Retrospective Monoinstitutional 2000–2010	1837	31 (1.7%)	Synchronous: 25.8%; Metachronous: 74.2%	NR	NR	Age <65: 51.6%; multiple metastatic sites (bone and visceral): 79.5%; multiple bone metastasis: 79.5%; ECOG PS 0–1: 58.1%	Undifferentiated: 67.8%	mOS: 3.3 months

Table 1. Cont.

Author and year *	Study Design, Timeline, Country	N Patients Analyzed	N Patient with Bone Metastasis (%)	Onset	Type	Distribution	Main Patients' Characteristics	Main Tumor's Characteristics	Outcomes
Mikami et al., 2017 [61]	Retrospective Monoinstitutional 2010–2015	NR	34 (100%)	Synchronous: 29.4%; Metachronous: 70.6%	NR	Thoracic vertebrae: 55.9%; Pelvic bones: 41.2%; Lumbar vertebrae: 38.2%; Ribs: 29.4%	multiple metastatic sites (bone and visceral): 76.5%; multiple bone metastasis: 64.7%	Undifferentiated: 55.9%	mOS: 7.5 months
Qiu et al., 2018 [58]	Retrospective Multicenter 2010–2014	19022	966 (5.1%)	NR	NR	NR	NR	Intestinal: 62%; G3: 60.7%; located to the cardia: 38%	mOS: 4 months; 5 year CSS: 1.27%
Wen L et al., 2019 [56]	Retrospective Monoinstitutional 2008–2018 China	884	66 (11.3%)	Synchronous: 45.5%; Metachronous: 54.5%	NR	Spine: 78.5%; pelvic bones: 68.2%; ribs: 47.0%; lower extremity: 34.8%; sternum: 33.3%; scapula: 31.8%; upper extremity: 21.2%; skull: 19.7%	young (median age 53 years old) male: 68.2%; ECOG PS 0–1: 68.2%; multiple metastatic sites (bone and visceral): 84.9%; multiple bone metastasis: 84.8%	G3/mucinous/ signet ring cells: 71.2%; located to the antrum: 30.3%	mOS: 6.5 months; mOS metachronous: 11.8 months synchronous: 4.1 months
Liang C et al., 2020 [57]	Retrospective Multicenter 2010–2016	42966	1798 (4.2%)	NR	NR	NR	multiple metastatic sites (bone and visceral): 52.6%	Intestinal: 60.8%; G3: 62.2%; located to the cardia: 38.4%	mOS: 3 months
Imura et al., 2020 [62]	Retrospective Monoinstitutional 2005–2017	NR	60 (100%)	NR	NR	NR	Age >60: 56.7%; multiple metastatic sites (bone and visceral): 61.7%; multiple bone metastasis: 83.3%; ECOG PS 0–2: 70%	NR	mOS: 9 months

* listed by year. Abbreviations: N: number; ECOG PS: performance status according to ECOG scale; G3: grade 3; mOS: median overall survival; SRE: skeletal-related events; NR: not reported.

A subsequent Chinese retrospective analysis evaluated the clinicopathological characteristics of bone metastases in 66 patients with GC treated at one institution over a period of 10 years (2008–2018), representing 11.3% of the entire metastatic GC patients population evaluated in the study (884 patients) [56]. Among them, 45.5% and 54.5% had synchronous and metachronous bone metastases, respectively. The majority of those patients were young male (68.2%) with ECOG PS 0–1 (68.2%), multiple metastatic sites involved (bone and visceral: 84.9%), and multiple bone metastases (84.8%) with prevalent axial distribution (spine: 78.5%; pelvic bones: 68.2%; ribs: 47.0%; lower extremity: 34.8%; sternum: 33.3%; scapula: 31.8%; upper extremity: 21.2%; skull: 19.7%). However, this analysis did not report the type of metastasis (osteolytic, osteoblastic, or mixed). Finally, the majority of tumors was poor differentiated/mucinous/signet ring cells (71.2%) and were located in the antrum (30.3%).

Recently, another Chinese retrospective analysis showed the data from 42,966 GC collected in the American population by Surveillance, Epidemiology, and End Results (SEER) database over a period of six years (2010–2016) [57]. Of them, 1798 patients had bone involvement (4.18%). In addition, in this case bone metastases were more commonly reported in young patients (7.3% in 20–39 years old range), with an inverse correlation with age (5.45% in 40–59 years older, 4.09% in 60–79 years older, and 2.39% in >80 years older subgroup). Additionally, they were more common in men and in tumors showing the following characteristics: grade 3 (odd ratio (OR): 3.93, $p < 0.001$), located to the stomach (antrum versus proximal location: OR = 0.81; $p = 0.02$), diffuse according to Lauren classification [63] (OR: 1.46, $p < 0.001$), with signet ring cells or with nodal involvement (OR: 2.09, $p < 0.001$). These data regarding tumor and patients' characteristics were consistent with those showed by Qiu MZ et al. in another retrospective analysis from the SEER database including GC treated between 2010 and 2014 [58]. Of note, Liang C et al. [56] reported that the patients who underwent to surgical resection of primary tumors had a lower incidence of bone metastases if compared to the patients who did not receive a surgical approach (0.36% versus 7.6%). Finally, also in this case, patients with bone metastases had concurrent extra-bone metastatic sites and multiple bone sites involved. However, this analysis evaluated neither the type of the lesions and their distribution nor their onset time.

Finally, few anecdotal cases of GC patients with bone metastasis located to the bones of the hand were reported [64–68].

For a summary of the incidence of bone involvement according to different skeletal sites, see Figure 1.

Additionally, there are few reports in the literature regarding the appearance of bone lesions related to early GC [69,70]. When the primary tumor is an early lesion, the presence of metastases to the bone is often underdiagnosed, because bone involvement is investigated only in case of symptoms (e.g., pain). Park et al. focused on the incidence and risk factors of bone recurrence in 1683 GC patients who received a curative resection between 1989 and 2008 [71]. Therefore, this retrospective study analyzed only metachronous bone disease. The incidence of bone involvement was 1.8% in the entire study population, with a higher rate in case of advanced primary tumor at diagnosis (0.4% in case of early GC versus 3.4% in the more advanced stages). The median time from the surgery to the detection of bone metastases was 28 months (range: 4–111 months) and the majority of patients had multiple metastases located to the axial skeleton (spine: 93.3%, pelvic bone: 40% and ribs: 36.6%).

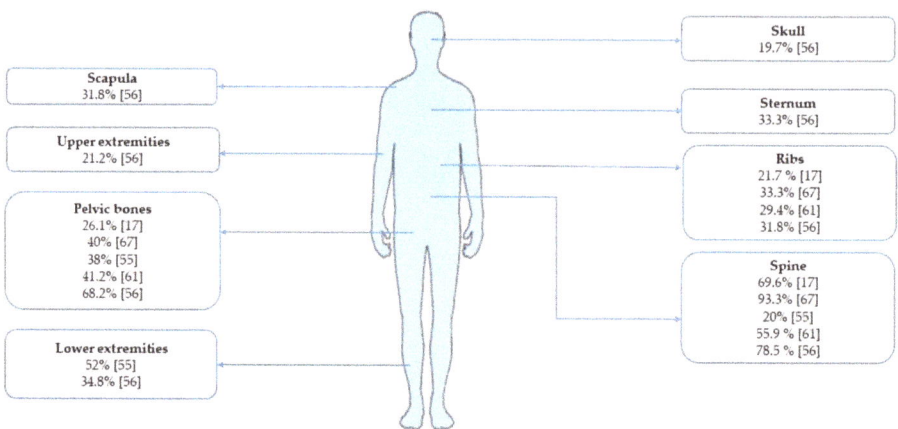

Figure 1. Incidence of bone metastases from gastric cancer according to skeletal sites.

Lastly, even if the majority of the GC recurrence occur into the first two years after curative resection, anecdotal cases of late relapses have been reported in the literature [72,73]. In particular, Iovino et al. reported the case of a 49-year-old patient who showed a tumor relapse from GC after 11 years from the curative surgical resection [73]. The patient had severe neurological signs from a diffuse vertebral involvement and marrow infiltration without detection of any other metastatic lesions or primary tumor; the biopsy of the soft tissue near the lumbar vertebra confirmed the metastatic nature of the lesion, which spread from GC. The authors explained the long latency with the tumor dormancy theory, according to that few tumor cells could be present in the organs in a state of cell-cycle arrest; thus, there is a balance between tumor cells growth and apoptosis that could persist over many years [34]. Even if the entire process is still poorly understood, the tumor cells could reactivate after the variable time, leading to a tumor relapse.

3.2. Prognostic Implications of Bone Metastasis in GC Patients

Unfortunately, unlike in other types of tumors, such as renal cancer [74,75], up to date, no prospective dedicated trials regarding GC patients with bone metastases exist in the literature. Additionally, no data about the outcomes of these patients were reported in the landmark phase II and III trials in the metastatic GC setting (see above). Therefore, the most representative data regarding the prognosis of patients with GC and bone metastasis came from the same retrospective analysis already cited in the previous Section 3.1 [17,49–62] (Table 1).

More in detail, Silvestris et al. reported a median overall survival (OS) of 14 months in the entire study population (95% confidence interval (CI): 12–15.9 months), with a median time of 8 months for the first diagnosis of bone involvement (95% CI: 6.1–9.8 months) and a median OS of 6 months from that diagnosis (95% CI: 5–6.9 months) [55]. Of note, they included in the analysis only GC patients with bone metastases who died, whereas they did not evaluate alive patients with documented metastases to the bone. Additionally, they showed that the appearance of skeletal-related events (SREs) impacts on the prognosis (for additional details regarding SRE see the next Section 4.2.2). This analysis showed that a D2 lymph node dissection was an independent prognostic factor of both shorter time to the diagnosis of bone involvement in GC patients (hazard ratio (HR): 2.7, p: 0.013) and worse survival in case of bone metastases recognition (HR: 2.285, p: 0.008). Finally, there was no difference in median OS in patients diagnosed with synchronous or metachronous bone disease (5 months in each subgroup). This may be related to the worse prognosis linked to the mere diagnosis of bone metastatic involvement. Finally, the authors evaluated only the use of zoledronic acid, whereas there is no mention of the type of chemotherapy used or its impact on survival.

Wen et al. [56] showed a median OS of 6.5 months in the entire population (95% CI: 4.2–8.7 months), with 69.7%, 41.5%, and 13.3% patients alive at 6, 12, and 24 months, respectively. Unlike the previous Italian analysis [55], the author showed a worse OS in case of synchronous disease if compared to metachronous one (4.1 versus 11.8 months, $p = 0.032$). Additionally, they reported a better survival in patients who had received an active chemotherapy (p: 0.004) as well as in patients who showed a good PS ECOG (8 months versus 3.6 months in the ECOG 0–1 and ECOG 2 subgroup, respectively; $p = 0.001$). However, the authors did not show the type of active treatment used and the study population was deeply heterogeneous, which was mainly due to the retrospective nature of the study design and the rarity of bone involvement in metastatic GC.

The risk of developing bone metastases was higher in patients affected by metastatic GC with lung involvement (20.24% versus 4.06%, $p < 0.001$) as reported by Qiu et al. [58]. In this analysis, they showed a median OS of 4 months in case of bone metastases, with a case-specific survival rate of 1.27% (versus 29.86% in patients without bone involvement). Therefore, they concluded that even if it is hard to routinely assess a metastatic disease to the bone or the brain from GC, due to the rarity of their involvement and the risk of overlook, it could be feasible to evaluate those sites in patients who have risk factors (e.g., lung or liver metastasis).

The recent analysis by Liang et al. underlined the impact of surgery of the primary tumor site and of the chemotherapy on the outcome of GC patients with bone involvement [57]. In fact, they reported a median OS of 3 months in the entire study population, improved to 9 months in patients who received surgery (versus 3 months in case of no resection, HR: 0.54, 95% CI: 0.40–0.72; $p < 0.001$) and to 7 months in patients who received chemotherapy (versus one month, $p < 0.001$). Of note, this analysis did not show any benefit by adding radiotherapy to the treatment ($p > 0.05$). However, also in this case, the authors did not describe the type of surgery or chemotherapy used, due to the nature of the analysis (retrospective design on data collected in the SEER database). Additionally, they reported the following limitations of the analysis: the underestimation of bone involvement in GC, since they recorded only symptomatic diagnosed cases, the lack of data regarding peritoneal metastasis, and the inaccurate evaluation of death-related causes.

In conclusion, the presence of bone metastases seems to be related to worse prognosis in metastatic GC patients. However, due to the retrospective design of the analysis, the heterogeneity of the study populations, and the rarity of bone involvement, further investigations are needed in order to evaluate the prognostic role of bone metastases and to confirm these findings.

4. Clinical Management of Metastatic Gastric Cancer Patients with Bone Involvement

4.1. Radiological Assessment

Unlike others cancer types with higher incidence of bone metastases, the European Society of Medical Oncology (ESMO) [3] and National Comprehensive Cancer Network (NCCN) guidelines [76] do not recommend skeletal screening with bone scintigraphy in patients with GC at the time of diagnosis or during treatment. Therefore, the incidence of asymptomatic bone lesions is likely underestimated, and approximately 14% of GC patients are diagnosed with bone metastasis only during autopsy [52].

Chest-abdomen-pelvis computed tomography (CT) scan is the most commonly used imaging technique in the initial diagnostic workup; however, in the follow-up setting, it is recommended only in case of symptoms suspicious for bone recurrence, such as pain [77].

The elevated serum levels of alkaline phosphatase (ALP), which is known to be the most predictive biological marker for the presence of bone metastases in GC, together with the presence of elevated tumor markers, such as carcinoembryonic antigen (CEA) and CA19-9, suggest the need for skeletal screening [78].

In case of recurrence of disease, it has been demonstrated that more aggressive tumor phenotypes, including the presence of lymph node metastasis, are associated with higher risk of bone recurrence. In particular, Park et al. showed that the N2/N3 stage has a risk of bone recurrence significantly higher than N0/N1 (HR: 1.44, 95% CI: 1.217–1.694) [64]. Additionally, Liang et al. have recently described some clinical and histological features than could help the oncologists to identify the "patients with high risk of bone metastases": Gastro Esophageal Junction (GEJ) cancer, younger age, white race, poor differentiated tumor grade, higher lymph nodes stage, and diffuse histology according to Lauren classification [57,63]. They might suggest the use of radiological bone assessment in this population as standard at baseline.

^{18}Fluorodeoxiglucose Positron Emission Tomography (^{18}FDG-PET) scan can be useful for the evaluation of lymph nodes involvement as well as for distant metastases including bone metastases. Nevertheless, it is well known that it has a lower sensitivity in GC patients with diffuse histological type, due to the lower glucose transporter 1 (GLUT1) expression in these cells [79].

Finally, the role of magnetic resonance imaging is limited to the evaluation of medullary involvement in the presence of neurological symptoms. Additionally, it is very sensitive for the study of vertebral and pelvic metastatic disease [80].

A "Tricky" Evaluation of the Response on Bone Metastases during Treatment: Focus on the Bone Flare

Patients with bone metastases from GC require periodic bone evaluation with a CT scan with a bone window in order to assess the response to therapy according to Response evaluation criteria in solid tumors (RECIST) 1.1 criteria [81]. Additionally, a bone scintigraphy or ^{18}FDG-PET could be performed. However, unlike the visceral sites, the response evaluation in case of bone metastases might be difficult due to the existence of strict criteria in this setting [81] and the possibility to detect the bone flair.

The bone flare is a radiological phenomenon, which refers to an increased radiotracer uptake (i.e., 99mTc-labeled bisphosphonates used in the bone scintigraphy) in the bones of the patients with metastatic cancer and bone metastases at baseline, despite the clinical and radiological findings of response to treatment in the other metastatic districts of the body. This phenomenon was firstly studied in prostate cancer patients in the mid-1980s [82]. Indeed, learning from the experiences in prostate cancer, a worsening in bone scan during the first months of systemic treatment for bone metastases could be caused by an intense osteoblastic response and not by a progression of disease [83]. Therefore, it is important to note that we can refer to the bone flair only in case of osteoblastic lesions, whereas an increased isotope uptake by osteolytic metastases should always be considered as a progression of disease. However, often it could be difficult to discriminate bone flare from progressive bone metastases, with a concrete risk of wrong response assessment. In prostate cancer, a prospective study on treatment-naïve metastatic patients showed that bone flare can occur in patients with positive baseline bone scan in a high percentage of cases but also in patients with no abnormalities at the scintigraphy performed at the baseline. Interestingly, these patients were confirmed to have skeletal metastases at follow-up [84].

Bone flare phenomenon has been also reported in other kind of tumors [85–88], including GC. Up to date, only two case reports about bone flare in GC patients have been published. More in detail, Amoroso et al. reported the case of a 43-year-old man who started chemotherapy for advanced disease. Despite of the appearance of new osteoblastic lesions, treatment was continued, and the second radiological evaluation confirmed the presence of stable osteoblastic lesions [89]. The other case is about a 54-year-old male with baseline bone metastases from GC who showed an increased intensity at bone scan after three cycles of chemotherapy, despite an improvement in skeletal pain. Nevertheless, after additional three cycles of chemotherapy, the bone scan revealed a decrease in the intensity of the signal in the same areas [90].

In conclusion, even if rare, bone flare should be taken into account in metastatic GC patients with osteoblastic lesions who show progression of disease only to the skeleton. In these cases, especially if the patients do not show a clinical worsening, the clinicians should be aware about this phenomenon, since it could be misinterpreted as progression of disease, leading to a change in the chemotherapy regimen. Therefore, a multidisciplinary framework in distinguishing the two conditions is critical also in GC patients.

4.2. How to Treat Metastatic Gastric Cancer Patients with Bone Metastases

The treatment of GC patients with metastases to the skeleton can be distinguished into two areas: treatment of metastatic GC disease per se and bone-related treatments.

4.2.1. Systemic Treatments

According to international guidelines [3,76], palliative chemotherapy—with or without targeted agents—is the standard of care in the treatment of metastatic GC. In fact, surgery is not an option in case of metastatic disease, especially to the bone. A detailed description of the currently recommended treatments for metastatic GC disease and/or future perspectives is not in the aim of this review; however, you can refer to dedicated literature and guidelines [3–5,12,76] for detailed coverage.

To date, there is a lack of specific data regarding bone involvement in the landmark phase II and III trials in GC. In fact, among ≈50 clinical trials investigating the role of chemotherapy, target therapies, and immunotherapies in advanced GC (first-, second-, ≥third lines) over the last two decades, only seven trials showed specific data for GC patients with skeletal metastases (Table 2).

In particular, among chemotherapy trials, in 2008, Al-Batran S et al. compared the efficacy of FLO (fluorouracil, leucovorin, and oxaliplatin) and FLP (fluorouracil, leucovorin, and cisplatin) regimen as first-line treatment for 220 metastatic GC patients, reporting the data of 6.8% of patients with bone involvement [91]. However, the trial did not show the subgroup analysis for those patients and did not report the outcomes accordingly. In 2009, the non-inferiority phase III ML17032 trial, which compared CX (cisplatin and capecitabine) versus CF (cisplatin and fluorouracil) as first-line treatment in 316 metastatic GC patients, showed a bone involvement in 6.3% of patients; additionally, the authors evaluated the impact of bone metastases on survival outcome (subgroup analysis), showing a benefit by using the CX regimen in these patients (see Table 2 for additional details) [92]. Finally, the phase III SOS trial reported 3.2% prevalence of bone metastases in 625 Asian patients receiving Cisplatin+S-1 every five weeks versus Cisplatin+S-1 every three weeks as first-line treatment [93]. However, no data regarding the impact of bone involvement on the prognosis were shown in this trial as well.

The Korean trial is the only second-line chemotherapy trial reporting the rate of bone involvement in the study population (6%) [94]. No data about the prognosis are available from this trial.

In the context of target therapies trials, the AVATAR [95] and INTEGRATE [96] are the only studies reporting the rate of skeletal metastases. The phase III AVATAR trial investigated the efficacy of the addition of bevacizumab (anti-vascular endothelial growth factor agent) to chemotherapy (CX regimen) as first-line treatment in 202 Asian patients with metastatic GC [95]. The phase II INTEGRATE trial evaluated the activity of regorafenib versus best supportive care as second or third-line treatment for 147 metastatic GC patients [96]. The trials showed that 3.5% [95] and 10.8% [96] of patients had metastatic bone disease, respectively. However, unfortunately, there are no data regarding the prognostic effect of bone involvement in both trials.

Regarding the trials investigating the role of immunotherapy in metastatic GC, the Asian phase III ATTRACTION-2 trial, which tested the efficacy of nivolumab in highly pretreated patients, is the only one showing data about the rate of bone metastases (2.2%) [97,98]. However, also in this case, no data about the outcomes are available for these patients.

Table 2. Data regarding bone metastases according to the landmark phase II/III trials in metastatic gastric cancer.

Trial and Year of Publication	Phase	Setting	N Patients	Type of Metastatic Sites Reported (% of Patients)	N Patients with Bone Metastases (%)	Arms and Eventual Target	Outcomes in Patients with Bone Metastases
Chemotherapy *							
V325 trial, 2006 [99]	III	First line	445	NR	NR	TCF versus CF	NR
Dank M et al., 2008 [100]	III	First line	333	Lung: 8.7%; Liver: 49%; Lymph node: 62.1%; Peritoneum: 24.3%; Pleura: 8.1%; Adrenal: 6.3%	NR	CF versus Folfiri	NR
REAL-2, 2008 [101]	III	First-line	1002	NR	NR	ECF/ECX versus EOF/EOX (non-inferiority)	NR
Al-Batran et al., 2008 [91]	III	First-line	220	Lung: 12.7%; Liver: 50.4%; Lymph node: 47.7%; Peritoneum: 30.4%; Pleura: 8.1%; Other: 28.6%	14 (6.8%)	FLO versus FLP	NR
ML17032, 2009 [92]	III	First line	316	Lung: 7.9%; Liver: 48.4%; Peritoneum: 18.7%; Pleura: 3.1%; Soft tissue: 3.8%; Skin: 0.6%	20 (6.3%)	CX versus CF (non-inferiority)	OS: Bone metastases: HR: 1, no bone: HR ≈0.8 (favor CX) PFS: Bone metastases: HR ≈0.6, no bone: HR ≈0.85 (favor CX)
FLAGS trial, 2010 [102]	III	First line	1053	NR	NR	Cisplatin+S-1 versus CF	NR
GC0301/TOP-002 trial, 2011 [103]	III	First line	326	Liver: 33.7%; Peritoneum: 32.2%	NR	S-1 versus S-1+ irinotecan	NR
FFCD trial, 2014 [104]	III	First line	416	NR	NR	ECX versus Folfiri	NR
Yamada et al., 2015 [105]	III	First line	685	Lung: 10.3%; Liver: 36.9%; Lymph node: 84.2%; Peritoneum: 18.2%	NR	Oxaliplatin+S-1 versus Cisplatin+S-1 (non-inferiority)	NR
SOS trial, 2015 [93]	III	First line	625	Lung: 6.8%; Liver: 35.3%; Lymph node: 67.7%; Peritoneum: 37.3%	20 (3.2%)	Cisplatin+S-1 q5 weeks versus q3 weeks	NR
AIO, 2011 [106]	III	Second line	40	Lung: 10%; Liver: 45%; Lymph node: 35%; Peritoneum: 45%; Other: 35%	NR	Irinotecan versus BSC	NR

Table 2. Cont.

Trial and Year of Publication	Phase	Setting	N Patients	Type of Metastatic Sites Reported (% of Patients)	N Patients with Bone Metastases (%)	Arms and Eventual Target	Outcomes in Patients with Bone Metastases
Korean trial, 2012 [94]	III	Second line	202	Peritoneum: 45%; Lung: 9%;; Liver: 28%; Lymph node: 44%	12 (6%)	Docetaxel or irinotecan versus BSC	NR
WJOG4007, 2013 [107]	III	Second line	223	Peritoneum: 25.1%	NR	Weekly paclitaxel versus irinotecan (non-inferiority)	NR
COUGAR-02, 2013 [108]	III	Second line	168	Lung: 26%; Liver: 44% Lymph node: 65%; Local: 31% Other: 34%	NR	Docetaxel versus BSC	NR
ABSOLUTE, 2017 [109]	III	Second line	741	Peritoneum: 35.2%	NR	nab-paclitaxel every 3 weeks versus weekly nab-paclitaxel versus weekly paclitaxel	NR
TAGS, 2018 [110]	III	≥ Third line	507	Peritoneum: 27.6%	NR	Trifluridin/tipiracil versus placebo	NR
Target therapy *							
AVAGAST, 2011 [111]	III	First line	774	NR	NR	CX ± Bevacizumab; VEGF	NR
ToGA, 2013 [112]	III	First line	594	NR	NR	CF/CX ± Trastuzumab; HER-2	NR
EXPAND, 2013 [113]	III	First line	904	Peritoneum: 25%	NR	CX ± Cetuximab; EGFR	NR
REAL-3, 2013 [114]	III	First line	553	NR	NR	EOC ± Panitumumab; EGFR	NR
AVATAR, 2015 [95]	III	First line	202	Liver: 39.1%	7 (3.5%)	CX ± Bevacizumab; VEGF	NR
FAST, 2016 [115]	IIb	First line	161	NR (only abstract available)	NR (only abstract available)	EOX ± Claudiximab; claudin 18.2	NR (only abstract available)
LOGIC, 2016 [116]	III	First line	545	NR	NR	CapeOX ± Lapatinib; HER-2	NR

Table 2. Cont.

Trial and Year of Publication	Phase	Setting	N Patients	Type of Metastatic Sites Reported (% of Patients)	N Patients with Bone Metastases (%)	Arms and Eventual Target	Outcomes in Patients with Bone Metastases
METGastric, 2017 [117]	III	First line	562	NR	NR	Folfox ± Onartuzumab; MET	NR
RILOMET-1, 2017 [118]	III	First line	609	Liver: 41.7%	NR	ECX ± Rilotumumab; MET	NR
HELOISE, 2017 [119]	IIIb	First line	248	NR	NR	CF/CX+ trastuzumab (two doses as mantainance); HER-2	NR
JACOB, 2018 [120]	III	First line	780	NR	NR	CF/CX+ Trastuzumab ± Pertuzumab; HER-2	NR
RAINFALL, 2019 [121]	III	First line	645	Peritoneum: 37.4%; Liver: 29.3%	NR	CF/CX+ ramucirumab; VEGFR-2	NR
GRANITE-1, 2013 [122]	III	Second line Third line	656	Lung: 19.6%; Liver: 45.5%	NR	Everolimus versus placebo; mTOR	NR
REGARD, 2014 [123]	III	Second line	355	Peritoneum: 30.7%	NR	Ramucirumab versus Placebo; VEGFR-2	NR
RAINBOW, 2014 [124]	III	Second line	665	Peritoneum: 47.3%	NR	Paclitaxel ± Ramucirumab; VEGFR-2	NR
TyTAN, 2014 [125]	III	Second line	261	No visceral: 98.8%	NR	Paclitaxel ± Lapatinib; HER-2	NR
INTEGRATE, 2016 [96]	II	Second line Third line	147	Lung: 20.4%; Liver: 53.7%; Lymph node: 51%; Peritoneum: 32%; Other: 36%	16 (10.8%)	Regorafenib versus placebo; multikinase inhibitor	NR
SHINE, 2017 [126]	II	Second line	71	Liver: 56.3%; Lung: 21.1% Peritoneum: 25.4%; Lymph nodes: 54.9%	NR	Paclitaxel ± AZD4546; FGFR-2	NR
GATSBY, 2017 [127]	II/III	Second line	345	Visceral (lung or liver): 100%	NR	Taxanes ± TDM-1; HER-2	NR
GOLD, 2017 [128]	III	Second line	643	NR	NR	paclitaxel ± olaparib; PARP	NR

Table 2. Cont.

Trial and Year of Publication	Phase	Setting	N Patients	Type of Metastatic Sites Reported (% of Patients)	N Patients with Bone Metastases (%)	Arms and Eventual Target	Outcomes in Patients with Bone Metastases
ANGEL, 2019 [129]	III	≥ Third line	460	NR	NR	Rivoceranib (apatinib) versus best supportive care; VEGFR-2	NR (abstract only)
DESTINY-Gastric 01, 2020 [130]	II	≥ Third line	187	NR	NR	Trastuzumab deruxtecan versus chemotherapy (paclitaxel or irinotecan); HER-2	NR
Immunotherapy (single agent and combinations) *							
Janjigian et al., 2020 [131]	II	First line	37	NR	NR	CF/CX or Folfox/Xelox + pembrolizumab + trastuzumab; PD-1, HER-2	NR
KEYNOTE-062, 2020 [7]	III	First line	763	NR	NR	CF/CX± pembrolizumab or pembrolizumab; PD-1	NR
CHECKMATE 649, 2020 [6]	III	First line	1581	NR (only abstract available)	NR (only abstract available)	Folfox/Xelox± nivolumab; PD-1	NR (only abstract available)
ATTRACTION-4, 2020 [132]	III	First line	724	NR (only abstract available)	NR (only abstract available)	chemotherapy± nivolumab; PD-1	NR (only abstract available)
KEYNOTE-590, 2020 [133]	III	First line	749	NR (only abstract available)	NR (only abstract available)	CF± pembrolizumab; PD-1	NR (only abstract available)
JAVELIN-100, 2020 [134]	III	First line maintenance	805	NR	NR	Folfox/Xelox versus avelumab; PD-L1	NR
EPOC1706, 2020 [135]	II	First line Second line	29	Lymph node: 90%; Liver: 45% Lung: 10%; Peritoneum: 31%	NR	Lenvatinib + pembrolizumab; TKI, PD-1	NR
KEYNOTE-061, 2018 [136]	III	Second line	592	Peritoneum: 28%	NR	Paclitaxel versus pembrolizumab; PD-1	NR

Table 2. Cont.

Trial and Year of Publication	Phase	Setting	N Patients	Type of Metastatic Sites Reported (% of Patients)	N Patients with Bone Metastases (%)	Arms and Eventual Target	Outcomes in Patients with Bone Metastases
ATTRACTION-2, 2017 [97]	III	≥Third line	493	Liver: 21.5%; Lung: 4.9%; Peritoneum: 21.3%; Lymph nodes: 85.8%; Pleural: 1.2%; Adrenal: 0.2%; Other: 10.7%	11 (2.2%)	Nivolumab versus placebo; PD-1	NR
JAVELIN-300, 2018 [137]	III	≥Third line	371	NR	NR	Chemotherapy (paclitaxel or irinotecan) versus avelumab; PD-L1	NR
KEYNOTE-059, 2019 [138]	II	≥Third line	259	Peritoneum: 1.5%	NR	Pembrolizumab; PD-1	NR

* listed by line of treatment and by year of publication. Abbreviations: N: number; NR: not reported; TCF: taxotere/cisplatin/5-fluorouracil; CF: cisplatin/5-fluorouracil; ECF: epirubicin/cisplatin/5-fluorouracil; ECX: epirubicin/cisplatin/capecitabine; EOF: epirubicin/oxaliplatin//5-fluorouracil; EOX: epirubicin/oxaliplatin/capecitabine; FLO: 5-fluorouracil/leucovorin/oxaliplatin; FLP: 5-fluorouracil/leucovorin/cisplatin; CX: cisplatin/capecitabine; CF: cisplatin/5-fluorouracil; OS: overall survival; PFS: progression free survival; BSC: best supportive care; VEGF: vascular endothelial growth factor; HER2: epithelial growth factor receptor 2; VEGFR-2: vascular endothelial growth factor receptor 2; FGFR-2: fibroblastic growth factor receptor 2; PARP: poli ADP ribose polymerase; PD-1: programmed death 1; PD-L1: programmed death ligand 1; TKI: tyrosine kinase inhibitor.

In conclusion, even if retrospective evidence seems to suggest a possible worse prognosis in patients with metastatic GC and bone disease, there are no randomized prospective trials confirming these findings. Additionally, no specific data regarding targeted-bone treatments in metastatic GC are available. Therefore, to date, the treatment of metastatic disease does not change according to the metastatic sites involved [3,76]. In particular, the data regarding the impact on bone involvement as well as the response of bone metastases to chemotherapy are limited, and further evaluations about the molecular mechanisms and landscape of bone invasions are needed in order to design specific trials. A multidisciplinary management of those patients, including bone-related treatments, is mandatory in order to palliate the symptoms and to preserve a good PS.

4.2.2. Skeletal-Related Events and Bone-Related Treatments

In general, the presence of bone metastases causes a reduction of physical functions of the patients and deterioration of their quality of life (QoL), especially in case of axial skeleton involvement with multiple osteolytic lesions. In fact, they are often the cause of consistent bone pain that requires opioid-based therapy [139]. Additionally, the presence of bone metastases results in significant morbidity for the patients, mainly because of the associated SREs, which are defined as "pathologic fractures, the need for radiotherapy or surgical interventions to treat or prevent an impending fracture, spinal cord compressions, and hypercalcemia" [59].

In the largest multicenter retrospective study on bone metastases in GC, 31% of patients with skeletal involvement experienced at least one SRE [55]. In this analysis, radiotherapy treatment of the bone lesions was the most common SRE (47.1% of all events), followed by pathologic fracture (22.4%), surgery to the bone sites (15.3%), spinal cord compression (10.6%), and hypercalcemia (4.7%).

Regarding the prognostic value of SREs, median survival in the whole population was 3 months after the development of the first SRE (versus 5 months in patients without SREs), suggesting that the poor prognosis of these patients is related not only to the presence of bone disease per se but also to the appearance of SREs.

Therefore, the bone-targeted treatments are important as well as the systemic therapies in order to improve the outcomes for metastatic patients, allowing them to control pain and to maintain a good PS and eventually receive multiple lines of treatment for metastatic disease ("continuum of care" concept). In this context, radiotherapy, surgery, and drug therapies represent the main options; there is no difference in those treatments according to the primary tumor site (e.g., prostate, breast, gastric, etc.) [140].

The use of radiotherapy has been shown to be very effective to control pain—especially with a neuropathic component—in patients with bone metastases after failure of or intolerance to opioid-based therapy as well as to prevent impending fractures. Several randomized trials have been conducted to assess the fraction schedule of the palliative radiotherapy; based on these analyses and a systematic review [141], a single dose of 8 Gy seems to be the best option for patients with poor prognosis, especially if they have vertebral involvement.

In selected cases, also, orthopedic surgery and neurosurgery can help to improve the QoL of these patients, to control incoercible pain, to prevent long bones and vertebral impending fractures and spinal cord compression.

The role of "bone-focused" drugs has been defined in the last years. Bisphosphonates and RANK-L inhibitors are the most important agents in this field. Bisphosphonates-based treatments, such as zoledronic acid at the dose of 4 mg every 3 or 4 weeks as intravenous infusion, is able to modify the bone homeostasis, with the inhibition of osteoclast-mediated bone resorption; they are useful to prevent and delay SREs in solid tumors, including GC [142]. Silvestris et al. showed a significant extension of the time to the first SRE and an increase in the median survival by using zoledronic acid after the diagnosis of bone metastases in GC patients [55]. These interesting retrospective data may support the beneficial effects of zoledronic acid in GC patients with bone involvement, especially in case of osteolytic lesions. However, further prospective analyses are needed in order to confirm this assumption. Denosumab is a well-studied agent among RANK-L inhibitors. Recently, a combined analysis of three randomized phase III trials has shown that the receptor activator of NF-κB ligand inhibitor Denosumab—used at the dose of 120 mg as subcutaneous injection every 4 weeks—is superior to zoledronic acid in delaying the time to first SRE appearance and in reducing the risk of SRE itself, also in patients with bone metastases caused by cancers different from breast, prostate, lung, and kidney [143]. The optimal duration of treatment with bone-related drugs is not well-established.

Another important issue in the management of bone metastases is the risk of hypercalcemia. In this case, the patient should receive a medical treatment according to guidelines for hypercalcemia stratified for serum calcium levels [144].

Finally, the "hungry bone" syndrome is worth mentioning. This syndrome typically occurs after curative surgery for hyperparathyroidism [145]. However, it could be diagnosed also in anecdotal cases of osteoblastic bone metastases by the occurrence of severe hypocalcemia, which is mainly related to excessive calcium apposition into the osteoblastic massive lesions. Recently, Sakai et al. reported the case of an 87-year-old man diagnosed with GC and bone involvement due to the appearance of hypocalcemia [146]. The treatment of the hungry bone syndrome is the correction of hypocalcemia.

In conclusion, although there are limited evidences regarding the efficacy of zoledronic acid and denosumab in patients with bone metastases from GC, the use of these drugs could be helpful also in GC in order to control the spread of the disease, to improve the life expectancy and QoL, and to reduce the probability of occurrence of SREs. Since no specific data are available up to date, the choice of the best drug should be based on the cost–benefit ratio and toxicity profile.

5. Conclusions and Future Perspectives

GC is a very heterogeneous disease; this quite recent concept has become diffusely accepted today. However, the journey to discover the molecular mechanisms that control GC behavior has just started. Recently, the molecular classifications of GC have depicted a very complex landscape [13,14] and multiple molecules, which could be eventually targeted by specific treatments, have been identified [4,5]. Among those molecules, the investigation regarding the role of antiangiogenic agents and multikinase inhibitors, such as cabozantinib, might be interesting future frontiers in the control of bone metastasis also in GC, as shown in other types of tumors, such as renal cancer [147]. However, at the moment, these classifications are hardly applicable in clinical practice. Additionally, there is a lack of knowledge about the molecular mechanisms that control the process of GC metastatization.

In this context, the bone metastases from GC represent still a challenge for the research in this field. In fact, they are rare and often underdiagnosed due to the lack of specific recommendation for their detection according to international guidelines [3,76]. However, bone involvement should be evaluated not only in patients with bone pain or neurological symptoms but also in metastatic GC patients with risk factors, such as aggressive disease or lung metastases. Additionally, there is a lack of prospective evidences regarding specific treatments for patients with bone metastases as well as data showing the outcomes of patients with skeletal metastases from GC or the response of those lesions to standard therapies. Therefore, since the majority of the data in the literature are retrospective and based on a very heterogeneous populations, further prospective studies are needed in order to define the best treatment for GC with bone metastases. Additionally, a better understanding of the underlying molecular mechanisms, by analyzing tumor cells as well as inflammatory tumor infiltrating cells or bone matrix compounds into the bone lesions specimens, could be useful in order to design specific trials.

Author Contributions: Conceptualization, A.P. (Angelica Petrillo); Topic, A.P. (Angelica Petrillo), D.B.; resources, A.P. (Angelica Petrillo), E.F.G., A.P. (Annalisa Pappalardo); writing—original draft preparation, A.P. (Angelica Petrillo), E.F.G., A.P. (Annalisa Pappalardo); writing of particular sections:

all authors; writing—review and editing, all authors; supervision, A.P. (Angelica Petrillo), B.D., L.A., C.C., A.D., A.F., T.F., P.G., M.O., M.R., A.S., P.F. All authors have read and agreed to the published version of the manuscript.

Funding: This research received no external funding.

Institutional Review Board Statement: Not applicable.

Informed Consent Statement: Not applicable.

Data Availability Statement: Not applicable.

Conflicts of Interest: Angelica Petrillo received personal fee from Eli-Lilly, Servier and MSD; EFG had personal fees from Novartis; L.A. received personal fee from GSK; A.D. received personal fees from Roche, Gentili, Italfarmaco, Ipsen, Novartis; B.D. received personal fee from Ipsen, Eisai, Eli Lilly, Astra Zeneca, Sanofi, MSD, Bayer, Roche, Amgen. No fees are connected with the submitted paper. The other authors declare no conflict of interest. The funders had no role in the design, writing of the manuscript, or in the decision to publish the paper.

References

1. Bray, F.; Ferlay, J.; Soerjomataram, I.; Siegel, R.L.; Torre, L.A.; Jemal, A. Global cancer statistics 2018: GLOBOCAN estimates of incidence and mortality worldwide for 36 cancers in 185 countries. *CA Cancer J. Clin.* **2018**, *68*, 394–424. [CrossRef]
2. Surveillance, Epidemiology, and End Results (SEER) Database. Available online: https://seer.cancer.gov/statfacts/html/stomach.html (accessed on 19 December 2020).
3. Smyth, E.C.; Verheij, M.; Allum, W.; Cunningham, D.; Cervantes, A.; Arnold, D.; ESMO Guidelines Committee. Gastric cancer: ESMO Clinical Practice Guidelines for diagnosis, treatment and follow-up. *Ann. Oncol.* **2016**, *27* (Suppl. S5), v38–v49. [CrossRef]
4. Tirino, G.; Pompella, L.; Petrillo, A.; Laterza, M.M.; Pappalardo, A.; Caterino, M.; Orditura, M.; Ciardiello, F.; Galizia, G.; De Vita, F. What's New in Gastric Cancer: The Therapeutic Implications of Molecular Classifications and Future Perspectives. *Int. J. Mol. Sci.* **2018**, *19*, 2659. [CrossRef] [PubMed]
5. Gambardella, V.; Fleitas, T.; Tarazona, N.; Papaccio, F.; Huerta, M.; Roselló, S.; Gimeno-Valiente, F.; Roda, D.; Cervantes, A. Precision Medicine to Treat Advanced Gastroesophageal Adenocarcinoma: A Work in Progress. *J. Clin. Med.* **2020**, *9*, 3049. [CrossRef]
6. Moehler, M.; Shitara, K.; Garrido, M.; Salman, P.; Shen, L.; Wyrwicz, L.; Yamaguchi, K.; Skoczylas, T.; Bragagnoli, A.C.; Liu, T.; et al. LBA6_PR Nivolumab (nivo) plus chemotherapy (chemo) versus chemo as first-line (1L) treatment for advanced gastric cancer/gastroesophageal junction cancer (GC/GEJC)/esophageal adenocarcinoma (EAC): First results of the CheckMate 649 study. *Ann. Oncol.* **2020**, *31* (Suppl. S4), S1142–S1215. [CrossRef]
7. Shitara, K.; Van Cutsem, E.; Bang, Y.-J.; Fuchs, C.; Wyrwicz, L.; Lee, K.-W.; Kudaba, I.; Garrido, M.; Chung, H.C.; Lee, J.; et al. Efficacy and Safety of Pembrolizumab or Pembrolizumab Plus Chemotherapy vs Chemotherapy Alone for Patients with First-line, Advanced Gastric Cancer: The KEYNOTE-062 Phase 3 Randomized Clinical Trial. *JAMA Oncol.* **2020**, *6*, 1571–1580. [CrossRef]
8. Boku, N.; Ryu, M.H.; Oh, D.; Oh, S.C.; Chung, H.C.; Lee, K.; Omori, T.; Shitara, K.; Sakuramoto, S.; Chung, I.J.; et al. LBA7_PR—Nivolumab plus chemotherapy versus chemotherapy alone in patients with previously untreated advanced or recurrent gastric/gastroesophageal junction (G/GEJ) cancer: ATTRACTION-4 (ONO-4538-37) study. *Ann. Oncol.* **2020**, *31* (Suppl. S4), S1142–S1215. [CrossRef]
9. Fanotto, V.; Fornaro, L.; Bordonaro, R.; Rosati, G.; Rimassa, L.; Di Donato, S.; Santini, D.; Tomasello, G.; Leone, F.; Silvestris, N.; et al. Second-line treatment efficacy and toxicity in older vs. non-older patients with advanced gastric cancer: A multicentre real-world study. *J. Geriatr. Oncol.* **2019**, *10*, 591–597. [CrossRef] [PubMed]
10. Davidson, M.; Cafferkey, C.; Goode, E.F.; Kouvelakis, K.; Hughes, D.; Reguera, P.; Kalaitzaki, E.; Peckitt, C.; Rao, S.; Watkins, D.; et al. Survival in Advanced Esophagogastric Adenocarcinoma Improves With Use of Multiple Lines of Therapy: Results From an Analysis of More Than 500 Patients. *Clin. Color. Cancer* **2018**, *17*, 223–230. [CrossRef] [PubMed]
11. Antoniotti, C.; Moretto, R.; Rossini, D.; Masi, G.; Falcone, A.; Cremolini, C. Treatments after first progression in metastatic colorectal cancer. A literature review and evidence-based algorithm. *Cancer Treat. Rev.* **2020**, *92*, 102135. [CrossRef]
12. Smyth, E.C.; Nilsson, M.; Grabsch, H.I.; van Grieken, N.C.; Lordick, F. Gastric cancer. *Lancet* **2020**, *396*, 635–648. [CrossRef]
13. Cancer Genome Atlas Research Network. Comprehensive molecular characterization of gastric adenocarcinoma. *Nature* **2014**, *513*, 202–209. [CrossRef]
14. Cristescu, R.; Lee, J.; Nebozhyn, M.; Kim, K.-M.; Ting, J.C.; Wong, S.S.; Liu, J.; Yue, Y.G.; Wang, J.; Yu, K.; et al. Molecular analysis of gastric cancer identifies subtypes associated with distinct clinical outcomes. *Nat. Med.* **2015**, *21*, 449–456. [CrossRef]
15. Petrillo, A.; Smyth, E.C. Biomarkers for Precision Treatment in Gastric Cancer. *Visc. Med.* **2020**, *36*, 364–372. [CrossRef] [PubMed]
16. Chau, I.; Norman, A.R.; Cunningham, D.; Waters, J.S.; Oates, J.; Ross, P.J. Multivariate prognostic factor analysis in locally advanced and metastatic esophago-gastric cancer—Pooled analysis from three multicenter, randomized, controlled trials using individual patient data. *J. Clin. Oncol.* **2004**, *22*, 2395–2403. [CrossRef] [PubMed]
17. Yoshikawa, K.; Kitaoka, H. Bone metastasis of gastric cancer. *Jpn. J. Surg.* **1983**, *13*, 173–176. [CrossRef] [PubMed]

18. Shupp, A.B.; Kolb, A.D.; Mukhopadhyay, D.; Bussard, K.M. Cancer Metastases to Bone: Concepts, Mechanisms, and Interactions with Bone Osteoblasts. *Cancers* **2018**, *10*, 182. [CrossRef]
19. Turajlic, S.; Xu, H.; Litchfield, K.; Rowan, A.; Chambers, T.; Lopez, J.I.; Nicol, D.; O'Brien, T.; Larkin, J.; Horswell, S.; et al. Tracking Cancer Evolution Reveals Constrained Routes to Metastases: TRACERx Renal. *Cell* **2018**, *173*, 581–594.e12. [CrossRef]
20. Capulli, M.; Paone, R.; Rucci, N. Osteoblast and osteocyte: Games without frontiers. *Arch. Biochem. Biophys.* **2014**, *561*, 3–12. [CrossRef]
21. Florencio-Silva, R.; Sasso, G.R.; Sasso-Cerri, E.; Simões, M.J.; Cerri, P.S. Biology of Bone Tissue: Structure, Function, and Factors That Influence Bone Cells. *BioMed Res. Int.* **2015**, *2015*, 421746. [CrossRef]
22. Guise, T.A.; Yin, J.J.; Taylor, S.D.; Kumagai, Y.; Dallas, M.; Boyce, B.F.; Yoneda, T.; Mundy, G.R. Evidence for a causal role of parathyroid hormone-related protein in the pathogenesis of human breast cancer-mediated osteolysis. *J. Clin. Investig.* **1996**, *98*, 1544–1549. [CrossRef]
23. Boyce, B.F.; Xing, L. Biology of RANK, RANKL, and osteoprotegerin. *Arthritis Res. Ther.* **2007**, *9* (Suppl. S1), S1. [CrossRef]
24. Armstrong, A.P.; Tometsko, M.E.; Glaccum, M.; Sutherland, C.L.; Cosman, D.; Dougall, W.C. A RANK/TRAF6-dependent signal transduction pathway is essential for osteoclast cytoskeletal organization and resorptive function. *J. Biol. Chem.* **2002**, *277*, 44347–44356. [CrossRef] [PubMed]
25. Campbell, J.P.; Karolak, M.R.; Ma, Y.; Perrien, D.S.; Masood-Campbell, S.K.; Penner, N.L.; Munoz, S.A.; Zijlstra, A.; Yang, X.; Sterling, J.A.; et al. Stimulation of host bone marrow stromal cells by sympathetic nerves promotes breast cancer bone metastasis in mice. *PLoS Biol.* **2012**, *10*, e1001363. [CrossRef] [PubMed]
26. Wan, X.; Song, Y.; Fang, H.; Xu, L.; Che, X.; Wang, S.; Zhang, X.; Zhang, L.; Li, C.; Fan, Y.; et al. RANKL/RANK promotes the migration of gastric cancer cells by interacting with EGFR. *Clin. Transl. Med.* **2020**, *9*, 3. [CrossRef]
27. Simonet, W.S.; Lacey, D.L.; Dunstan, C.R.; Kelley, M.; Chang, M.-S.; Lüthy, R.; Nguyen, H.Q.; Wooden, S.; Bennett, L.; Boone, T.; et al. Osteoprotegerin: A novel secreted protein involved in the regulation of bone density. *Cell* **1997**, *89*, 309–319. [CrossRef]
28. Ono, T.; Nakashima, T. Recent advances in osteoclast biology. *Histochem. Cell Biol.* **2018**, *149*, 325–341. [CrossRef]
29. Maurizi, A.; Rucci, N. The Osteoclast in Bone Metastasis: Player and Target. *Cancers* **2018**, *10*, 218. [CrossRef] [PubMed]
30. Eriksen, E.F. Cellular mechanisms of bone remodeling. *Rev. Endocr. Metab. Disord.* **2010**, *11*, 219–227. [CrossRef] [PubMed]
31. Boskey, A.L.; Coleman, R. Aging and Bone. *J. Dent. Res.* **2010**, *89*, 1333–1348. [CrossRef] [PubMed]
32. Demontiero, O.; Vidal, C.; Duque, G. Aging and bone loss: New insights for the clinician. *Ther. Adv. Musculoskelet. Dis.* **2011**, *4*, 61–76. [CrossRef]
33. Bussard, K.M.; Gay, C.V.; Mastro, A.M. The bone microenvironment in metastasis; what is special about bone? *Cancer Metastasis Rev.* **2008**, *27*, 41–55. [CrossRef]
34. Kusumbe, A.P. Vascular niches for disseminated tumour cells in bone. *J. Bone Oncol.* **2016**, *5*, 112–116. [CrossRef] [PubMed]
35. Sosa, M.S.; Bragado, P.; Aguirre-Ghiso, J.A. Mechanisms of disseminated cancer cell dormancy: An awakening field. *Nat. Rev. Cancer* **2014**, *14*, 611–622. [CrossRef]
36. Huang, J.-F.; Shen, J.; Li, X.; Rengan, R.; Silvestris, N.; Wang, M.; DeRosa, L.; Zheng, X.; Belli, A.; Zhang, X.-L.; et al. Incidence of patients with bone metastases at diagnosis of solid tumors in adults: A large population-based study. *Ann. Transl. Med.* **2020**, *8*, 482. [CrossRef] [PubMed]
37. D'Amico, L.; Satolli, M.A.; Mecca, C.; Castiglione, A.; Ceccarelli, M.; D'Amelio, P.; Garino, M.; De Giuli, M.; Sandrucci, S.; Ferracini, R.; et al. Bone metastases in gastric cancer follow a RANKL-independent mechanism. *Oncol. Rep.* **2013**, *29*, 1453–1458. [CrossRef] [PubMed]
38. Hsieh, H.-L.; Tsai, M.-M. Tumor progression-dependent angiogenesis in gastric cancer and its potential application. *World J. Gastrointest. Oncol.* **2019**, *11*, 686–704. [CrossRef]
39. Ammendola, M.; Marech, I.; Sammarco, G.; Zuccalà, V.; Luposella, M.; Zizzo, N.; Patruno, R.; Crovace, A.; Ruggieri, E.; Zito, A.F.; et al. Infiltrating mast cells correlate with angiogenesis in bone metastases from gastric cancer patients. *Int. J. Mol. Sci.* **2015**, *16*, 3237–3250. [CrossRef]
40. Richard, V.; Rosol, T.J.; Foley, J. PTHrP gene expression in cancer: Do all paths lead to Ets? *Crit. Rev. Eukaryot. Gene Expr.* **2005**, *15*, 115–132. [CrossRef]
41. Alipov, G.K.; Ito, M.; Nakashima, M.; Ikeda, Y.; Nakayama, T.; Ohtsuru, A.; Yamashita, S.; Sekine, I. Expression of parathyroid hor-mone-related peptide (PTHrP) in gastric tumours. *J. Pathol.* **1997**, *182*, 174–179. [CrossRef]
42. Ito, M.; Nakashima, M.; Alipov, G.K.; Matsuzaki, S.; Ohtsuru, A.; Yano, H.; Yamashita, S.; Sekine, I. Gastric cancer associated with overexpression of parathyroid hormone-related peptide (PTHrP) and PTH/PTHrP receptor in relation to tumor progression. *J. Gastroenterol.* **1997**, *32*, 396–400. [CrossRef]
43. Zhang, X.; Song, Y.; Song, N.; Zhang, L.; Wang, Y.; Li, D.; Wang, Z.; Qu, X.; Liu, Y. Rankl expression predicts poor prognosis in gastric cancer patients: Results from a retrospective and single-center analysis. *Braz. J. Med. Biol. Res.* **2018**, *51*, e6265. [CrossRef]
44. Katoh, M.; Terada, M. Overexpression of bone morphogenic protein (BMP)-4 mRNA in gastric cancer cell lines of poorly differentiated type. *J. Gastroenterol.* **1996**, *31*, 137–139. [CrossRef] [PubMed]
45. Lee, Y.-C.; Cheng, C.-J.; Bilen, M.A.; Lu, J.-F.; Satcher, R.L.; Yu-Lee, L.-Y.; Gallick, G.E.; Maity, S.N.; Lin, S.-H. BMP4 promotes prostate tumor growth in bone through osteogenesis. *Cancer Res.* **2011**, *71*, 5194–5203. [CrossRef] [PubMed]
46. Deng, G.; Chen, Y.; Guo, C.; Yin, L.; Han, Y.; Li, Y.; Fu, Y.; Cai, C.; Shen, H.; Zeng, S. BMP4 promotes the metastasis of gastric cancer by inducing epithelial–mesenchymal transition via ID1. *J. Cell Sci.* **2020**, *133*, jcs237222. [CrossRef] [PubMed]

47. Brook, N.; Brook, E.; Dharmarajan, A.; Dass, C.R.; Chan, A. Breast cancer bone metastases: Pathogenesis and therapeutic targets. *Int. J. Biochem. Cell Biol.* **2018**, *96*, 63–78. [CrossRef]
48. Rucci, N.; Angelucci, A. Prostate cancer and bone: The elective affinities. *BioMed Res. Int.* **2014**, *2014*, 167035. [CrossRef] [PubMed]
49. Riihimäki, M.; Hemminki, A.; Sundquist, K.; Sundquist, J.; Hemminki, K. Metastatic spread in patients with gastric cancer. *Oncotarget* **2016**, *7*, 52307–52316. [CrossRef] [PubMed]
50. Gomi, D.; Fukushima, T.; Kobayashi, T.; Sekiguchi, N.; Sakamoto, A.; Mamiya, K.; Koizumi, T. Gastric cancer initially presenting as bone metastasis: Two case reports and a literature review. *Oncol. Lett.* **2018**, *16*, 5863–5867. [CrossRef]
51. Guadagni, S.; Catarci, M.; Kinoshitá, T.; Valenti, M.; De Bernardinis, G.; Carboni, M. Causes of death and recurrence after surgery for early gastric cancer. *World J. Surg.* **1997**, *21*, 434–439. [CrossRef]
52. Turkoz, F.P.; Solak, M.; Kilickap, S.; Ulas, A.; Esbah, O.; Oksuzoglu, B.; Yalcin, S. Bone metastasis from gastric cancer: The incidence, clinicopathological features, and influence on survival. *J. Gastric Cancer* **2014**, *14*, 164–172. [CrossRef]
53. Ahn, J.B.; Ha, T.K.; Kwon, S.J. Bone metastasis in gastric cancer patients. *J. Gastric Cancer* **2011**, *11*, 38–45. [CrossRef]
54. Clézardin, P. Pathophysiology of bone metastases from solid malignancies. *Jt. Bone Spine* **2017**, *84*, 677–684. [CrossRef]
55. Silvestris, N.; Pantano, F.; Ibrahim, T.; Gamucci, T.; De Vita, F.; Di Palma, T.; Pedrazzoli, P.; Barni, S.; Bernardo, A.; Febbraro, A.; et al. Natural history of malignant bone disease in gastric cancer: Final results of a multicenter bone metastasis survey. *PLoS ONE* **2013**, *8*, e74402. [CrossRef]
56. Wen, L.; Li, Y.-Z.; Zhang, J.; Zhou, C.; Yang, H.-N.; Chen, X.-Z.; Xu, L.-W.; Kong, S.-N.; Wang, X.-W.; Zhang, H.-M. Clinical analysis of bone metastasis of gastric cancer: Incidence, clinicopathological features and survival. *Future Oncol.* **2019**, *15*, 2241–2249. [CrossRef]
57. Liang, C.; Chen, H.; Yang, Z.; Han, C.; Ren, C. Risk factors and prognosis of bone metastases in newly diagnosed gastric cancer. *Future Oncol.* **2020**, *16*, 733–748. [CrossRef]
58. Qiu, M.-Z.; Shi, S.-M.; Chen, Z.-H.; Yu, H.-E.; Sheng, H.; Jin, Y.; Wang, D.-S.; Wang, F.-H.; Li, Y.-H.; Xie, D.; et al. Frequency and clinicopathological features of metastasis to liver, lung, bone, and brain from gastric cancer: A SEER-based study. *Cancer Med.* **2018**, *7*, 3662–3672. [CrossRef]
59. Park, H.S.; Rha, S.Y.; Kim, H.S.; Hyung, W.J.; Park, J.S.; Chung, H.C.; Noh, S.H.; Jeung, H.-C. A prognostic model to predict clinical outcome in gastric cancer patients with bone metastasis. *Oncology* **2011**, *80*, 142–150. [CrossRef] [PubMed]
60. Nakamura, K.; Tomioku, M.; Nabeshima, K.; Yasuda, S. Clinicopathologic features and clinical outcomes of gastric cancer patients with bone metastasis. *Tokai J. Exp. Clin. Med.* **2014**, *39*, 193–198. [PubMed]
61. Mikami, J.; Kimura, Y.; Makari, Y.; Fujita, J.; Kishimoto, T.; Sawada, G.; Nakahira, S.; Nakata, K.; Tsujie, M.; Ohzato, H. Clinical outcomes and prognostic factors for gastric cancer patients with bone metastasis. *World J. Surg. Oncol.* **2017**, *15*, 8. [CrossRef] [PubMed]
62. Imura, Y.; Tateiwa, D.; Sugimoto, N.; Inoue, A.; Wakamatsu, T.; Outani, H.; Tanaka, T.; Tamiya, H.; Yagi, T.; Naka, N.; et al. Prognostic factors and skeletal-related events in patients with bone metastasis from gastric cancer. *Mol. Clin. Oncol.* **2020**, *13*, 31. [CrossRef]
63. Laurén, P. The two histological main types of gastric carcinoma: Diffuse and so-called intestinal-type carcinoma. An attempt at a histo-clinical classification. *Acta Pathol. Microbiol. Scand.* **1965**, *64*, 31–49. [CrossRef]
64. Miyamoto, W.; Yamamoto, S.; Uchio, Y. Metastasis of gastric cancer to the fifth metacarpal bone. *Hand Surg.* **2008**, *13*, 193–195. [CrossRef] [PubMed]
65. Harris, H.; Khan, M.; Jaunoo, S. Distal phalanx: An unusual site for a gastric adenocarcinoma metastasis. *BMJ Case Rep.* **2020**, *13*, e236259. [CrossRef] [PubMed]
66. Okamoto, M.; Yamazaki, H.; Yoshimura, Y.; Aoki, K.; Tanaka, A.; Kato, H. Massive trapezial metastasis from gastric adenocarcinoma resected and reconstructed with a vascularized scapular bone graft. A case report. *Medicine* **2017**, *96*, e9294. [CrossRef] [PubMed]
67. Chang, H.C.; Lew, K.H.; Low, C.O. Metastasis of an adenocarcinoma of the stomach to the 4th metacarpal bone. *Hand Surg.* **2001**, *6*, 239–242. [CrossRef]
68. Kumar, A. Acrometastases to the hand in stomach carcinoma: A rare entity. *BMJ Case Rep.* **2019**, *12*, e229390. [CrossRef]
69. Gurzu, S.; Jung, I.; Kádár, Z. Aberrant metastatic behavior and particular features of early gastric cancer. *APMIS* **2015**, *123*, 999–1006. [CrossRef]
70. Fujita, I.; Toyokawa, T.; Makino, T.; Matsueda, K.; Omote, S.; Horii, J. Small early gastric cancer with synchronous bone metastasis: A case report. *Mol. Clin. Oncol.* **2020**, *12*, 202–207. [CrossRef]
71. Park, J.M.; Song, K.Y.; O, J.H.; Kim, W.C.; Choi, M.-G.; Park, C.H. Bone recurrence after curative resection of gastric cancer. *Gastric Cancer* **2013**, *16*, 362–369. [CrossRef]
72. Blanchette, P.; Lipton, J.; Barth, D.; Mackay, H. Case Report of very late gastric cancer recurrence. *Curr. Oncol.* **2013**, *20*, 161–164. [CrossRef] [PubMed]
73. Iovino, F.; Orditura, M.; Auriemma, P.P.; Ciorra, F.R.; Giordano, G.; Orabona, C.; Bara, F.; Sergio, R.; Savastano, B.; Fabozzi, A.; et al. Vertebral carcinomatosis eleven years after advanced gastric cancer resection: A case report. *Oncol. Lett.* **2015**, *9*, 1403–1405. [CrossRef]

74. Di Nunno, V.; Mollica, V.; Schiavina, R.; Nobili, E.; Fiorentino, M.; Brunocilla, E.; Ardizzoni, A.; Massari, F. Improving IMDC Prognostic Prediction Through Evaluation of Initial Site of Metastasis in Patients with Metastatic Renal Cell Carcinoma. *Clin. Genitourin. Cancer* **2020**, *18*, e83–e90. [CrossRef]
75. Massari, F.; Di Nunno, V.; Guida, A.; Silva, C.A.C.; Derosa, L.; Mollica, V.; Colomba, E.; Brandi, G.; Albiges, L. Addition of Primary Metastatic Site on Bone, Brain, and Liver to IMDC Criteria in Patients with Metastatic Renal Cell Carcinoma: A Validation Study. *Clin. Genitourin. Cancer* **2021**, *19*, 32–40. [CrossRef] [PubMed]
76. National Comprehensive Cancer Network (NCCN). Clinical Practice Guidelines in Oncology. *Gastric Cancer, Version 1*. 2020. Available online: https://www.nccn.org/guidelines/guidelines-detail?category=1&id=1434 (accessed on 15 November 2020).
77. Nilsson, M. Postgastrectomy follow-up in the West: Evidence base, guidelines, and daily practice. *Gastric Cancer* **2017**, *20* (Suppl. S1), 135–140. [CrossRef]
78. Lim, S.M.; Kim, Y.N.; Park, K.H.; Kang, B.; Chon, H.J.; Kim, C.; Kim, J.H.; Rha, S.Y. Bone alkaline phosphatase as a surrogate marker of bone metastasis in gastric cancer patients. *BMC Cancer* **2016**, *16*, 385. [CrossRef] [PubMed]
79. Kawamura, T.; Kusakabe, T.; Sugino, T.; Watanabe, K.; Fukuda, T.; Nashimoto, A.; Honma, K.; Suzuki, T. Expression of glucose transporter-1 in human gastric carcinoma: Association with tumor aggressiveness, metastasis, and patient survival. *Cancer* **2001**, *92*, 634–641. [CrossRef]
80. Grillo, A.; Capasso, R.; Petrillo, A.; De Vita, F.; Conforti, R. An intramedullary "flame" recognized as being an intramedullary spinal cord metastasis from esophageal cancer. *J. Radiol. Case Rep.* **2019**, *13*, 14–20. [CrossRef]
81. Eisenhauer, E.A.; Therasse, P.; Bogaerts, J.; Schwartz, L.H.; Sargent, D.; Ford, R.; Dancey, J.; Arbuck, S.; Gwyther, S.; Mooney, M.; et al. New response evaluation criteria in solid tumours: Revised RECIST guideline (version 1.1). *Eur. J. Cancer* **2009**, *45*, 228–247. [CrossRef]
82. Pollen, J.J.; Witztum, K.F.; Ashburn, W.L. The flare phenomenon on radionuclide bone scan in metastatic prostate cancer. *Am. J. Roentgenol.* **1984**, *142*, 773–776. [CrossRef]
83. Fogelman, I. The flare phenomenon: Still learning after 35 years. *Eur. J. Nucl. Med. Mol. Imaging* **2011**, *38*, 5–6. [CrossRef]
84. Cook, G.J.; Venkitaraman, R.; Sohaib, A.S.; Lewington, V.J.; Chua, S.C.; Huddart, R.A.; Parker, C.C.; Dearnaley, D.D.; Horwich, A. The diagnostic utility of the flare phenomenon on bone scintigraphy in staging prostate cancer. *Eur. J. Nucl. Med. Mol. Imaging* **2011**, *38*, 7–13. [CrossRef]
85. De Bondt, C.; Snoeckx, A.; Raskin, J. A Flare for the Unexpected: Bone Flare as Response to Tyrosine Kinase Inhibitor Treatment in a Lung Cancer Patient: New osteoblastic bone lesions in a lung cancer patient may represent bone flare and should not be misdiagnosed as disease progression. *J. Belg. Soc. Radiol.* **2020**, *104*, 18. [CrossRef]
86. Harisankar, C.N.B.; Preethi, R.; John, J. Metabolic flare phenomenon on 18 fluoride-fluorodeoxy glucose positron emission tomography-computed tomography scans in a patient with bilateral breast cancer treated with second-line chemotherapy and bevacizumab. *Indian J. Nucl. Med.* **2015**, *30*, 145–147. [CrossRef]
87. Hashisako, M.; Wakamatsu, K.; Ikegame, S.; Kumazoe, H.; Nagata, N.; Kajiki, A. Flare phenomenon following gefitinib treatment of lung adenocarcinoma with bone metastasis. *Tohoku J. Exp. Med.* **2012**, *228*, 163–168. [CrossRef] [PubMed]
88. Lu, M.-C.; Chuang, T.-L.; Lee, M.-S.; Chiou, W.-Y.; Lin, H.-Y.; Hung, S.-K. The Super-scan and Flare Phenomena in a Nasopharyngeal Cancer Patient: A Case Report. *J. Clin. Med. Res.* **2012**, *4*, 221–223. [CrossRef]
89. Amoroso, V.; Pittiani, F.; Grisanti, S.; Valcamonico, F.; Simoncini, E.; Ferrari, V.D.; Marini, G. Osteoblastic flare in a patient with advanced gastric cancer after treatment with pemetrexed and oxaliplatin: Implications for response assessment with RECIST criteria. *BMC Cancer* **2007**, *7*, 94. [CrossRef] [PubMed]
90. Lee, S.; Shi, H.; Sohn, S.; Park, S.; Wang, S.; Song, J.; Jang, G. The Flare Phenomenon in a Patient with Advanced Gastric Cancer with Bone Metastases. *Korean J. Med.* **2016**, *91*, 321–324. [CrossRef]
91. Al-Batran, S.-E.; Hartmann, J.T.; Probst, S.; Schmalenberg, H.; Hollerbach, S.; Hofheinz, R.; Rethwisch, V.; Seipelt, G.; Homann, N.; Wilhelm, G.; et al. Phase III trial in metastatic gastroesophageal adenocarcinoma with fluorouracil, leucovorin plus either oxaliplatin or cisplatin: A study of the arbeitsgemeinschaft internistische onkologie. *J. Clin. Oncol.* **2008**, *26*, 1435–1442. [CrossRef]
92. Kang, Y.; Kang, W.K.; Shin, D.B.; Chen, J.; Xiong, J.; Wang, J.; Lichinitser, M.; Philco, M.; Suarez, T.; Santamaria, J. Randomized phase III trial of capecitabine/cisplatin (XP) vs. continuous infusion of 5-FU/cisplatin (FP) as first-line therapy in patients (pts) with advanced gastric cancer (AGC): Efficacy and safety results. *J. Clin. Oncol.* **2006**, *24* (Suppl. S18), LBA4018. [CrossRef]
93. Ryu, M.-H.; Baba, E.; Lee, K.H.; Park, Y.I.; Boku, N.; Hyodo, I.; Nam, B.-H.; Esaki, T.; Yoo, C.; Ryoo, B.-Y.; et al. Comparison of two different S-1 plus cisplatin dosing schedules as first-line chemotherapy for metastatic and/or recurrent gastric cancer: A multicenter, randomized phase III trial (SOS). *Ann. Oncol.* **2015**, *26*, 2097–2101. [CrossRef] [PubMed]
94. Kang, J.H.; Lee, S.I.; Lim, D.H.; Park, K.-W.; Oh, S.Y.; Kwon, H.-C.; Hwang, I.G.; Lee, S.-C.; Nam, E.; Shin, D.B.; et al. Salvage chemotherapy for pretreated gastric cancer: A randomized phase III trial comparing chemotherapy plus best supportive care with best supportive care alone. *J. Clin. Oncol.* **2012**, *30*, 1513–1518. [CrossRef]
95. Shen, L.; Li, J.; Xu, J.; Pan, H.; Dai, G.; Qin, S.; Wang, L.; Wang, J.; Yang, Z.; Shu, Y.; et al. Bevacizumab plus capecitabine and cisplatin in Chinese patients with inoperable locally advanced or metastatic gastric or gastroesophageal junction cancer: Randomized, double-blind, phase III study (AVATAR study). *Gastric Cancer* **2015**, *18*, 168–176. [CrossRef] [PubMed]
96. Pavlakis, N.; Sjoquist, K.M.; Martin, A.J.; Tsobanis, E.; Yip, S.; Kang, Y.-K.; Bang, Y.-J.; Alcindor, T.; O'Callaghan, C.J.; Burnell, M.J.; et al. Regorafenib for the Treatment of Advanced Gastric Cancer (INTEGRATE): A Multinational Placebo-Controlled Phase II Trial. *J. Clin. Oncol.* **2016**, *34*, 2728–2735. [CrossRef] [PubMed]

97. Kang, Y.-K.; Boku, N.; Satoh, T.; Ryu, M.-H.; Chao, Y.; Kato, K.; Chung, H.C.; Chen, J.-S.; Muro, K.; Kang, W.K.; et al. Nivolumab in patients with advanced gastric or gastro-oesophageal junction cancer refractory to, or intolerant of, at least two previous chemotherapy regimens (ONO-4538-12, ATTRACTION-2): A randomised, double-blind, placebo-controlled, phase 3 trial. *Lancet* **2017**, *390*, 2461–2471. [CrossRef]
98. Chen, L.-T.; Satoh, T.; Ryu, M.-H.; Chao, Y.; Kato, K.; Chung, H.C.; Chen, J.-S.; Muro, K.; Kang, W.K.; Yeh, K.-H.; et al. A phase 3 study of nivolumab in previously treated advanced gastric or gastroesophageal junction cancer (ATTRACTION-2): 2-year update data. *Gastric Cancer* **2020**, *23*, 510–519. [CrossRef]
99. Van Cutsem, E.; Moiseyenko, V.M.; Tjulandin, S.; Majlis, A.; Constenla, M.; Boni, C.; Rodrigues, A.; Fodor, M.; Chao, Y.; Voznyi, E.; et al. V325 Study Group. Phase III study of docetaxel and cisplatin plus fluorouracil compared with cisplatin and fluorouracil as first-line therapy for advanced gastric cancer: A report of the V325 Study Group. *J. Clin. Oncol.* **2006**, *24*, 4991–4997. [CrossRef]
100. Dank, M.; Zaluski, J.; Barone, C.; Valvere, V.; Yalcin, S.; Peschel, C.; Wenczl, M.; Goker, E.; Cisar, L.; Wang, K.; et al. Randomized phase III study comparing irinotecan combined with 5-fluorouracil and folinic acid to cisplatin combined with 5-fluorouracil in chemotherapy naive patients with advanced adenocarcinoma of the stomach or esophagogastric junction. *Ann. Oncol.* **2008**, *19*, 1450–1457. [CrossRef] [PubMed]
101. Cunningham, D.; Starling, N.; Rao, S.; Iveson, T.; Nicolson, M.; Coxon, F.; Middleton, G.; Daniel, F.; Oates, J.; Norman, A.R. Capecitabine and Oxaliplatin for Advanced Esophagogastric Cancer. *New Engl. J. Med.* **2008**, *358*, 36–46. [CrossRef]
102. Ajani, J.A.; Rodriguez, W.; Bodoky, G.; Moiseyenko, V.; Lichinitser, M.; Gorbunova, V.; Vynnychenko, I.; Garin, A.; Lang, I.; Falcon, S. Multicenter Phase III Comparison of Cisplatin/S-1 With Cisplatin/Infusional Fluorouracil in Advanced Gastric or Gastroesophageal Adenocarcinoma Study: The FLAGS Trial. *J. Clin. Oncol.* **2010**, *28*, 1547–1553. [CrossRef]
103. NaraharaHiroyasu, H.; Iishi, H.; Imamura, H.; Tsuburaya, A.; Chin, K.; Imamoto, H.; Esaki, T.; Furukawa, H.; Hamada, C.; Sakata, Y. Randomized phase III study comparing the efficacy and safety of irinotecan plus S-1 with S-1 alone as first-line treatment for advanced gastric cancer (study GC0301/TOP-002). *Gastric Cancer* **2011**, *14*, 72–80. [CrossRef]
104. Guimbaud, R.; Louvet, C.; Ries, P.; Ychou, M.; Maillard, E.; André, T.; Gornet, J.-M.; Aparicio, T.; Nguyen, S.; Azzedine, A.; et al. Prospective, Randomized, Multicenter, Phase III Study of Fluorouracil, Leucovorin, and Irinotecan Versus Epirubicin, Cisplatin, and Capecitabine in Advanced Gastric Adenocarcinoma: A French Intergroup (Fédération Francophone de Cancérologie Digestive, Fédération Nationale des Centres de Lutte Contre le Cancer, and Groupe Coopérateur Multidisciplinaire en Oncologie) Study. *J. Clin. Oncol.* **2014**, *32*, 3520–3526. [CrossRef] [PubMed]
105. Yamada, Y.; Higuchi, K.; Nishikawa, K.; Gotoh, M.; Fuse, N.; Sugimoto, N.; Nishina, T.; Amagai, K.; Chin, K.; Niwa, Y.; et al. Phase III study comparing oxaliplatin plus S-1 with cisplatin plus S-1 in chemotherapy-naïve patients with advanced gastric cancer. *Ann. Oncol.* **2015**, *26*, 141–148. [CrossRef] [PubMed]
106. Thuss-Patience, P.C.; Kretzschmar, A.; Bichev, D.; Deist, T.; Hinke, A.; Breithaupt, K.; Dogan, Y.; Gebauer, B.; Schumacher, G.; Reichardt, P. Survival advantage for irinotecan versus best supportive care as second-line chemotherapy in gastric cancer—A randomised phase III study of the Arbeitsgemeinschaft Internistische Onkologie (AIO). *Eur. J. Cancer* **2011**, *47*, 2306–2314. [CrossRef] [PubMed]
107. Hironaka, S.; Ueda, S.; Yasui, H.; Nishina, T.; Tsuda, M.; Tsumura, T.; Sugimoto, N.; Shimodaira, H.; Tokunaga, S.; Moriwaki, T.; et al. Randomized, Open-Label, Phase III Study Comparing Irinotecan With Paclitaxel in Patients With Advanced Gastric Cancer Without Severe Peritoneal Metastasis After Failure of Prior Combination Chemotherapy Using Fluoropyrimidine Plus Platinum: WJOG 4007 Trial. *J. Clin. Oncol.* **2013**, *31*, 4438–4444. [CrossRef] [PubMed]
108. Ford, H.E.R.; Marshall, A.; A Bridgewater, J.; Janowitz, T.; Coxon, F.Y.; Wadsley, J.; Mansoor, W.; Fyfe, D.; Madhusudan, S.; Middleton, G.W.; et al. Docetaxel versus active symptom control for refractory oesophagogastric adenocarcinoma (COUGAR-02): An open-label, phase 3 randomised controlled trial. *Lancet Oncol.* **2014**, *15*, 78–86. [CrossRef]
109. Shitara, K.; Takashima, A.; Fujitani, K.; Koeda, K.; Hara, H.; Nakayama, N.; Hironaka, S.; Nishikawa, K.; Makari, Y.; Amagai, K.; et al. Nab-paclitaxel versus solvent-based paclitaxel in patients with previously treated advanced gastric cancer (ABSOLUTE): An open-label, randomised, non-inferiority, phase 3 trial. *Lancet Gastroenterol. Hepatol.* **2017**, *2*, 277–287. [CrossRef]
110. Shitara, K.; Doi, T.; Dvorkin, M.; Mansoor, W.; Arkenau, H.-T.; Prokharau, A.; Alsina, M.; Ghidini, M.; Faustino, C.; Gorbunova, V.; et al. Trifluridine/tipiracil versus placebo in patients with heavily pretreated metastatic gastric cancer (TAGS): A randomised, double-blind, placebo-controlled, phase 3 trial. *Lancet Oncol.* **2018**, *19*, 1437–1448. [CrossRef]
111. Ohtsu, A.; Shah, M.A.; Van Cutsem, E.; Rha, S.Y.; Sawaki, A.; Park, S.R.; Lim, H.Y.; Yamada, Y.; Wu, J.; Langer, B.; et al. Bevacizumab in Combination With Chemotherapy As First-Line Therapy in Advanced Gastric Cancer: A Randomized, Double-Blind, Placebo-Controlled Phase III Study. *J. Clin. Oncol.* **2011**, *29*, 3968–3976. [CrossRef]
112. Bang, Y.-J.; Van Cutsem, E.; Feyereislova, A.; Chung, H.C.; Shen, L.; Sawaki, A.; Lordick, F.; Ohtsu, A.; Omuro, Y.; Satoh, T.; et al. Trastuzumab in combination with chemotherapy versus chemotherapy alone for treatment of HER2-positive advanced gastric or gastro-oesophageal junction cancer (ToGA): A phase 3, open-label, randomised controlled trial. *Lancet* **2010**, *376*, 687–697. [CrossRef]
113. Lordick, F.; Kang, Y.-K.; Chung, H.-C.; Salman, P.; Oh, S.C.; Bodoky, G.; Kurteva, G.; Volovat, C.; Moiseyenko, V.M.; Gorbunova, V.; et al. Capecitabine and cisplatin with or without cetuximab for patients with previously untreated advanced gastric cancer (EXPAND): A randomised, open-label phase 3 trial. *Lancet Oncol.* **2013**, *14*, 490–499. [CrossRef]

114. Waddell, T.; Chau, I.; Cunningham, D.; Gonzalez, D.; Okines, A.F.C.; Wotherspoon, A.; Saffery, C.; Middleton, G.; Wadsley, J.; Ferry, D.; et al. Epirubicin, oxaliplatin, and capecitabine with or without panitumumab for patients with previously untreated advanced oesophagogastric cancer (REAL3): A randomised, open-label phase 3 trial. *Lancet Oncol.* **2013**, *14*, 481–489. [CrossRef]
115. Al-Batran, S.-E.; Schuler, M.H.; Zvirbule, Z.; Manikhas, G.; Lordick, F.; Rusyn, A.; Vynnyk, Y.; Vynnychenko, I.; Fadeeva, N.; Nechaeva, M.; et al. FAST: An international, multicenter, randomized, phase II trial of epirubicin, oxaliplatin, and capecitabine (EOX) with or without IMAB362, a first-in-class anti-CLDN18.2 antibody, as first-line therapy in patients with advanced CLDN18.2+ gastric and gastroesophageal junction (GEJ) adenocarcinoma. *J. Clin. Oncol.* **2016**, *34*, LBA4001. [CrossRef]
116. Hecht, J.R.; Bang, Y.-J.; Qin, S.K.; Chung, H.C.; Xu, J.M.; Park, J.O.; Jeziorski, K.; Shparyk, Y.; Hoff, P.M.; Sobrero, A.; et al. Lapatinib in Combination With Capecitabine Plus Oxaliplatin in Human Epidermal Growth Factor Receptor 2–Positive Advanced or Metastatic Gastric, Esophageal, or Gastroesophageal Adenocarcinoma: TRIO-013/LOGiC—A Randomized Phase III Trial. *J. Clin. Oncol.* **2016**, *34*, 443–451. [CrossRef]
117. Shah, M.A.; Bang, Y.-J.; Lordick, F.; Alsina, M.; Chen, M.; Hack, S.P.; Bruey, J.M.; Smith, D.; McCaffery, I.; Shames, D.S.; et al. Effect of Fluorouracil, Leucovorin, and Oxaliplatin With or Without Onartuzumab in HER2-Negative, MET-Positive Gastroesophageal Adenocarcinoma. *JAMA Oncol.* **2017**, *3*, 620–627. [CrossRef]
118. Cunningham, D.; Al-Batran, S.-E.; Davidenko, I.; Ilson, D.H.; Murad, A.M.; Tebbutt, N.C.; Jiang, Y.; Loh, E.; Dubey, S. RILOMET-1 investigators RILOMET-1: An international phase III multicenter, randomized, double-blind, placebo-controlled trial of rilotumumab plus epirubicin, cisplatin, and capecitabine (ECX) as first-line therapy in patients with advanced MET-positive gastric or gastroesophageal junction (G/GEJ) adenocarcinoma. *J. Clin. Oncol.* **2013**, *31*, TPS4153. [CrossRef]
119. Shah, M.A.; Xu, R.-H.; Bang, Y.-J.; Hoff, P.M.; Liu, T.; Herráez-Baranda, L.A.; Xia, F.; Garg, A.; Shing, M.; Tabernero, J. HELOISE: Phase IIIb Randomized Multicenter Study Comparing Standard-of-Care and Higher-Dose Trastuzumab Regimens Combined With Chemotherapy as First-Line Therapy in Patients With Human Epidermal Growth Factor Receptor 2–Positive Metastatic Gastric or Gastroesophageal Junction Adenocarcinoma. *J. Clin. Oncol.* **2017**, *35*, 2558–2567. [CrossRef]
120. Tabernero, J.; Hoff, P.M.; Shen, L.; Ohtsu, A.; A Shah, M.; Cheng, K.; Song, C.; Wu, H.; Eng-Wong, J.; Kim, K.; et al. Pertuzumab plus trastuzumab and chemotherapy for HER2-positive metastatic gastric or gastro-oesophageal junction cancer (JACOB): Final analysis of a double-blind, randomised, placebo-controlled phase 3 study. *Lancet Oncol.* **2018**, *19*, 1372–1384. [CrossRef]
121. Fuchs, C.S.; Shitara, K.; Di Bartolomeo, M.; Lonardi, S.; Al-Batran, S.-E.; Van Cutsem, E.; Ilson, D.H.; Alsina, M.; Chau, I.; Lacy, J.; et al. Ramucirumab with cisplatin and fluoropyrimidine as first-line therapy in patients with metastatic gastric or junctional adenocarcinoma (RAINFALL): A double-blind, randomised, placebo-controlled, phase 3 trial. *Lancet Oncol.* **2019**, *20*, 420–435. [CrossRef]
122. Ohtsu, A.; Ajani, J.A.; Bai, Y.-X.; Bang, Y.-J.; Chung, H.-C.; Pan, H.-M.; Sahmoud, T.; Shen, L.; Yeh, K.-H.; Chin, K.; et al. Everolimus for Previously Treated Advanced Gastric Cancer: Results of the Randomized, Double-Blind, Phase III GRANITE-1 Study. *J. Clin. Oncol.* **2013**, *31*, 3935–3943. [CrossRef]
123. Fuchs, C.S.; Tomasek, J.; Yong, C.J.; Dumitru, F.; Passalacqua, R.; Goswami, C.; Safran, H.; dos Santos, L.V.; Aprile, G.; Ferry, D.R.; et al. Ramucirumab monotherapy for previously treated advanced gastric or gastro-oesophageal junction adenocarcinoma (REGARD): An international, randomised, multicentre, placebo-controlled, phase 3 trial. *Lancet* **2014**, *383*, 31–39. [CrossRef]
124. Wilke, H.; Muro, K.; Van Cutsem, E.; Oh, S.-C.; Bodoky, G.; Shimada, Y.; Hironaka, S.; Sugimoto, N.; Lipatov, O.; Kim, T.-Y.; et al. Ramucirumab plus paclitaxel versus placebo plus paclitaxel in patients with previously treated advanced gastric or gastro-oesophageal junction adenocarcinoma (RAINBOW): A double-blind, randomised phase 3 trial. *Lancet Oncol.* **2014**, *15*, 1224–1235. [CrossRef]
125. Satoh, T.; Xu, R.-H.; Chung, H.C.; Sun, G.-P.; Doi, T.; Xu, J.-M.; Tsuji, A.; Omuro, Y.; Li, J.; Wang, J.-W.; et al. Lapatinib Plus Paclitaxel Versus Paclitaxel Alone in the Second-Line Treatment ofHER2-Amplified Advanced Gastric Cancer in Asian Populations: TyTAN—A Randomized, Phase III Study. *J. Clin. Oncol.* **2014**, *32*, 2039–2049. [CrossRef]
126. Van Cutsem, E.; Bang, Y.-J.; Mansoor, W.; Petty, R.D.; Chao, Y.; Cunningham, D.; Ferry, D.R.; Smith, N.R.; Frewer, P.; Ratnayake, J.; et al. A randomized, open-label study of the efficacy and safety of AZD4547 monotherapy versus paclitaxel for the treatment of advanced gastric adenocarcinoma with FGFR2 polysomy or gene amplification. *Ann. Oncol.* **2017**, *28*, 1316–1324. [CrossRef] [PubMed]
127. Thuss-Patience, P.C.; A Shah, M.; Ohtsu, A.; Van Cutsem, E.; Ajani, J.A.; Castro, H.; Mansoor, W.; Chung, H.C.; Bodoky, G.; Shitara, K.; et al. Trastuzumab emtansine versus taxane use for previously treated HER2-positive locally advanced or metastatic gastric or gastro-oesophageal junction adenocarcinoma (GATSBY): An international randomised, open-label, adaptive, phase 2/3 study. *Lancet Oncol.* **2017**, *18*, 640–653. [CrossRef]
128. Bang, Y.-J.; Xu, R.-H.; Chin, K.; Lee, K.-W.; Park, S.H.; Rha, S.Y.; Shen, L.; Qin, S.; Xu, N.; Im, S.-A.; et al. Olaparib in combination with paclitaxel in patients with advanced gastric cancer who have progressed following first-line therapy (GOLD): A double-blind, randomised, placebo-controlled, phase 3 trial. *Lancet Oncol.* **2017**, *18*, 1637–1651. [CrossRef]
129. Kang, Y.-K.; Kang, W.; Di Bartolomeo, M.; Chau, I.; Yoon, H.; Cascinu, S.; Ryu, M.-H.; Kim, J.; Lee, K.-W.; Oh, S.; et al. Randomized phase III ANGEL study of rivoceranib (apatinib) + best supportive care (BSC) vs placebo + BSC in patients with advanced/metastatic gastric cancer who failed ≥2 prior chemotherapy regimens. *Ann. Oncol.* **2019**, *30*, v877–v878. [CrossRef]
130. Shitara, K.; Bang, Y.-J.; Iwasa, S.; Sugimoto, N.; Ryu, M.-H.; Sakai, D.; Chung, H.-C.; Kawakami, H.; Yabusaki, H.; Lee, J.; et al. Trastuzumab Deruxtecan in Previously Treated HER2-Positive Gastric Cancer. *New Engl. J. Med.* **2020**, *382*, 2419–2430. [CrossRef]

131. Janjigian, Y.Y.; Maron, S.B.; Chatila, W.K.; Millang, B.; Chavan, S.S.; Alterman, C.; Chou, J.F.; Segal, M.F.; Simmons, M.Z.; Momtaz, P.; et al. First-line pembrolizumab and trastuzumab in HER2-positive oesophageal, gastric, or gastro-oesophageal junction cancer: An open-label, single-arm, phase 2 trial. *Lancet Oncol.* **2020**, *21*, 821–831. [CrossRef]
132. Chen, L.; Kang, Y.; Tanimoto, M.; Boku, N. 43544—ATTRACTION-04 (ONO-4538-37): A Randomized, Multicenter, Phase 2/3 Study of Nivolumab (Nivo) Plus chemotherapy in Patients (Pts) with Previously Untreated Advanced or Recurrent Gastric (G) or Gastroesophageal Junction (GEJ) Cancer. *Ann. Oncol.* **2017**, *28* (Suppl. S5), v209–v268. [CrossRef]
133. Kato, K.; Sun, J.; Shah, M.J.; Enzinger, P.C.; Adenis, A.; Doi, T.; Kojima, T.; Metges, J.; Li, Z.; Kim, S.; et al. LBA8_PR—Pembrolizumab plus chemotherapy versus chemotherapy as first-line therapy in patients with advanced esophageal cancer: The phase 3 KEYNOTE-590 study. *Ann. Oncol.* **2020**, *31* (Suppl. S4), S1142–S1215. [CrossRef]
134. Moehler, M.; Dvorkin, M.; Boku, N.; Özgüroğlu, M.; Ryu, M.H.; Muntean, A.S.; Lonardi, S.; Nechaeva, M.; Bragagnoli, A.C.; Coşkun, H.S.; et al. Phase III Trial of Avelumab Maintenance After First-Line Induction Chemotherapy Versus Continuation of Chemotherapy in Patients With Gastric Cancers: Results From JAVELIN Gastric 100. *J Clin Oncol.* **2021**, *39*, 966–977. [CrossRef]
135. Kawazoe, A.; Fukuoka, S.; Nakamura, Y.; Kuboki, Y.; Wakabayashi, M.; Nomura, S.; Mikamoto, Y.; Shima, H.; Fujishiro, N.; Higuchi, T.; et al. Lenvatinib plus pembrolizumab in patients with advanced gastric cancer in the first-line or second-line setting (EPOC1706): An open-label, single-arm, phase 2 trial. *Lancet Oncol.* **2020**, *21*, 1057–1065. [CrossRef]
136. Shitara, K.; Özgüroğlu, M.; Bang, Y.-J.; Di Bartolomeo, M.; Mandalà, M.; Ryu, M.-H.; Fornaro, L.; Olesiński, T.; Caglevic, C.; Chung, H.C.; et al. Pembrolizumab versus paclitaxel for previously treated, advanced gastric or gastro-oesophageal junction cancer (KEYNOTE-061): A randomised, open-label, controlled, phase 3 trial. *Lancet* **2018**, *392*, 123–133. [CrossRef]
137. Bang, Y.-J.; Ruiz, E.; Van Cutsem, E.; Lee, K.-W.; Wyrwicz, L.; Schenker, M.; Alsina, M.; Ryu, M.-H.; Chung, H.-C.; Evesque, L.; et al. Phase III, randomised trial of avelumab versus physician's choice of chemotherapy as third-line treatment of patients with advanced gastric or gastro-oesophageal junction cancer: Primary analysis of JAVELIN Gastric 300. *Ann. Oncol.* **2018**, *29*, 2052–2060. [CrossRef]
138. Bang, Y.-J.; Kang, Y.-K.; Catenacci, D.V.; Muro, K.; Fuchs, C.S.; Geva, R.; Hara, H.; Golan, T.; Garrido, M.; Jalal, S.I.; et al. Pembrolizumab alone or in combination with chemotherapy as first-line therapy for patients with advanced gastric or gastroesophageal junction adenocarcinoma: Results from the phase II nonrandomized KEYNOTE-059 study. *Gastric Cancer* **2019**, *22*, 828–837. [CrossRef]
139. Lipton, A.; Cook, R.; Brown, J.; Body, J.; Smith, M.; Coleman, R. Skeletal-related events and clinical outcomes in patients with bone metastases and normal levels of osteolysis: Exploratory analyses. *Clin. Oncol.* **2013**, *25*, 217–226. [CrossRef]
140. National Comprehensive Cancer Network (NCCN). Prostate Cancer Guidelines Version 3. 2020. Available online: https://www.nccn.org/guidelines/guidelines-detail?category=1&id=1459 (accessed on 15 November 2020).
141. Rich, S.E.; Chow, R.; Raman, S.; Zeng, K.L.; Lutz, S.; Lam, H.; Silva, M.F.; Chow, E. Update of the systematic review of palliative radiation therapy fractionation for bone metastases. *Radiother. Oncol.* **2018**, *126*, 547–557. [CrossRef] [PubMed]
142. Rosen, L.S.; Gordon, D.; Tchekmedyian, S.; Yanagihara, R.; Hirsh, V.; Krzakowski, M.; Pawlicki, M.; De Souza, P.; Zheng, M.; Urbanowitz, G.; et al. Zoledronic acid versus placebo in the treatment of skeletal metastases in patients with lung cancer and other solid tumors: A phase III, double-blind, randomized trial—The Zoledronic Acid Lung Cancer and Other Solid Tumors Study Group. *J. Clin. Oncol.* **2003**, *21*, 3150–3157. [CrossRef] [PubMed]
143. Lipton, A.; Fizazi, K.; Stopeck, A.T.; Henry, D.H.; Brown, J.E.; Yardley, D.A.; Richardson, G.E.; Siena, S.; Maroto, P.; Clemens, M.; et al. Superiority of denosumab to zoledronic acid for prevention of skeletal-related events: A combined analysis of 3 pivotal, randomised, phase 3 trials. *Eur. J. Cancer* **2012**, *48*, 3082–3092. [CrossRef] [PubMed]
144. Associazione Italiana Oncologi Medici. Linee Guida AIOM 2018, Disordini Elettrolitici. Available online: https://www.aiom.it/disordini-elettrolitici-raccomandazioni-per-liter-diagnostico-terapeutico-nel-paziente-oncologico (accessed on 3 November 2020).
145. Witteveen, J.E.; Van Thiel, S.; Romijn, J.A.; Hamdy, N.A. Hungry bone syndrome: Still a challenge in the post-operative management of primary hyperparathyroidism: A systematic review of the literature. *Eur. J. Endocrinol.* **2013**, *168*, R45–R53. [CrossRef] [PubMed]
146. Sakai, K.; Tomoda, Y.; Saito, H.; Tanaka, K. Hungry Bone Syndrome and Osteoblastic Bone Metastasis from Gastric Cancer. *QJM: Int. J. Med.* **2020**, *113*, 903–904. [CrossRef] [PubMed]
147. Di Nunno, V.; Cimadamore, A.; Santoni, M.; Scarpelli, M.; Fiorentino, M.; Ciccarese, C.; Iacovelli, R.; Cheng, L.; Lopez-Beltran, A.; Massari, F.; et al. Biological issues with cabozantinib in bone metastatic renal cell carcinoma and castration-resistant prostate cancer. *Future Oncol.* **2018**, *14*, 2559–2564. [CrossRef] [PubMed]

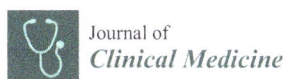

Review

Precision Medicine to Treat Advanced Gastroesophageal Adenocarcinoma: A Work in Progress

Valentina Gambardella [1,2,†], **Tania Fleitas** [1,2,†], **Noelia Tarazona** [1,2], **Federica Papaccio** [1], **Marisol Huerta** [1], **Susana Roselló** [1], **Francisco Gimeno-Valiente** [1], **Desamparados Roda** [1,2] and **Andrés Cervantes** [1,*]

1. Department of Medical Oncology, Biomedical Research Institute INCLIVA, University of Valencia, Blasco Ibañez 17, 46010 Valencia, Spain; vgambardella@incliva.es (V.G.); tfleitas@incliva.es (T.F.); noetalla@incliva.es (N.T.); fede.papaccio@yahoo.it (F.P.); mhuerta@incliva.es (M.H.); srosello@incliva.es (S.R.); fgimenovaliente@gmail.com (F.G.-V.); droda@incliva.es (D.R.)
2. Instituto de Salud Carlos III, CIBERONC, 28000 Madrid, Spain
* Correspondence: andres.cervantes@uv.es; Tel.: +34-9-61-97-35-43; Fax: +34-9-61-97-39-82
† These authors equally contributed to the article.

Received: 3 August 2020; Accepted: 14 September 2020; Published: 22 September 2020

Abstract: Gastroesophageal adenocarcinoma (GEA) represents a heterogeneous disease and, when diagnosed as locally advanced or metastatic, it is characterized by poor prognosis. During the last few years, several molecular classifications have been proposed to try to personalize treatment for those patients diagnosed with advanced disease. Nevertheless, despite the great effort, precision medicine is still far from being a reality. The improvement in the molecular analysis due to the application of high throughput technologies based on DNA and RNA sequencing has opened a novel scenario leading to the personalization of treatment. The possibility to target epidermal growth factor receptor (HER)2, Claudine, Fibroblast Growth Factor Receptors (FGFR), and other alterations with a molecular matched therapy could significantly improve clinical outcomes over advanced gastric cancer patients. On the other hand, the development of immunotherapy could also represent a promising strategy in a selected population. In this review, we sought to describe the novel pathways implicated in GEA progression and the results of the molecular matched therapies.

Keywords: advanced gastric cancer; precision medicine; new drug development

1. Introduction

Gastroesophageal adenocarcinoma (GEA) represents the fifth most frequent tumor and the third leading cause of cancer-related deaths worldwide. In 2018 GEA was diagnosed in about 1,000,000 people, causing death in 783,000 patients [1]. GEA is characterized by a worldwide variation in incidence, with a peak in Japan and South Korea, and lower incidence observed in the United States, Canada, India, and Middle Eastern countries. Beyond their higher rates of gastric cancer, Asian patients tend to have more distal gastric tumors, often associated with H. pylori, with less frequent gastroesophageal junction (GEJ) tumors, adenocarcinomas of the esophagus or Barrett's esophagus disease [2]. This geographical distribution is a reflection of multifactorial etiology related mainly to genetic susceptibility, diverse strains of H. pylori, dietary factors, and principally differences in the tumor–immune microenvironment [3,4]. As symptoms during early cancer development are generally mild and unspecific, late diagnosis is frequent, contributes to the high mortality observed in countries without screening programs [5,6]. GEA is recognized as a highly heterogeneous disease. Despite concerted efforts to develop comprehensive molecular classifications for GEA aimed at offering a precision approach to patients, only a few drugs have been approved. The aim of this article is to review the state of the art in precision medicine for advanced GEA.

2. From Morphological to Molecular Classifications

Historically, Lauren classified gastric cancers into intestinal, diffuse, and indeterminate/mixed histology [7]. The most common type is intestinal, which tends to form glandular structures and is often associated with intestinal metaplasia and H. pylori infection. Conversely, diffuse-type tumors are characterized by non-cohesive scattered cells, sometimes associated with the presence of signet-ring cells. These tumors trends to be locally aggressive with a higher rate of peritoneum invasion and a lower response rate in neoadjuvant studies, when treated with platinum-based therapies without taxanes [8,9]. The World Health Organization (WHO) further classified gastric cancer into tubular, papillary, mucinous, poorly cohesive (including Lauren diffuse type), and mixed variants. Nevertheless, neither stratification has helped characterize patient outcomes or guide treatment approach.

Further research focus has been directed at analyzing predictive biomarkers and targetable drivers. Molecular studies have been led by The Cancer Genome Atlas (TCGA) and also by the Asian Cancer Research Group (ACRG) [10,11]. TCGA studied both adenocarcinoma and squamous cell carcinoma spanning the stomach and esophagus while the ACRG focused on gastric adenocarcinoma across the Asian population. TCGA proposed a comprehensive molecular classification of GEA according to genomic, transcriptomic and proteomic data into four different subgroups, respectively, named as chromosomally instability (CIN), genomically stable (GS), Epstein–Barr Virus (EBV) and microsatellite instability (MSI). More than 50% of tumors belong to the CIN subgroup, which is mainly characterized by receptor tyrosine kinase (RTK) alterations [10]. Despite this, apart from epidermal growth factor receptor (HER)2 amplification, MSI and EBV, no other molecular alterations have been used in the clinic as effective predictors for treatment decision-making (Table 1).

Table 1. Molecular features of GEA subgroups of TCGA analysis.

GS	EBV	MSI	CIN
CDH1 and *RHOA* mutations	DNA hypermethylation	Hypermutation	RTK-RAS activation
CLDN18-ARHGAP 26 fusion	*PIK3CA* and *ARID1A* mutations	*MLH1* silencing	*TP53* mutation
Cell adhesion	*JAK2* amplification	*RAS* activation	Cell cycle activation
	CDKN2 silencing		
	Immune activation	Mitotic pathway	

GEA: Gastroesophageal adenocarcinoma; TCGA: The Cancer Genome Atlas.

The ACRG [11] group developed a different classification, considering also four groups based on array-based gene-expression profiling: MSI (22.7%), microsatellite stable with epithelial-to-mesenchymal transition (MSS/EMT; 15.3%), MSS with TP53 mutations (26.3%), and MSS without TP53 mutations (35.7%). The MSS/EMT class was enriched in diffuse-type tumors classified as GS by TCGA, and MSS/TP53+ was enriched for EBV+ tumors. ACRG analysis found inferior survival among the MSS/EMT+ group. Although no survival associations were seen in the TCGA study, potentially owing to the therapeutic heterogeneity of the internationally diverse sample set, subsequent studies applying the TCGA classes to two large independent cohorts demonstrated that EBV+ tumors have superior survival and GS tumors have inferior survival [12].

Tumor heterogeneity is the main obstacle to progress in precision medicine for GEA patients. Comprehensive molecular assessment sequencing primary and metastatic GEA has revealed marked differences in genomic aberrations, with frequent discrepancies between findings in primary versus metastatic tumors. When gene mutations were specifically analyzed, 20% could be found only in the primary tumor, while a similar proportion was found only in metastatic tumors. The rest (60%) of mutations detected were shared by both primary and metastatic. Turning to gene amplifications, 32% are seen only in primary tumors, 31% in metastatic tumors and only 37% were shared by both. This observed discrepancy in genomic aberrations led to treatment modification in almost a third of patients [13,14]. Liquid biopsies assessing cell-free DNA have the potential to help optimize therapy selection.

3. Targeting HER2 beyond Trastuzumab: Novel Steps towards Precision Medicine

HER2 receptor is a member of the epidermal growth factor receptor (HER) family consisting of four members (HER1 (ErbB1, EGFR), HER2 (ErbB2), HER3 (ErbB3) and HER4 (ErbB4)), activated by spontaneous homo/heterodimerization [15]. HER2 is amplified in several tumors, such as breast, colorectal and GEA [16], where it accounts for about 7–34% of all cases. HER2 overexpression is more highly detected among tumors of the GE junction (GEJ) and varies across different histological subtypes and differentiation grades [17]. HER2-amplified tumors are mostly well- or moderately-differentiated intestinal subtypes [18]. Despite identification of HER2 amplification in GEA, the use of HER2 blocking agents has not achieved the outstanding results shown in breast cancer (Table 2.). Trastuzumab, a monoclonal antibody inhibiting HER2 activation by binding to the extracellular domain IV of HER2, improves clinical outcomes over HER2-amplified localized and advanced breast cancer, both as a single agent and in combination with chemotherapy.

A randomized multicenter trial (ToGA) assessed the addition of trastuzumab to platinum-based chemotherapy in HER2-amplified patients with locally advanced or metastatic GEA [19]. Patients were randomized to receive trastuzumab plus platinum-based chemotherapy (capecitabine or 5-fluorouracil plus cisplatin) versus chemotherapy alone. In the experimental arm, patients experienced a substantial improvement in all outcomes and particularly in overall survival (OS). Median OS was increased by 2.7 months in the trastuzumab-containing arm (13.8 versus 11.1 months, Hazard ratio (HR) 0.74, P.0.0046) [19]. Based on these results, the combination of trastuzumab plus platinum-based chemotherapy represents the gold standard for advanced HER2-amplified GEA. The extent of improvement was related to the degree of amplification, as demonstrated in an exploratory post-hoc analysis. The subset of tumors with HER2 immunohistochemistry (IHC) 3 or IHC2/FISH+ reached a median OS of 16 months in the trastuzumab group versus only 11.8 months in the chemotherapy control arm (HR 0.68, 95% CI 0.5–0.83). These results suggest that trastuzumab provides the best therapeutic benefit in strongly HER2-amplified patients [20].

These findings highlight the need for adequate patient selection. HER2 amplification is highly heterogeneous across patients and even intratumorally [21], a phenomenon that could account for the general lack of benefit when anti-HER2 drugs are administered without correct scoring by a dedicated pathologist. The level of HER2 amplification in metastatic GEA by FISH has been shown to predict response to trastuzumab [22]. Beyond IHC and FISH, when HER2 amplification was determined by next-generation sequencing (NGS) in tumor samples or in plasma, analyzing cell-free circulating tumor DNA, response to antiHER2 agents directly correlated with level of expression observed in plasma samples.

Other HER2 blocking drugs were successively tested to evaluate their potential in HER2-amplified and advanced GEA patients (Table 2). Disappointingly, no benefit in overall survival was achieved in patients diagnosed with locally advanced or metastatic GEA when treated with lapatinib, either as a single agent or in combination with platinum-based chemotherapy (CT) pertuzumab or TDM-1. Lapatinib, a dual EGFR/HER2 small tyrosine kinase inhibitor, was tested as first-line treatment in a phase III, double-blinded study (LoGic Trial) and failed to demonstrate OS improvement [23]. Lapatinib also failed to improve OS in a second-line trial in Asian patients (TyTAN trial) despite a significant increase in response rate. [24]. Based on the good results achieved in advanced HER2-amplified breast cancer patients, we also tested pertuzumab, a humanized monoclonal HER2-targeted antibody that binds to a different epitope on the HER2 receptor than trastuzumab. In a phase III trial (JACOB), the combination of trastuzumab, pertuzumab and platinum-based (CT) was tested as a first-line treatment in HER2 amplified GEA patients [25] and failed to improve survival.

Trastuzumab emtansine (TDM-1), an antibody-drug conjugate, was also tested as second line versus paclitaxel in patients progressing after first-line trastuzumab-containing treatment, showing no benefit in OS in the phase II/III GATSBY trial [26]. Similarly, when trastuzumab was tested in combination with paclitaxel beyond tumor progression in a phase II trial enrolling patients who experienced progression on first line with trastuzumab and platinum-based CT, no benefit was found.

In this phase II randomized trial, trastuzumab beyond progression, a common approach used in HER2 amplified BC did not improve progression free-survival (PFS) in advanced HER amplified GEA patients [27]. One possible cause of treatment failure could have been the significant loss of HER2 amplification after trastuzumab blockade, already described in HER2 amplified BC [22,28]. Several other mechanisms of resistance have been addressed to explain the lack of benefit of other antiHER2 agents. Among them, the most significant could be intratumor heterogeneity, as well as the presence of emerging molecular alterations, such as PI3K, MAPK activation and MET or FGFR aberrations [13,17,29–31].

Interestingly, an elegant translational study found that oral pan-HER inhibitor afatinib could rescue patients progressing after trastuzumab when they co-expressed HER2, EGFR or MET amplifications, paving the way for multi-targeted agents according to personalized profiles [13].

Among other antiHER2 agents under development, margetuximab, an Fc-modified chimeric monoclonal antibody, has shown promising results in early-phase clinical studies for HER2-expressing solid tumors, including low HER2-expressing gastric cancer [32]. In a phase 1b–2 trial in locally advanced HER2-amplified, PD-L1 unselected GEJ, patients who experienced disease progression to trastuzumab and at least two previous lines of CT were enrolled to receive margetuximab and pembrolizumab. This combination showed acceptable safety and tolerability and objective responses were observed in 18.4% of evaluable patients, suggesting synergistic anti-tumor activity with checkpoint inhibitors [33]. Preclinical and clinical evidence support combining pembrolizumab with trastuzumab and cytotoxic chemotherapy to treat HER2-positive cancers [34]. In several analyses performed in tumor samples of GEA patients treated with trastuzumab, it was possible to observe upregulation of PD-1 and enhanced gene expression signatures of immune infiltration, [35] which could suggest a potential benefit deriving from checkpoint inhibitors. Moreover, the combination of trastuzumab with pembrolizumab could increase T-cell response [36,37]. On the strength of these findings, this combination has a promising biological rationale.

In a phase II trial, patients diagnosed with locally advanced or metastatic HER2-amplified GEA were treated with pembrolizumab, trastuzumab, fluoropyrimidine and platinum as first-line therapy. Twenty-six (70%) of 37 patients were progression-free at 6 months and 17% achieved a complete response. The 91% response rate and median overall survival of 27.3 months were also higher than previously reported for chemotherapy plus trastuzumab, the existing first-line standard [19]. Treatment-related adverse events were similar as with combinations of trastuzumab with chemotherapy and pembrolizumab with chemotherapy [38,39]. PD-L1 combined positive score was not predictive of outcome in this study population; nevertheless, patients with HER2 amplification had more durable responses to trastuzumab-based combination therapy than HER2-positive patients who did not have HER2 gene amplification by next-generation sequencing. A phase III trial of pembrolizumab versus placebo in combination with trastuzumab and chemotherapy is ongoing.

Interesting results have recently been achieved with another antibody-drug conjugate. Trastuzumab deruxtecan (DS-8201) consists of a humanized, monoclonal, anti-HER2 antibody binding a cytotoxic topoisomerase I inhibitor by means of a cleavable, tetrapeptide-based linker [40]. This drug is stable in plasma [41], but is highly cleaved in cancer cells [42]. The most appealing characteristic of this conjugate is that it binds even to cells with lower levels of HER2 expression [43] due to the ability of the released payload to diffuse across cell membranes. Probably owing to this dynamic feature, trastuzumab deruxtecan represents a good strategy for heterogeneous tumors, such as gastric cancer in which HER2 overexpression may vary from cell to cell or even across different metastatic locations within the same patient [19,44]. In a phase II trial design, after encouraging results obtained in a previous phase I, patients diagnosed with advanced GEA who had received at least two previous lines were stratified into high and low HER2 and were randomized 2:1 to receive trastuzumab deruxtecan versus the treating physician's choice of irinotecan or paclitaxel [45,46]. Objective response was significantly higher in the experimental group than with chemotherapy (51% versus 14%). Ten patients (8%) in the experimental arm had a confirmed complete response versus none in the chemotherapy arm.

Patients on trastuzumab deruxtecan gained significantly in overall survival (median OS, 12.5 months versus 8.4 months. HR = 0.59; p = 0.01). Greater efficacy of trastuzumab deruxtecan over chemotherapy was confirmed in patients with the highest level of HER2 expression (Response Rate 58% versus 29%) [46]. However, in tumors with lower HER2 expression levels, a lower response rate was determined. The more efficient linker-payload system of trastuzumab deruxtecan, ten-fold more potent than SN-38, may contribute to the differing treatment outcomes versus TDM-1 [47,48]. Interstitial lung disease has been observed in 10% of patients receiving trastuzumab deruxtecan, most classified as grade II, although some were severe. Monitoring this trend and understanding ways of preventing and treating it is vital before recommending this drug-conjugate antibody for general use.

Table 2. Randomized clinical trials testing anti-epidermal growth factor receptor (HER)2 blocking agents in HER2-amplified advanced GEA.

TRIAL	Phase	Experimental Drug	Chemotherapy Backbone	Line of Therapy	Number of Included Patients	HR for OS	p Value	Response Rate	Increase in Median Survival
ToGA [19]	III	Trastuzumab	Cisplatin+5-FU/ capecitabine	First	584	0.74	0.04	51% vs. 37% p = 0.0017	+2.8 months
LOGiC [20]	III	Lapatinib	Oxaliplatin/ capecitabine +/−Lapatinib	First	545	0.91	0.35	53% vs. 39% p = 0.031	+1.7 months
TyTAN [21]	III	Lapatinib	Paclitaxel+/− Lapatinib	Second	261	0.84	0.20	27% vs. 9% p = 0.001	+2.1 months
GATSBY [20]	II/III	TDM-1	TDM-1 vs. Taxane	Second	345	1.15	0.85	NP	−0.7 months
JACOB [21]	III	Pertuzumab	Cisplatin+5-FU/ capecitabine /Trastuzumab +/− Pertuzumab	First	780	0.84	0.056	56% vs. 48% p = 0.026	3.3 months
DESTINY-Gastric01 [46]	II	Trastuzumab Deruxtecan	Trastuzumab Deruxtecan vs. Paclitaxel or Irinotecan	Third	187	0.59	0.01	51% vs. 14%	4.1 months

GEA: Gastroesophageal adenocarcinoma. HR: Hazard Ratio. OS: Overall survival. 5FU: 5-fluorouracile.

4. Targeting MET, EGFR, PI3K/AKT/mTOR Pathways and NTRK Fusions

Phase III trials with other targeted therapies based on molecular features other than HER2 have achieved disappointing results in GEA (Table 3) [2,49]. The epidermal growth factor receptor (EGFR) is amplified in about 5% and the receptor is overexpressed in between 30–50% of cases [50]. Both cetuximab and panitumumab, approved anti-EGFR monoclonal antibodies in advanced colon cancer, have been tested. However, in two randomized phases III trials, no improvement in clinical outcomes was detected when the anti-EGFR treatment was added to a first line of a platinum-based chemotherapy [51,52]. These anti-EGFR antibodies might have decreased the tolerance of the backbone CT in first line, leading to dose delays and reduction which could have had a detrimental effect. Beyond first line, the anti-EGFR tyrosine kinase inhibitor gefitinib showed no clinical benefit versus placebo in tests [53]. As a general limitation, no molecular patient selection was properly performed. The subset analysis of both COG [53] and EXPAND trials [51] underlined a potential effect in EGFR-amplified patients. Nevertheless, these results should be confirmed prospectively.

The results of MET inhibition have also been discouraging. MET amplification is detectable in about 6% and overexpressed in 25–60% of GEA [10,49]. When monoclonal antibodies such as onartuzumab [54] and rilotumumab [55] were added to first-line chemotherapy, no clinical benefit was observed. Moreover, similarly negative results were obtained when tyrosine kinase inhibitors such as AMG 337 were administered in a heavily treated population of MET-amplified patients. Another molecular alteration widely present across GEA patients is activation of the PI3K–AKT–mTOR pathway. Everolimus, a mTOR inhibitor approved in breast cancer, was tested on unselected patients, showing no clinical benefit in OS beyond the first line [56].

Given the evidence of the complex molecular landscape of GEA, an umbrella platform [57] has been designed with preplanned genomic biomarker analyses to assign advanced GEA patients to molecularly matched therapies. Several biomarker groups were identified based on RAS alterations, TP53, PIK3CA mutations, MET and PIK3CA amplification, etc. Of the whole screened population, only 14.7%

received biomarker-assigned drug treatment. The highest response rate was observed in patients with MET amplification treated with savolitinib, a potent small-molecule reversible MET kinase inhibitor. This strategy obtained encouraging response rates and survival when compared with conventional second-line standard chemotherapy, especially in patients presenting high MET expression enriched for higher MET copy number. Circulating tumor (ctDNA) analysis demonstrated good correlation between high MET copy number by ctDNA and response to MET inhibitors. Further results are awaited.

As NTRK has been recently identified as a relevant molecular driver over solid tumors, despite the low incidence over GEA, the molecular evaluation searching for NTRK fusion, could be an option in patients with a good performance status [58].

5. The Role of Stemness and Metalloprotease in GEA

As interesting preclinical data suggested the potential role of stemness pathways in GEA development and progression, the inhibition of STAT3, a principal actor of this pathway, was also tested. Nevertheless, when NAPA, a STAT3 inhibitor, was added to Paclitaxel, no clinical benefit was demonstrated in a phase III trial enrolling pre-treated GEA patient [58]. Disappointing results were also observed in a phase III trial randomizing patients to receive andecaliximab, a monoclonal antibody targeting matrix metalloproteinase 9 (MMS9), combined with CT in pretreated GEA patients. Despite the potential role of MMS9 in GEA development and progression, the inhibition of this target was no longer able to increase PFS or OS [59]. The lack of predictive biomarker could have negatively influenced the potential role of these drugs.

6. Angiogenesis-Targeting Drugs

Although antiangiogenic therapies are the current standard of care in other gastrointestinal tumors, addition of these agents did not show a benefit in unselected patients with GEA. In first line, bevacizumab improved overall response rate and PFS, but not OS, when added to chemotherapy for the first-line treatment of advanced gastric cancer [60]. In the same setting, ramucirumab was not able to improve clinical outcomes, yet demonstrated significant albeit modest OS benefit in the second line, both as monotherapy and combined with docetaxel [61–63]. In an Asian population, apatinib, a tyrosine kinase inhibitor of VEGFR2, showed improvement in PFS and OS when used in patients who experienced disease progression to two or more lines [64]. No biomarkers able to predict response to antiangiogenics have been so far identified.

Table 3. Randomized trials targeting angiogenesis, EGFR and MET pathways in first line in GEA.

Trial	Chemotherapy	Experimental Drug	HR	Trial	Chemotherapy
AVAGAST [62]	Cisplatin+ capecitabine	Bevacizumab	0.87	0.10	+2.0 months
RAINFALL [63]	Cisplatin+5-FU/ capecitabine	Ramucirumab	0.96	0.68	0.5 month
EXPAND [51]	Cisplatin+ capecitabine	Cetuximab	1.00	0.95	−1.3 months
REAL-3 [52]	Oxaliplatin+ epi- + capecitabine	Panitumumab	1.37	0.013	−2.5 months
RILOMET-1 [55]	Cisplatin+ epi+capecitabine	Rilotumumab	–	–	Stopped in futility analysis
METGASTRIC [54]	FOLFOX6	Onartuzumab	1.06	0.83	−0.6 months

GEA: Gastroesophageal adenocarcinoma. HR: Hazard Ratio, OS: Overall Survival, EGFR: Epidermal Growth Factor Receptor. 5FU: 5-Fluorouracile.

7. The Search for Biomarkers for Precision Immunotherapy

Immunotherapy has revolutionized the treatment of many solid tumors; nonetheless, no biomarker for patient selection has been clearly identified as yet [65,66]. Among GEA patients, the PD-L1 combined positivity score (CPS), consisting of immunohistochemistry-detected protein in at least 1% of cells in the tumor or surrounding stroma, is often used for candidate selection in pembrolizumab-related trials. In the phase II KEYNOTE-059 trial, evaluating pembrolizumab as third-line treatment for metastatic gastric cancer, the overall response rate was 22.7% in PD-L1–positive tumors, with a median response duration of 8.1 months [38]. However, response rate was only 16.2% in PD-L1-negative tumors. On the other hand, results obtained testing another anti-PD-1 inhibitor, nivolumab, were similar to pembrolizumab, yet no relation with PD-L1 expression was found. In the phase III ATTRACTION-2 trial including Asian patients, nivolumab monotherapy led to an overall response rate ORR of 11% and significantly increased 12-month OS to 27% versus 11% with a placebo (HR: 0.63; $p = 0.0001$). This survival benefit was independent of PD-L1 positivity [65]. When nivolumab was tested in a western population as a single agent or added to ipilimumab, ORR was higher in PDL1-positive tumors (27%) than in PDL1-negative tumors (12%) [66].

MSI-H and EBV-positive tumors each comprise approximately 5% of metastatic and 20–30% of localized gastric cancers [10]. The MSI-H subtype is characterized by hypermutation, frequently on *KRAS, PI3K, PTEN, mTOR, ALK,* and *ARID1A*, resulting from silenced DNA mismatch repair proteins, such as MLH1. EBV-positive gastric cancer is characterized by high PD-L1 and 2 expression, *PIK3CA* and *CDKN2A* mutations, and *JAK2* amplification. Both MSI-H and EBV-positive types, regardless of histology, are considered the most immunogenic subtypes, susceptible to treatment with checkpoint inhibitors [67]. A recent phase II study testing pembrolizumab in metastatic gastric cancer patients described a notable, durable response in the MSI and EBV subtypes [68]. In MSI tumors, checkpoint inhibitor antitumor activity is associated with high tumor mutation load and neoantigen formation [68], with response rates for MSI gastric cancer ranging from 57% to 86% [67,68]. EBV subtype tumors are associated with tumor immune-cell infiltration and high expression of PD-L1, and in a subgroup analysis of a phase II study, all EBV-positive gastric cancer patients responded to pembrolizumab [67].

Furthermore, correlation between gene expression profile and response to checkpoint inhibitors was assessed in two different cohorts of advanced GEA patients treated with immunotherapy, used as a test and validation cohort. High alternate promoter utilization tumors exhibited decreased markers of T-cell anti-cancer activity, causing immune evasion and lower responses to checkpoint inhibitors (8% versus 42%, $p = 0.03$). This alternative promoter utilization was confirmed in multivariate analysis as an independent predictor of survival in patients receiving checkpoint inhibitors, indicating the potential role of alternate promoter utilization as a predictive biomarker for immunotherapy [69,70].

The GEA tumor microenvironment is directly involved in tumor development and progression [71] and, for this reason, the combinations of checkpoint inhibitors and antiangiogenetic drugs is being tested. In a small phase II trial, the use of the combination of pembrolizumab and levantinib as I or II line showed, across HER2 negative Asiatic GEA, an objective response recorded in 69% of patients with an acceptable toxicity suggesting a potential role of the combination also in the MSS population that should be further explored [72,73]. The combination of nivolumab and regorafenib is also under evaluation [74]. Further results are awaited.

8. Novel Potentially Druggable Pathways: Tight Junction Proteins, Fibroblast Growth Factor Pathway and DNA Damage Repair Response

8.1. Claudin 18.2

Tight junction protein Claudin (CLDN) 18.2 has recently been identified as a possible target for GEA patients [75]. Physiologically, CLDN18.2 is buried in the tight junction supramolecular complex. However, due to changes occurring in the malignant transformation, tight junctions expose CLDN18.2 epitopes on the surface of tumor cells [75], making it possible to target it. Zolbetuximab is a chimeric IgG1 monoclonal antibody that binds to CLDN18.2 on the surface of tumor cells inhibiting cell survival and proliferation through antibody-dependent cellular cytotoxicity (ADCC) and complement-dependent cytotoxicity (CDC) [76].

In a phase II trial, patients diagnosed with advanced GEA who had progressed to at least one previous chemotherapy line, whose tumors expressed CLDN18.2 (moderate–intense membrane staining intensity in >50% of cancer cells) were treated with zolbetuximab as monotherapy [77]. A total of 54 patients were enrolled. Zolbetuximab monotherapy was found to be well tolerated with only mild gastrointestinal adverse events and exhibited anti-tumor activity in patients with CLDN18.2-positive advanced gastric or GEJ adenocarcinomas, as already demonstrated when it was used as a single agent. Despite the small number included, among 43 evaluable patients, 4 achieved partial response (ORR 9%) and 6 (14%) had stable disease for a clinical benefit rate of 23%. In the subgroup of patients whose tumors expressed moderate or high CLDN18.2 level in >70% of tumor cells, ORR was 14%. Moreover, a randomized exploratory phase II trial (FAST) showed that zolbetuximab combined with platinum-based chemotherapy (EOX) confers a survival benefit over EOX alone in patients with CLDN18.2þ positive advanced gastric/GEJ cancer. These results warrant validation in a prospective randomized phase III design. Several phase III trials among Caucasian and Asian patients are currently underway to evaluate the role of zolbetuximab in improving OS in locally advanced and metastatic GEA in combination with a platinum-based chemotherapy.

8.2. FGFR Pathway

FGFR signaling is made up of four highly conserved transmembrane tyrosine kinases receptors (FGFR1–4) and FGFR5, which lack the intracellular kinase domain. All these receptors are activated by FGF, and participate in cell survival and proliferation [78,79]. Multiple trials studying diverse solid tumors have proposed the aberrant FGFR signaling pathway as a potential therapeutic target, and several inhibitors are under development (Table 4) [80–89]. The FGFR2 splice variant FGFR2b [89] is overexpressed in 2.5–31.1% of GEA [10]. In in vitro and in vivo models of GEA, FGFR2b overexpression has been related to both amplification and aberrant transcriptional upregulation of the FGFR2 gene [78], and in GEA, both FGFR2b overexpression and FGFR2 gene amplification have been associated with worse prognosis. FGFR2 gene amplification is associated with both chromosomal instability and genomically stable molecular subtypes [71].

In a phase II trial, patients diagnosed with advanced GEA presenting FGFR2 amplification or polysomy were randomized to receive AZD4547, an FGFR tyrosine kinase inhibitor, or paclitaxel. AZD4547 did not improve PFS over standard CT [88]. The lack of benefit could relate to the notorious intratumor heterogeneity for FGFR2 gene amplification and poor concordance between FGFR2 amplification/polysomy and FGFR2 expression [88]. Bemarituzumab (FPA144), is a humanized IgG1 monoclonal antibody that specifically inhibits cancer cells presenting the splice-variant FGFR2b binding of the ligands FGF7, FGF10, and FGF22 (25). In a phase I basket trial enrolling patients with advanced solid tumors and a specific cohort for GEA, it demonstrated single-agent activity as late-line therapy in patients with advanced-stage GEA, achieving partial response in 5 out of 28 patients. Bemarituzumab is currently being evaluated in combination with chemotherapy in a phase III trial as front-line therapy for patients with high FGFR2b-overexpressing advanced-stage GEA [89]. Apart from amplification, FGFR may exhibit other molecular alterations, and several novel drugs have been tested in solid tumors harboring mutations and gene rearrangements. The specific role of each one and their contribution in predicting drug response seems different for each specific molecular alteration presented in each of the four genes involved in the FGFR family [85]. Table 4 shows different FGFR inhibitors under development, describing their mechanisms of action as well as other characteristics including availability of predictive biomarkers.

Table 4. FGFR inhibitors under development.

Compound	Type	Mechanisms of Action	Predictive Biomarkers	Clinical Phase of Development
Bemarituzumab	mAb	Inhibitor of FGF7, FGF10, and FGF22 ligand of the splice-variant FGFR2b		II, III
AZD4547	TKi	Potent and selective inhibitor of FGFR 1, 2, and 3		II
Infigratinib	TKi	Selective, ATP-competitive inhibitor of FGFR1, 2, and 3		I
E-7090	TKi	Oral and selective inhibitor of FGFR1, 2, and 3		I
LY2874455	TKi	Potent Pan FGFR inhibitor		I
Pemigatinib [81]	TKi	Potent inhibitor of FGFR1, 2, and 3	FGFR2 fusions	II
Rogaratinib [82]	TKi	Potent Pan FGFR inhibitor	FGFR1-3 mRNA expression	I
Futibatinib [83]	TKi	Potent and highly specific against wildtype FGFR1–4 as well as against some FGFR2 kinase domain mutations	FGFR2 fusions, FGFR1 mutations	I
Fisogatinib	TKi	Potent and selective inhibitor of FGFR4		I
H3B-6527	TKi	Selective and covalent inhibitor of FGFR4		I
Roblitinib	TKi	Potent and selective, reversible-covalent small-molecule inhibitor of FGFR4		I
Erdafitinib	TKi	Potent Pan FGFR inhibitor	FGFR3 mutations, FGFR2/3 fusions	II

mAb: monoclonal antibody; TKi: Tyrosine Kinase inhibitors.

8.3. DNA Damage Response Pathway in GEA

The identification of a molecular subgroup characterized by chromosomal instability (CIN) and aneuploidy underlines the possible role of DNA damage in GEA. In light of this, several trials have studied the use of PARP inhibitors. Despite promising phase II data [90], the phase III GOLD trial failed to show benefit from adding the PARP inhibitor olaparib to paclitaxel in the second-line setting [91]. These negative results across the overall unselected population might be explained by the lack of appropriate predictive biomarkers indicating PARP-dependency or homologous recombination defects (HRD). Unexpectedly, patients in whom immunohistochemistry detected loss of ATM expression causing potential sensitivity to PARP inhibitors, saw no benefit from olaparib either. Potential explanations include immature follow-up of the ATM-negative subgroup, and confounding of treatment by favorable prognostic factors enriched in ATM-low tumors, such as PD-L1 expression [91]. The data also underline the need for additional evaluation of HRD and replication stress as predictive biomarkers of response to PARP inhibitors. Platinum sensitivity may itself be a predictive biomarker, a concept that has led to a phase III trial of PARP inhibition versus placebo as maintenance therapy in locally advanced or metastatic gastric cancer that experienced response to a first line of platinum-based chemotherapy.

Maintenance strategies are also ongoing. In a phase III trial, advanced GEA patients, who have responded to first-line, platinum-based chemotherapy for at least 8 weeks, are randomized to placebo versus pamiparib, a novel PARP inhibitor. Other experimental agents, such as CHEK1, ATR, and WEE1 inhibitors are also under clinical testing. Among the CIN subgroup, some GEAs presented high amplification of KRAS or other alterations in cell-cycle regulators, and consequently several studies evaluating inhibition of RAS downstream effectors and CDK2 inhibitors are underway.

9. Conclusions

GEA presents as a very heterogeneous disease. The high number of molecular alterations, as reflected in the percentage of tumors belonging to the CIN subtype, makes a precision approach complicated. Nevertheless, the possibility of identifying certain drivers due to the implementation of omics in recent years has opened up novel opportunities in cancer patients. Among HER2-amplified tumors, more active molecules are leading to significantly improved benefits in these patients.

The growing interest in tumor microenvironment, together with development of novel immunotherapies and combinations could also herald new approaches. The road towards a personalized approach is long, requiring further studies and breakthroughs in current knowledge.

Author Contributions: V.G., T.F., N.T., F.P., M.H., S.R., F.G.-V., D.R.: conceptualization, writing—original draft preparation, writing—editing and reviewing. A.C.: writing—editing and reviewing. All authors have read and agreed to the published version of the manuscript.

Funding: This study was supported by grants from the Instituto de Salud Carlos III (PI15/02180 and PI18/01909 to AC; PI18/01508 to TF). V.G. was supported by Rio Hortega contract CM18/00241 from the Carlos III Health Institute; T.F. is supported by Joan Rodes contract 17/00026 from the Carlos III Health Institute. N.T. was supported by Rio Hortega contract CM15/00246 from the Instituto de Salud Carlos III; F.P. is supported by a ESMO Fellowship Contract 2019. D.R. was supported by Joan Rodes contract 16/00040 from the Instituto de Salud Carlos III.

Conflicts of Interest: A.C. declares institutional research funding from Genentech, Merck Serono, BMS, MSD, Roche, Beigene, Bayer, Servier, Lilly, Novartis, Takeda, Astellas and Fibrogen and advisory board or speaker fees from Merck Serono, Roche, Servier, Takeda and Astellas in the last 5 years. All remaining authors have declared no conflicts of interest.

References

1. Bray, F.; Ferlay, J.; Soerjomataram, I.; Siegel, R.L.; Torre, L.A.; Jemal, A. Global Cancer Statistics 2018: GLOBOCAN Estimates of Incidence and Mortality Worldwide for 36 Cancers in 185 Countries. *CA Cancer J. Clin.* **2018**, 394–424. [CrossRef] [PubMed]
2. Nagaraja, A.K.; Kikuchi, O.; Bass, A.J. Genomics and Targeted Therapies in Gastroesophageal Adenocarcinoma. *Cancer Discov.* **2019**. [CrossRef] [PubMed]
3. Anderson, W.F.; Rabkin, C.S.; Turner, N.; Fraumeni, J.F.J.; Rosenberg, P.S.; Camargo, M.C. The Changing Face of Noncardia Gastric Cancer Incidence among US Non-Hispanic Whites. *J. Natl. Cancer Inst.* **2018**, *110110*, 608–615. [CrossRef] [PubMed]
4. Lin, S.J.; Gagnon-bartsch, J.A.; Tan, I.B.; Earle, S.; Ruff, L.; Pettinger, K.; Ylstra, B.; van Grieken, N.; Rha, S.Y.; Chung, Y.C.; et al. Signatures of tumour immunity distinguish Asian and non-Asian gastric adenocarcinomas. *Gut* **2015**, *64*, 1721–1731. [CrossRef]
5. Cervantes, A.; Roda, D.; Tarazona, N.; Roselló, S. Current questions for the treatment of advanced gastric cancer. *Cancer Treat. Rev.* **2013**, *3939*, 60–67. [CrossRef]
6. Lordick, F.; Allum, W.; Carneiro, F.; Mitryd, E.; Tabernero, J.; Tan, P.; Van Cutsem, E.; van de Veldeh, C.; Cervantes, A. Unmet needs and challenges in gastric cancer: The way forward. *Cancer Treat. Rev.* **2014**, *4040*, 692–700. [CrossRef]
7. Lauren, P. The two Histological Main Types of Gastric Carcinoma: Diffuse and So-Called Intestinal-Type Carcinoma. An Attempt at a Histo-Clinical Classification. *Acta Pathol. Microbiol. Scand.* **1965**, *64*, 31–49. [CrossRef]
8. Cunningham, D.; Allum, W.H.; Stenning, S.P.; Thompson, J.N.; Van de Velde, C.; Nicolson, M.; Scarffe, J.H.; Lofts, F.J.; Falk, S.J.; Iveson, T.J.; et al. Perioperative chemotherapy versus surgery alone for resectable gastroesophageal cancer. *N. Engl. J. Med.* **2006**, *355355*, 11–20. [CrossRef]
9. Al-Batran, S.-E.; Homann, N.; Pauligk, C.; Goetze, T.G.; Meiler, J.; Kasper, S.; Kopp, H.-G.; Mayer, F.; Haag, G.H.; Luley, K. Perioperative chemotherapy with fluorouracil plus leucovorin, oxaliplatin, and docetaxel versus fluorouracil or capecitabine plus cisplatin and epirubicin for locally advanced, resectable gastric or gastro-oesophageal junction adenocarcinoma (FLOT4): A randomised, phase 2/3 trial. *Lancet* **2019**, *393393*, 1948–1957. [CrossRef]
10. Cancer Genome Atlas Research Network. Comprehensive molecular characterization of gastric adenocarcinoma. *Nature* **2014**, *513*, 202–209. [CrossRef]
11. Cristescu, R.; Lee, J.; Nebozhyn, M.; Aggwarl, A. Molecular analysis of gastric cancer identifies subtypes associated with distinct clinical outcomes. *Nat. Med.* **2015**, *21*, 449–456. [CrossRef] [PubMed]
12. Sohn, B.H.; Hwang, J.-E.; Jang, H.-J.; Lee, H.S.; Oh, S.C.; Shim, J.J.; Lee, K.W.; Kim, E.H.; Yim, S.Y.; Lee, S.H.; et al. Clinical Significance of Four Molecular Subtypes of Gastric Cancer Identified by The Cancer Genome Atlas Project. *Clin. Cancer Res. J. Am. Assoc. Cancer Res.* **2017**. [CrossRef] [PubMed]

13. Pectasides, E.; Stachler, M.D.; Derks, S.; Liu, Y.; Maron, S.; Islam, M.; Alpert, L.; Kwak, H.; Kindler, H.; Polite, B.; et al. Genomic Heterogeneity as a Barrier to Precision Medicine in Gastroesophageal Adenocarcinoma. *Cancer Discov.* **2018**, *8*, 37–48. [CrossRef]
14. Arteaga, C.L.; Engelman, J.A. ERBB receptors: From oncogene discovery to basic science to mechanism-based cancer therapeutics. *Cancer Cell.* **2014**, *25*, 282–303. [CrossRef] [PubMed]
15. Yarden, Y.; Sliwkowski, M.X. Untangling the ErbB signalling network. *Nat. Rev. Mol. Cell Biol.* **2001**, *2*, 127–137. [CrossRef]
16. Gambardella, V.; Fleitas, T.; Tarazona, N.; Cejalvo, J.M.; Gimeno-Valiente, F.; Martinez-Ciarpaglini, C.; Huerta, M.; Roselló, S.; Castillo, J.; Roda, D.; et al. Towards precision oncology for HER2 blockade in gastroesophageal adenocarcinoma. *Ann. Oncol.* **2019**, *30*, 1254–1264. [CrossRef]
17. Wang, H.-B.; Liao, X.-F.; Zhang, J. Clinicopathological factors associated with HER2-positive gastric cancer: A meta-analysis. *Medicine (Baltimore)* **2017**, *96*, e8437. [CrossRef]
18. Bang, Y.-J.; Van Cutsem, E.; Feyereislova, A.; Chung, H.; Shen, L.; Sawaki, A.; Lordick, F.; Ohtsu, A.; Omuro, Y.; Satoh, T.; et al. Trastuzumab in combination with chemotherapy versus chemotherapy alone for treatmentof HER2-positive advanced gastric or gastro-oesophageal junction cancer (ToGA): A phase 3, open-label, randomised controlled trial. *Lancet* **2010**, *376*, 687–697. [CrossRef]
19. Tarazona, N.; Gambardella, V.; Huerta, M.; Roselló, S.; Cervantes, A. Personalised Treatment in Gastric Cancer: Myth or Reality? *Curr. Oncol. Rep.* **2016**, *18*, 41. [CrossRef]
20. Sicklick, J.K.; Kato, S.; Okamura, R.; Schwaederle, M.; Hahn, M.E.; Williams, C.B.; De, P.; Krie, A.; Piccioni, D.E.; Miller, V.A.; et al. Molecular profiling of cancer patients enables personalized combination therapy: The I-PREDICT study. *Nat. Med.* **2019**. [CrossRef]
21. Gomez-Martin, C.; Plaza, J.C.; Pazo-Cid, R.; Pons, F.; Fonseca, P.; Leon, A.; Alsina, M.; Visa, L.; Rivera, F.; Galan, M.C.; et al. Level of HER2 gene amplification predicts response and overall survival in HER2-positive advanced gastric cancer treated with trastuzumab. *J. Clin. Oncol. J. Am. Soc. Clin. Oncol.* **2013**, *31*, 4445–4452. [CrossRef] [PubMed]
22. Hecht, J.R.; Bang, Y.-J.; Qin, S.K.; Chung, H.C.; Xu, J.M.; Park, J.O.; Jeziorski, K.; Shparyk, Y.; Hoff, P.M.; Sobrero, A.; et al. Lapatinib in Combination with Capecitabine Plus Oxaliplatin in Human Epidermal Growth Factor Receptor 2-Positive Advanced or Metastatic Gastric, Esophageal, or Gastroesophageal Adenocarcinoma: TRIO-013/LOGiC—A Randomized Phase III Trial. *J. Clin. Oncol. J. Am. Soc. Clin. Oncol.* **2016**, *34*, 443–451. [CrossRef] [PubMed]
23. Satoh, T.; Xu, R.-H.; Chung, H.C.; Sun, G.P.; Doi, T.; Xu, J.M.; Tsuji, A.; Omuro, Y.; Li, J.; Wang, J.W.; et al. Lapatinib plus paclitaxel versus paclitaxel alone in the second-line treatment of HER2-amplified advanced gastric cancer in Asian populations: TyTAN—A randomized, phase III study. *J. Clin. Oncol. J. Am. Soc. Clin. Oncol.* **2014**, *32*, 2039–2049. [CrossRef] [PubMed]
24. Tabernero, J.; Hoff, P.M.; Shen, L.; Ohtsu, A.; Shah, M.A.; Cheng, K.; Song, C.; Wu, H.; Eng-Wong, J.; Kim, K.; et al. Pertuzumab plus trastuzumab and chemotherapy for HER2-positive metastatic gastric or gastro-oesophageal junction cancer (JACOB): Final analysis of a double-blind, randomised, placebo-controlled phase 3 study. *Lancet Oncol.* **2018**, *19*, 1372–1384. [CrossRef]
25. Thuss-Patience, P.C.; Shah, M.A.; Ohtsu, A.; Van Cutsem, E.; Ajani, J.A.; Castro, H.; Mansoor, W.; Chung, H.C.; Bodoky, G.; Shitara, K.; et al. Trastuzumab emtansine versus taxane use for previously treated HER2-positive locally advanced or metastatic gastric or gastro-oesophageal junction adenocarcinoma (GATSBY): An international randomised, open-label, adaptive, phase 2/3 study. *Lancet Oncol.* **2017**, *18*, 640–653. [CrossRef]
26. Makiyama, A.; Sukawa, Y.; Kashiwada, T.; Kawada, J. Original reports abstract Randomized Phase II Study of Trastuzumab Beyond Progression in Patients with HER2-Positive Advanced Gastric or Gastroesophageal Junction Cancer: WJOG7112G (T-ACT Study). *J. Clin. Onciol.* **2020**, *38*, 1919–1928. [CrossRef]
27. Pietrantonio, F.; Caporale, M.; Morano, F.; Sugimoto, N.; Ryu, M.H.; Sakai, D.; Chung, H.C.; Kawakami, H.; Yabusaki, H.; Lee, J.; et al. HER2 loss in HER2-positive gastric or gastroesophageal cancer after trastuzumab therapy: Implication for further clinical research. *Int. J. Cancer* **2016**, *139*, 2859–2864. [CrossRef]
28. Gambardella, V.; Gimeno-Valiente, F.; Tarazona, N.; Martinez-Ciarpaglini, C.; Roda, D.; Fleitas, T.; Tolosa, P.; Cejalvo, J.M.; Huerta, M.; Roselló, S.; et al. Nrf2 through RPs6 activation is related to anti-HER2 drug resistance in HER2-amplified gastric cancer. *Clin. Cancer Res.* **2019**, *25*, 1639–1649. [CrossRef]

29. Janjigian, Y.Y.; Sanchez-Vega, F.; Jonsson, P.; Chatila, W.C.; Hechtman, J.F.; Ku, G.Y.; Riches, J.C.; Tuvy, Y.; Kundra, R.; Bouvie, N.; et al. Genetic Predictors of Response to Systemic Therapy in Esophagogastric Cancer. *Cancer Discov.* **2018**, *8*, 49–58. [CrossRef]
30. Kim, S.T.; Banks, K.C.; Pectasides, E.; Kim, S.Y.; Kim, K.; Lanman, R.B.; Talasaz, A.; An, J.; Choi, M.G.; Lee, J.H.; et al. Impact of genomic alterations on lapatinib treatment outcome and cell-free genomic landscape during HER2 therapy in HER2+ gastric cancer patients. *Ann. Oncol. J. Eur. Soc. Med. Oncol.* **2018**, *29*, 1037–1048. [CrossRef]
31. Bang, Y.J.; Giaccone, G.; Im, S.A.; Oh, Y.D.; Bauer, T.M.; Nordstrom, J.L.; Li, H.; Chichili, G.R.; Moore, P.A.; Hong, S.; et al. First-in-human phase 1 study of margetuximab antibody, in patients with HER2-positive advanced solid tumors. *Ann. Oncol.* **2017**, *28*, 855–861. [CrossRef] [PubMed]
32. Catenacci, D.V.; Kang, Y.K.; Park, H.; Uronis, H.E.; Lee, K.W.; Ng, M.C.; Enzinger, P.C.; Park, S.H.; Gold, P.J.; Lacy, J.; et al. Articles Margetuximab plus pembrolizumab in patients with previously treated, HER2-positive gastro-oesophageal phase 1b-2 trial. *Lancet Oncol.* **2020**, *2045*, 1–11. [CrossRef]
33. Loi, S.; Giobbie-Hurder, A.; Gombos, A.; Bachelot, T.; Hui, R.; Curigliano, G.; Campone, M.; Bingazoli, L.; Bonnefoi, H.; Jerusalem, G.; et al. Pembrolizumab plus trastuzumab in trastuzumab-resistant, advanced, HER2-positive breast cancer (PANACEA): A single-arm, multicentre, phase 1b-2 trial. *Lancet Oncol.* **2019**, *20*, 371–382. [CrossRef]
34. Varadan, V.; Gilmore, H.; Miskimen, K.L.S.; Tuck, D.; Parsai, S.; Awadallah, A.; Krop, I.E.; Winer, E.P.; Bossuyt, C.; Somlo, G.; et al. Immune Signatures Following Single Dose Trastuzumab Predict Pathologic Response to PreoperativeTrastuzumab and Chemotherapy in HER2-Positive Early Breast Cancer. *Clin. Cancer Res. J. Am. Assoc. Cancer Res.* **2016**, *22*, 3249–3259. [CrossRef]
35. Taylor, C.; Hershman, D.; Shah, N.; Suciu-Foca, N.; Petrylak, D.P.; Taub, R.; Vahdat, L.; Cheng, B.; Pegram, M.; Knutson, L.K.; et al. Augmented HER-2 specific immunity during treatment with trastuzumab and chemotherapy. *Clin. Cancer Res. J. Am. Assoc. Cancer Res.* **2007**, *13*, 5133–5143. [CrossRef]
36. Park, S.; Jiang, Z.; Mortenson, E.D.; Deng, L.; Radkevich-Brown, O.; Yang, X.; Sattar, H.; Wang, Y.; Brown, N.K.; Greene, M.; et al. The therapeutic effect of anti-HER2/neu antibody depends on both innate and adaptive immunity. *Cancer Cell* **2010**, *18*, 160–170. [CrossRef]
37. Fuchs, C.S.; Doi, T.; Jang, R.W.; Muro, K.; Satoh, T.; Machado, M.; Sun, W.; Jalal, S.I.; Shah, M.A.; Metges, J.P.; et al. Safety and Efficacy of Pembrolizumab Monotherapy in Patients With Previously Treated Advanced Gastric and Gastroesophageal Junction Cancer: Phase 2 Clinical KEYNOTE-059 Trial. *JAMA Oncol.* **2018**, *4*, e180013. [CrossRef]
38. Janjigian, Y.Y.; Maron, S.B.; Chatila, W.K.; Millang, B.; Chavan, S.; Alterman, C.; Chou, J.F.; Segal, M.F.; Simmons, M.Z.; Momtaz, P.; et al. First-line pembrolizumab and trastuzumab in HER2-positive oesophageal, gastric, or gastro-oesophageal junction cancer: An open-label, single-arm, phase 2 trial. *Lancet Oncol.* **2020**, *21*, 821–831. [CrossRef]
39. Ogitani, Y.; Aida, T.; Hagihara, K.; Yamaguchi, J.; Ishii, C.; Harada, N.; Soma, M.; Okamoto, H.; Oitate, M.; Arakawa, S.; et al. DS-8201a, A Novel HER2-Targeting ADC with a Novel DNA Topoisomerase I Inhibitor, Demonstrates a Promising Antitumor Efficacy with Differentiation from T-DM1. *Clin. Cancer Res. J. Am. Assoc. Cancer Res.* **2016**, *22*, 5097–5108. [CrossRef]
40. Nagai, Y.; Oitate, M.; Shiozawa, H.; Ando, O. Comprehensive preclinical pharmacokinetic evaluations of trastuzumab deruxtecan (DS-8201a), a HER2-targeting antibody-drug conjugate, in cynomolgus monkeys. *Xenobiotica* **2019**, *49*, 1086–1096. [CrossRef]
41. Mohamed, M.M.; Sloane, B.F. Cysteine cathepsins: Multifunctional enzymes in cancer. *Nat. Rev. Cancer* **2006**, *6*, 764–775. [CrossRef] [PubMed]
42. Ogitani, Y.; Hagihara, K.; Oitate, M.; Naito, H.; Agatsuma, T. Bystander killing effect of DS-8201a, a novel anti-human epidermal growth factor receptor 2 antibody-drug conjugate, in tumors with human epidermal growth factor receptor 2 heterogeneity. *Cancer Sci.* **2016**, *107*, 1039–1046. [CrossRef] [PubMed]
43. Grabsch, H.; Sivakumar, S.; Gray, S.; Gabbert, H.E.; Müller, W. HER2 expression in gastric cancer: Rare, heterogeneous and of no prognostic value—Conclusions from 924 cases of two independent series. *Cell Oncol. J. Int. Soc. Cell Oncol.* **2010**, *32*, 57–65. [CrossRef]

44. Doi, T.; Shitara, K.; Naito, Y.; Shimomura, A.; Fujiwara, Y.; Yanemori, K.; Shimizu, C.; Shimoi, T.; Kuboki, Y.; Matsubara, N.; et al. Safety, pharmacokinetics, and antitumour activity of trastuzumab deruxtecan (DS-8201), a HER2-targeting antibody–drug conjugate, in patients with advanced breast and gastric or gastro-oesophageal tumours: A phase 1 dose-escalation study. *Lancet Oncol.* **2017**, *18*, 1512–1522. [CrossRef]
45. Shitara, K.; Bang, Y.-J.; Iwasa, S.; Sugimoto, N.; Ryu, M.H.; Sakai, D.; Chung, H.C.; Kawakami, H.; Yabusaki, H.; Lee, J.; et al. Trastuzumab Deruxtecan in Previously Treated HER2-Positive Gastric Cancer. *N. Engl. J. Med.* **2020**, *382*, 2419–2430. [CrossRef]
46. Takegawa, N.; Tsurutani, J.; Kawakami, H.; Yonesaka, K.; Kato, R.; Haratani, K.; Hayashi, H.; Takeda, M.; Nonagase, Y.; Maenishi, O.; et al. [fam-] trastuzumab deruxtecan, antitumor activity is dependent on HER2 expression level rather than on HER2 amplification. *Int. J. Cancer* **2019**, *145*, 3414–3424. [CrossRef]
47. Marcoux, J.; Champion, T.; Colas, O.; Wagner-Rousset, E.; Corvaia, N.; Dorsselaer, A.V.; Beck, A.; Cianférani, S. Native mass spectrometry and ion mobility characterization of trastuzumab emtansine, a lysine-linked antibody drug conjugate. *Protein Sci.* **2015**, *24*, 1210–1223. [CrossRef]
48. Deng, N.; Goh, L.K.; Wang, H.; Das, K.; Tao, J.; Tan, I.B.; Zhang, S.; Lee, M.; Wu, J.; Lim, K.H.; et al. A comprehensive survey of genomic alterations in gastric cancer reveals systematic patterns of molecular exclusivity and co-occurrence among distinct therapeutic targets. *Gut* **2012**, *61*, 673–684. [CrossRef]
49. Maron, S.B.; Alpert, L.; Kwak, H.A.; Lomnicki, S.; Chase, L.; Xu, D.; O'Day, E.; Nagy, R.J.; Lanman, R.B.; Cecchi, F.; et al. Targeted Therapies for Targeted Populations: Anti-EGFR Treatment for EGFR-Amplified Gastroesophageal Adenocarcinoma. *Cancer Discov.* **2018**, *8*, 696–713. [CrossRef]
50. Lordick, F.; Kang, Y.-K.; Chung, H.-C.; Salman, P.; Oh, S.C.; Bodoky, G.; Kurteva, G.; Volovat, C.; Moiseyenko, V.M.; Gorbunova, V.; et al. Capecitabine and cisplatin with or without cetuximab for patients with previously untreated advanced gastric cancer (EXPAND): A randomised, open-label phase 3 trial. *Lancet Oncol.* **2013**, *14*, 490–499. [CrossRef]
51. Waddell, T.; Chau, I.; Cunningham, D.; Gonzalez, D.; Okines, A.F.C.; Okines, C.; Wotherspoon, A.; Saffery, C.; Middleton, G.; Wadsley, J.; et al. Epirubicin, oxaliplatin, and capecitabine with or without panitumumab for patients with previously untreated advanced oesophagogastric cancer (REAL3): A randomised, open-label phase 3 trial. *Lancet Oncol.* **2013**, *14*, 481–489. [CrossRef]
52. Dutton, S.J.; Ferry, D.R.; Blazeby, J.M.; Abbas, H.; Dahle-Smith, A.; Mansoor, W.; Thompson, J.; Harrison, M.; Chatterjee, A.; Falk, S.; et al. Gefitinib for oesophageal cancer progressing after chemotherapy (COG): A phase 3, multicentre, double-blind, placebo-controlled randomised trial. *Lancet Oncol.* **2014**, *15*, 894–904. [CrossRef]
53. Shah, M.A.; Bang, Y.-J.; Lordick, F.; Alsina, M.; Chen, M.; Hack, S.P.; Bruey, J.M.; Smith, D.; McCaffery, I.; Shames, D.S.; et al. Effect of Fluorouracil, Leucovorin, and Oxaliplatin With or Without Onartuzumab in HER2-Negative, MET-Positive Gastroesophageal Adenocarcinoma: The METGastric Randomized Clinical Trial. *JAMA Oncol.* **2017**, *3*, 620–627. [CrossRef] [PubMed]
54. Catenacci, D.V.T.; Tebbutt, N.C.; Davidenko, I.; Murad, A.M.; Al-Batran, S.-E.; Ilson, D.H.; Tjulandin, S.; Gotovkin, E.; Karaszewska, B.; Bondarenki, I.; et al. Rilotumumab plus epirubicin, cisplatin, and capecitabine as first-line therapy in advanced MET-positive gastric or gastro-oesophageal junction cancer (RILOMET-1): A randomised, double-blind, placebo-controlled, phase 3 trial. *Lancet Oncol.* **2017**, *18*, 1467–1482. [CrossRef]
55. Van Cutsem, E.; Karaszewska, B.; Kang, Y.-K.; Chung, H.C.; Shankaran, V.; Siena, S.; Go, N.F.; Yang, H.; Schupp, M.; Cunningham, D.; et al. A Multicenter Phase II Study of AMG 337 in Patients with MET-Amplified Gastric/Gastroesophageal Junction/Esophageal Adenocarcinoma and Other MET-Amplified Solid Tumors. *Clin. Cancer Res. J. Am. Assoc. Cancer Res.* **2019**, *25*, 2414–2423. [CrossRef]
56. Ohtsu, A.; Ajani, J.A.; Bai, Y.-X.; Bang, YJ.; Chung, H.C.; Sahmund, H.-M.; Shen, L.; Yeh, K.-H.; Chin, K.; Muro, K.; et al. Everolimus for previously treated advanced gastric cancer: Results of the randomized, double-blind, phase III GRANITE-1 study. *J. Clin. Oncol. J. Am. Soc. Clin. Oncol.* **2013**, *31*, 3935–3943. [CrossRef]
57. Lee, J.; Kim, S.T.; Kim, K.; Lee, H.; Kozarewa, I.; Mortimer, P.G.S.; Odegaard, J.I.; Harrington, E.A.; Lee, J.; Lee, T.; et al. Tumor Genomic Profiling Guides Patients with Metastatic Gastric Cancer to Targeted Treatment: The VIKTORY Umbrella Trial. *Cancer Discov.* **2019**, *9*, 1388–1405. [CrossRef]
58. Drilon, A.; Laetsch, T.W.; Kummar, S.; DuBois, S.G.; Lassen, U.N.; Demetri, G.D.; Nathenson, M.; Doebele, R.C.; Farago, A.F.; Pappo, A.S.; et al. Efficacy of larotrectinib in TRK fusion-positive cancers in adults and children. *N. Engl. J. Med.* **2018**, *378*, 731–739. [CrossRef]

59. Shah, M.A.; Starodub, A.; Sharma, S.; Berlin, J.; Patel, M.; Wainberg, Z.A.; Chaves, J.; Gordon, M.; Windsor, K.; Brachmann, C.B.; et al. Andecaliximab/GS-5745 Alone and Combined with mFOLFOX6 in Advanced Gastric and Gastroesophageal Junction Adenocarcinoma: Results from a Phase I Study. *Clin. Cancer Res.* **2018**, *24*, 3829–3837. [CrossRef]
60. Ohtsu, A.; Shah, M.A.; Van Cutsem, E.; Rha, S.Y.; Sawaki, A.; Park, S.R.; Lim, H.Y.; Yamada, Y.; Wu, J.; Langer, B.; et al. Bevacizumab in combination with chemotherapy as first-line therapy in advanced gastric cancer: A randomized, double-blind, placebo-controlled phase III study. *J. Clin. Oncol. J. Am. Soc. Clin. Oncol.* **2011**, *29*, 3968–3976. [CrossRef]
61. Fuchs, C.S.; Shitara, K.; Di Bartolomeo, M.; Lonardi, S.; Al-Batran, S.-E.; Van Cutsem, E.; Ilson, D.H.; Alsina, M.; Chau, I.; Lacy, J.; et al. Ramucirumab with cisplatin and fluoropyrimidine as first-line therapy in patients with metastatic gastric or junctional adenocarcinoma (RAINFALL): A double-blind, randomised, placebo-controlled, phase 3 trial. *Lancet Oncol.* **2019**, *20*, 420–435. [CrossRef]
62. Fuchs, C.S.; Tomasek, J.; Yong, C.J.; Dumitru, F.; Passalacqua, R.; Goswami, C.; Safran, H.; Vieira dos Santos, L.; Aprile, G.; Ferry, D.R.; et al. Ramucirumab monotherapy for previously treated advanced gastric or gastro-oesophageal junction adenocarcinoma (REGARD): An international, randomised, multicentre, placebo-controlled, phase 3 trial. *Lancet* **2014**, *383*, 31–39. [CrossRef]
63. Wilke, H.; Muro, K.; Van Cutsem, E.; Oh, S.-C.; Bodoky, G.; Shimada, Y.; Hironaka, S.; Sugimoto, N.; Lipatov, O.; Kim, T.-Y.; et al. Ramucirumab plus paclitaxel versus placebo plus paclitaxel in patients with previously treated advanced gastric or gastro-oesophageal junction adenocarcinoma (RAINBOW): A double-blind, randomised phase 3 trial. *Lancet Oncol.* **2014**, *15*, 1224–1235. [CrossRef]
64. Li, J.; Qin, S.; Xu, J.; Xiong, J.; Wu, C.; Bai, Y.; Liu, W.; Tong, J.; Liu, Y.; Xu, R.; et al. Randomized, Double-Blind, Placebo-Controlled Phase III Trial of Apatinib in Patients with Chemotherapy-Refractory Advanced or Metastatic Adenocarcinoma of the Stomach or Gastroesophageal Junction. *J. Clin. Oncol. J. Am. Soc. Clin. Oncol.* **2016**, *34*, 1448–1454. [CrossRef]
65. Kang, Y.-K.; Boku, N.; Satoh, T.; Ryu, M.-H.; Chao, Y.; Kato, K.; Chung, H.C.; Chen, J.S.; Muro, K.; Kang, W.K.; et al. Nivolumab in patients with advanced gastric or gastro-oesophageal junction cancer refractory to, or intolerant of, at least two previous chemotherapy regimens (ONO-4538-12, ATTRACTION-2): A randomised, double-blind, placebo-controlled, phase 3 trial. *Lancet* **2017**, *390*, 2461–2471. [CrossRef]
66. Janjigian, Y.Y.; Bendell, J.; Calvo, E.; Kim, J.W.; Ascierto, P.A.; Sharma, P.; Ott, P.A.; Peltola, K.; Jaeger, D.; Evans, J.; et al. CheckMate-032 Study: Efficacy and Safety of Nivolumab and Nivolumab Plus Ipilimumab in Patients With Metastatic Esophagogastric Cancer. *J. Clin. Oncol. J. Am. Soc. Clin. Oncol.* **2018**, *36*, 2836–2844. [CrossRef]
67. Kim, S.T.; Cristescu, R.; Bass, A.J.; Kim, K.M.; Odegaard, J.I.; Kim, K.; Liu, X.Q.; Sher, X.; Jung, H.; Lee, M.; et al. Comprehensive molecular characterization of clinical responses to PD-1 inhibition in metastatic gastric cancer. *Nat. Med.* **2018**, *24*, 1449–1458. [CrossRef]
68. Le, D.T.; Uram, J.N.; Wang, H.; Bartlett, B.R.; Kemberling, H.; Eyring, A.; Skora, A.; Luber, B.S.; Azad, N.S.; Laheru, D.; et al. PD-1 blockade in tumors with mismatch-repair deficiency. *N. Engl. J. Med.* **2015**, *372*, 2509–2520. [CrossRef]
69. Sundar, R.; Qamra, A.; Tan, A.L.K.; Zhang, S.; Ng, C.C.; Teh, B.T.; Lee, J.; Kim, K.M.; Tan, P. Transcriptional analysis of immune genes in Epstein-Barr virus-associated gastric cancer and association with clinical outcomes. *Gastric Cancer* **2018**, *21*, 1064–1070. [CrossRef]
70. Sundar, R.; Huang, K.K.; Qamra, A.; Kim, K.M.; Kim, S.T.; Kang, W.K.; Tan, A.L.K.; Lee, J.; Tan, P. Epigenomic promoter alterations predict for benefit from immune checkpoint inhibition in metastatic gastric cancer. *Ann. Oncol. J. Eur. Soc. Med. Oncol.* **2019**, *30*, 424–430. [CrossRef]
71. Gambardella, V.; Fleitas, T.; Cervantes, A. Understanding mechanisms of primary resistance to checkpoint inhibitors will lead to precision immunotherapy of advanced gastric cancer. *Ann. Oncol. J. Eur. Soc. Med. Oncol.* **2019**, *30*, 351–352. [CrossRef] [PubMed]
72. Kawazoe, A.; Fukuoka, S.; Nakamura, Y.; Kuboki, Y.; Wakabayashi, M.; Nomura, S.; Mikamoto, Y.; Shima, H.; Fujishiro, N.; Higuchi, T.; et al. Articles Lenvatinib plus pembrolizumab in patients with advanced gastric cancer in the first-line or second-line setting. *Lancet Oncol.* **2020**, *21*, 1057–1065. [CrossRef]
73. Cascinu, S. Comment Lenvatinib and pembrolizumab in advanced gastric cancer. *Lancet Oncol.* **2020**, *2045*, 1–2. [CrossRef]

74. Fukuoka, S.; Hara, H.; Takahashi, N.; Kojima, T.; Kawazoe, A.; Asayama, M.; Yoshii, T.; Kotani, D.; Tamura, H.; Mikamoto, Y.; et al. Regorafenib Plus Nivolumab in Patients With Advanced Gastric or Colorectal Cancer: An Open-Label, Dose-Escalation, and Dose-Expansion Phase Ib Trial (REGONIVO, EPOC1603). *J. Clin. Oncol. Off. J. Am. Soc. Clin. Oncol.* **2020**, *38*, 2053–2061. [CrossRef]
75. Sahin, U.; Koslowski, M.; Dhaene, K.; Usener, D.; Brandenburg, G.; Seitz, G.; Huber, C.; Türeci, O. Human Cancer Biology Claudin-18 Splice Variant 2 Is a Pan-Cancer Target Suitable for Therapeutic Antibody Development. *Clin. Cancer Res.* **2008**, *14*, 7624–7634. [CrossRef]
76. Sahin, U.; Schuler, M.; Richly, H.; Bauer, S.; Krilova, S.; Dechow, T.; Jerling, M.; Utsch, M.; Rohde, C.; Dhaene, K.; et al. ScienceDirect A phase I dose-escalation study of IMAB362 (Zolbetuximab) in patients with advanced gastric and gastro-oesophageal junction cancer *. *Eur. J. Cancer* **2018**, *100*, 17–26. [CrossRef]
77. Tu, O. Original article a multicentre, phase IIa study of zolbetuximab as a single agent in patients with recurrent or refractory advanced adenocarcinoma of the stomach or lower oesophagus: The MONO study. *Ann. Oncol.* **2019**, *30*, 1487–1495. [CrossRef]
78. Dienstmann, R.; Rodon, J.; Prat, A.; Perez-Garcia, J.; Adamo, B.; Felip, E.; Cortes, J.; Iafrate, A.J.; Nuciforo, P.; Tabernero, J. Genomic aberrations in the FGFR pathway: Opportunities for targeted therapies in solid tumors. *Ann. Oncol. J. Eur. Soc. Med. Oncol.* **2014**, *25*, 552–563. [CrossRef]
79. Babina, I.S.; Turner, N.C. Advances and challenges in targeting FGFR signalling in cancer. *Nat. Rev. Cancer* **2017**, *17*, 318–332. [CrossRef]
80. Gambardella, V.; Tarazona, N.; Cejalvo, J.M.; Lombardi, P.; Huerta, M.; Roselló, S.; Fleitas, T.; Roda, D.; Cervantes, A. Personalized Medicine: Recent Progress in Cancer Therapy. *Cancers* **2020**, *12*. [CrossRef]
81. Abou-Alfa, G.K.; Sahai, V.; Hollebecque, A.; Vaccaro, G.; Melisi, D.; Al-Rajabi, R.; Paulson, A.S.; Borad, M.J.; Gallinson, D.; Murphy, G.A.; et al. Pemigatinib for previously treated, locally advanced or metastatic cholangiocarcinoma: A multicentre, open-label, phase 2 study. *Lancet Oncol.* **2020**, *21*, 671–684. [CrossRef]
82. Schuler, M.; Cho, B.C.; Sayehli, C.M.; Navarro, A.; Soo, R.A.; Richly, H.; Cassier, P.A.; Tai, D.; Penel, N.; Nogova, L.; et al. Rogaratinib in patients with advanced cancers selected by FGFR mRNA expression: A phase 1 dose-escalation and dose-expansion study. *Lancet Oncol.* **2019**, *20*, 1454–1466. [CrossRef]
83. Bahleda, R.; Meric-Bernstam, F.; Goyal, L.; Tran, B.; He, Y.; Yamamiya, I.; Benhadji, K.A.; Matos, I.; Arkenau, H.T. Phase 1, First-in-Human Study of Futibatinib, a Highly Selective, Irreversible FGFR1-4 Inhibitor in Patients with Advanced Solid Tumors. *Ann. Oncol. J. Eur. Soc. Med. Oncol.* **2020**. [CrossRef] [PubMed]
84. Bahleda, R.; Italiano, A.; Hierro, C.; Mita, A.; Cervantes, A.; Chan, N.; Awad, M.; Calvo, E.; Moreno, V.; Ramaswamy, G.; et al. Multicenter Phase I Study of Erdafitinib (JNJ-42756493), Oral Pan-Fibroblast Growth Factor Receptor Inhibitor, in Patients with Advanced or Refractory Solid Tumors. *Clin. Cancer Res. J. Am. Assoc. Cancer Res.* **2019**, *25*, 4888–4897. [CrossRef] [PubMed]
85. Ahn, S.; Lee, J.; Hong, M.; Kim, S.; Park, S.H.; Choi, M.G.; Lee, J.-H.; Sohn, T.S.; Bae, J.M.; Kim, S.; et al. FGFR2 in gastric cancer: Protein overexpression predicts gene amplification and high H-index predicts poor survival. *Mod. Pathol.* **2016**, *29*, 1095–1103. [CrossRef]
86. Zhang, J.; Tang, P.M.K.; Zhou, Y.; Cheng, A.S.-L.; Yu, J.; Kang, W.; To, K.F. Targeting the Oncogenic FGF-FGFR Axis in Gastric Carcinogenesis. *Cells* **2019**, *8*. [CrossRef]
87. Paik, P.K.; Shen, R.; Berger, M.F.; Ferry, D.; Soria, J.-C.; Mathewson, A.; Rooney, C.; Smith, N.R.; Cullberg, M.; Kilgour, E.; et al. A phase Ib open-label multicenter study of AZD4547 in patients with advanced squamous cell lung cancers. *Clin. Cancer Res.* **2017**, *23*, 5366–5373. [CrossRef]
88. Van Cutsem, E.; Bang, Y.-J.; Mansoor, W.; Petty, R.D.; Chao, Y.; Cunningham, D.; Ferry, D.R.; Smith, N.R.; Frewer, P.; Ratnayake, J.; et al. A randomized, open-label study of the efficacy and safety of AZD4547 monotherapy versus paclitaxel for the treatment of advanced gastric adenocarcinoma with FGFR2 polysomy or gene amplification. *Ann. Oncol. J. Eur. Soc. Med. Oncol.* **2017**, *28*, 1316–1324. [CrossRef]
89. Catenacci, D.V.; Tesfaye, A.; Tejani, M.; Cheung, E.; Eisenberg, P.; Scott, A.J.; Eng, C.; Hnatyszyn, J.; Marina, N.; Powers, J.; et al. Bemarituzumab with modified FOLFOX6 for advanced FGFR2-positive gastroesophageal cancer: FIGHT Phase III study design. *Future Oncol.* **2019**, *15*, 2073–2082. [CrossRef]

90. Bang, Y.; Im, S.-A.; Lee, K.W.; Cho, J.Y.; Song, E.-K.; Kim, K.H.; Park, J.O.; Chun, H.J.; Zang, D.Y.; Fielding, A.; et al. Randomized, Double-Blind Phase II Trial With Prospective Classification by ATM Protein Level to Evaluate the Efficacy and Tolerability of Olaparib Plus Paclitaxel in Patients With Recurrent or Metastatic Gastric Cancer. *J. Clin. Oncol.* **2015**, *33*, 3858–3865. [CrossRef]
91. Bang, Y.; Xu, R.-H.; Chin, K.; Lee, K.-W.; Hoon Park, S.H.; Rha, S.Y.; Shen, L.; Qin, S.; Xu, N.; Im, S.A.; et al. Olaparib in combination with paclitaxel in patients with advanced gastric cancer who have progressed following first-line therapy (GOLD): A double-blind, randomised, placebo-controlled, phase 3 trial. *Lancet Oncol.* **2017**, *18*, 1637–1651. [CrossRef]

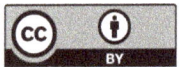

© 2020 by the authors. Licensee MDPI, Basel, Switzerland. This article is an open access article distributed under the terms and conditions of the Creative Commons Attribution (CC BY) license (http://creativecommons.org/licenses/by/4.0/).

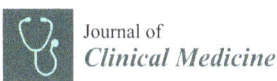

Journal of Clinical Medicine

Review

How to Best Exploit Immunotherapeutics in Advanced Gastric Cancer: Between Biomarkers and Novel Cell-Based Approaches

Michele Ghidini [1,*], Angelica Petrillo [2], Andrea Botticelli [3,4], Dario Trapani [5], Alessandro Parisi [6,7], Anna La Salvia [8], Elham Sajjadi [9,10], Roberto Piciotti [9,10], Nicola Fusco [9,10] and Shelize Khakoo [11]

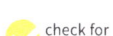

Citation: Ghidini, M.; Petrillo, A.; Botticelli, A.; Trapani, D.; Parisi, A.; La Salvia, A.; Sajjadi, E.; Piciotti, R.; Fusco, N.; Khakoo, S. How to Best Exploit Immunotherapeutics in Advanced Gastric Cancer: Between Biomarkers and Novel Cell-Based Approaches. J. Clin. Med. 2021, 10, 1412. https://doi.org/10.3390/jcm10071412

Academic Editor: Hidekazu Suzuki

Received: 14 February 2021
Accepted: 22 March 2021
Published: 1 April 2021

Publisher's Note: MDPI stays neutral with regard to jurisdictional claims in published maps and institutional affiliations.

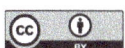

Copyright: © 2021 by the authors. Licensee MDPI, Basel, Switzerland. This article is an open access article distributed under the terms and conditions of the Creative Commons Attribution (CC BY) license (https://creativecommons.org/licenses/by/4.0/).

[1] Medical Oncology Unit, Fondazione IRCCS Ca' Granda Ospedale Maggiore Policlinico, 20122 Milan, Italy
[2] Medical Oncology Unit, Ospedale Del Mare, 80147 Naples, Italy; angelic.petrillo@gmail.com
[3] Department of Clinical and Molecular Medicine, Sapienza University, 00189 Rome, Italy; andrea.botticelli@uniroma1.it
[4] Medical Oncology (B), Policlinico Umberto I, 00161 Rome, Italy
[5] Division of Early Drug Development for innovative therapies, European Institute of Oncology, IRCCS, 20141 Milan, Italy; dario.trapani@ieo.it
[6] Department of Life, Health and Environmental Sciences, University of L'Aquila, 67100 L'Aquila, Italy; alexparis@hotmail.it
[7] Medical Oncology Unit, St. Salvatore Hospital, 67100 L'Aquila, Italy
[8] Department of Oncology, University Hospital 12 De Octubre, 28041 Madrid, Spain; alasalvi@ucm.es
[9] Division of Pathology, European Institute of Oncology, IRCCS, 20141 Milan, Italy; elham.sajjadi@ieo.it (E.S.); roberto.piciotti@unimi.it (R.P.); nicola.fusco@unimi.it (N.F.)
[10] Department of Oncology and Hemato-Oncology, University of Milan, 20122 Milan, Italy
[11] Department of Medicine, Royal Marsden Hospital, London and Surrey, Sutton SM25PT, UK; shelize.khakoo@rmh.nhs.uk
* Correspondence: michele.ghidini@policlinico.mi.it; Tel.: +39-02-5503-2660; Fax: +39-02-5503-2659

Abstract: Despite extensive research efforts, advanced gastric cancer still has a dismal prognosis with conventional treatment options. Immune checkpoint inhibitors have revolutionized the treatment landscape for many solid tumors. Amongst gastric cancer subtypes, tumors with microsatellite instability and Epstein Barr Virus positive tumors provide the strongest rationale for responding to immunotherapy. Various predictive biomarkers such as mismatch repair status, programmed death ligand 1 expression, tumor mutational burden, assessment of tumor infiltrating lymphocytes and circulating biomarkers have been evaluated. However, results have been inconsistent due to different methodologies and thresholds used. Clinical implementation therefore remains a challenge. The role of immune checkpoint inhibitors in gastric cancer is emerging with data from monotherapy in the heavily pre-treated population already available and studies in earlier disease settings with different combinatorial approaches in progress. Immune checkpoint inhibitor combinations with chemotherapy (CT), anti-angiogenics, tyrosine kinase inhibitors, anti-Her2 directed therapy, poly (ADP-ribose) polymerase inhibitors or dual checkpoint inhibitor strategies are being explored. Moreover, novel strategies including vaccines and CAR T cell therapy are also being trialed. Here we provide an update on predictive biomarkers for response to immunotherapy with an overview of their strengths and limitations. We discuss clinical trials that have been reported and trials in progress whilst providing an account of future steps needed to improve outcome in this lethal disease.

Keywords: immune checkpoint inhibitors; gastric cancer; Epstein Barr Virus; tumor mutational burden; microsatellite instability; predictive biomarkers; CAR T cell therapy; vaccines

1. Introduction

Overview of Gastric Cancer Classification and Relevance for Immunotherapy

Gastric cancer (GC) is a leading global cause of morbidity and mortality [1]. In 2020, over a million people were diagnosed with GC (representing almost 6% of all cancer diagnoses), and nearly 800,000 patients died due to this disease (representing 8.2% of all cancer deaths) [2]. Worldwide, GC is particularly prevalent in East Asia and central/Eastern Europe.

The Lauren classification, published in 1965, differentiates gastric adenocarcinoma into two distinct types, termed the intestinal and diffuse subtypes [3]. The intestinal type is most common, present in over half of the patients and characterized by microscopic glandular structures, with infiltrating capacity of the mesenchymal tissues [4]. The diffuse subtype accounts for a third of cases and is characterized by poor differentiation and poorly cohesive malignant cells with invasive capacity [5]. In general, the intestinal type is associated with exogenous risk factors such as Helicobacter pylori, while the diffuse subtype encompasses a hereditary familial pattern related to germline pathogenetic mutations of the E-cadherin (CDH1) and αE-catenin (CTNNA1) genes [6]. While these subtypes of GC are associated with different carcinogenesis mechanisms and disease biology, this classification, along with the subsequent World Health Organization classification of GC, has not translated into distinct subtype-driven treatment strategies [7,8]. More recently, following comprehensive molecular profiling, The Cancer Genome Atlas (TCGA) defined four distinct subtypes of gastric cancer: Epstein-Barr virus (EBV) positive, microsatellite unstable tumors (MSI), genomically stable tumors (GS) and tumors with chromosomal instability (CIN) [9]. Significant overlap was seen between the histologically determined Lauren's diffuse variant and the molecular GS TCGA subtype [10]. Interestingly, certain molecular subtypes were most commonly detected in specific anatomic locations with EBV positive tumors more likely to be in the gastric fundus or body and CIN tumors in the cardia [9]. Although the molecular classification of gastric cancer has not directly changed clinical practice, it has provided an important platform to identify novel molecular targets and pave the way for innovative clinical trial design with the incorporation of biomarker enrichment stratification strategies. EBV-positive and MSI tumors are associated with signatures suggestive of an immune responsive profile [11]. A hyper-mutated DNA phenotype is defined as 20.5 mutations/Mb in GC and is a phenotype typical of most MSI tumors [12]. The MSI high (MSI-H) phenotype is most commonly related to epigenetic silencing of the mismatch repair gene, MLH1, rather than germline mutation (i.e., Lynch syndrome) [13]. The presence of a higher number of somatic mutations has been associated with a better prognosis [14] and an increased susceptibility to immune-activating antineoplastic treatments [15]. Currently, patients with MSI gastric cancer can benefit from established immunotherapy approaches with anti-programmed death-1 (anti-PD-1) immune-checkpoint inhibitors [16]. Rather than a hypermutated phenotype, EBV-positive tumors (accounting for 9% of GC) have a profile favoring immunotherapy in view of their high expression of membrane immune-checkpoint molecules such as programmed death ligand-1 (PD-L1) and 2. Key molecular features of EBV-positive tumors include the expression of virus-associated antigens (e.g., nuclear antigen 1, latent membrane protein 2A), the extensive methylation of viral and host genome and the epigenetic regulation of specific cytosine-phosphatidyl-guanosine (CpG) DNA islands through methylation mechanisms [17]. The pattern of DNA methylation of CpG has been associated with anti-tumor immune-activation, with predictive and prognostic significance [18,19]. Therefore, MSI and EBV-positive tumors have been proposed as chief candidates for immunotherapy trials, though not exclusively, for their intrinsic immune-mediated biology [11]. The advent of immunotherapy in oncology has in fact been embraced in most if not all tumor types and disease settings [20]. The identification of an immune-signature or predictive factors of immune-response in patients with GC have been identified as a research priority given that it is a tumor type associated with poor prognosis when diagnosed at an advanced stage and any benefit derived from chemotherapy (CT) is very limited [21]. While advancements in the development of pharmacotherapies have improved overall survival (OS) and quality of life, the low proportion of patients alive after two years from the diagnosis of metastatic disease remains a cause for concern [22,23].

The strategies implemented to enhance the immune response against tumors, including GC, aim to re-orient the immune-system response, by dampening the suppressive regulatory molecules and enhancing a stimulating milieu [24]. This strategy has been pursued by developing a number of immune-checkpoint inhibitors [e.g., PD-1, cytotoxic T-lymphocyte antigen-4 (CTLA-4)], a class of molecules capable of acting on several immune cells and (re-)activating an effective antineoplastic response [25]. This strategy is particularly beneficial in tumors exerting immune-activating signatures and/or recognized by the immune-system as foreign, and therefore regulated by the immune-response [26].

Another therapeutic approach is based on the bioengineering of immune-competent cells against specific tumor- associated antigens [27]. The principal expression of this approach is represented by the Chimeric Antigen Receptor T-cells (CAR-T) constructs. CAR-T are genetically engineered T-cells designed to direct the specific immune-response against tumor- antigens, thereby inducing an artificial acquired antineoplastic immune response, through cytotoxic activity. Though still widely experimental in solid neoplasms, the clinical implementation of CAR-T cells for hematological malignancies has paved a new way of cancer immunotherapy, due to the durable responses seen in some cases, the different patterns of response observed [28] as well as the specific safety profile which needs to be considered and the structural efforts required to build and deliver cell-based treatments [29].

Here we review the clinical and translational landscape of the determinants of response to various immunotherapy agents in patients with GC, by elucidating the key findings from clinical trials and describing established and proposed predictive biomarkers throughout ongoing clinical studies incorporating immunotherapy.

2. Biomarkers of Response to Immunotherapy in Gastric Cancer

The characterization of immune-related biomarkers is becoming increasingly important in the multi-modality treatment of advanced GC (Figure 1) [30].

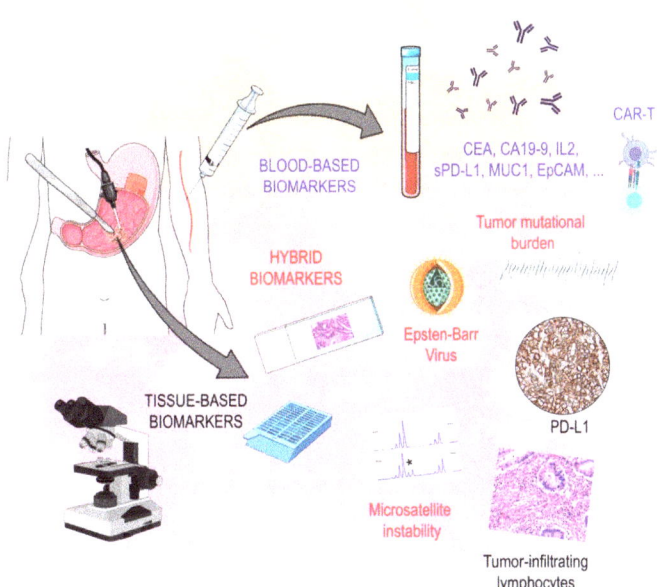

Figure 1. Biomarkers of response to immunotherapy: soluble, tissue based and hybrid. Legend: CAR-T: chimeric antigen receptor-T cell, CA 19.9: carbohydrate antigen 19.9, CEA: carcinoembryonic antigen, EPCAM: epithelial cell adhesion molecule, IL2: interleukin 2, MUC1: mucin 1, cell surface associated, PD-L1: programmed death-ligand 1, s PD-L1: serum programmed death-ligand.

2.1. Tissue Based Biomarkers

Currently, the most studied biomarkers include mismatch repair (MMR) status assessment, MSI identification, PD-L1 expression, tumor-infiltrating lymphocytes (TILs) assessment, and tumor mutational burden (TMB) quantification. However, there is currently a gap in knowledge regarding the reliability of these tests for clinical use in GC. MMR deficiency (dMMR) and/or MSI has been reported in approximately 14% and 22% of GCs, respectively [31,32]. The MMR system is able to identify and counteract unpaired DNA bases in order to preserve genome stability [33–35]. Alterations in this system, due to dMMR, are associated with the accumulation of alterations in microsatellite regions, resulting in variable degrees of MSI that are commonly defined as "low" (MSI-L) and "high" (MSI-H) [35]. MMR and MSI screening is recommended as a useful tool at all stages of GC to refine treatments and determine patient prognosis [36]. In GC, MSI is more common with older age, female sex, distal stomach location, lower number of lymph-node metastases and is associated with an overall better prognosis [36–38]. According to a meta-analysis which included 1556 resectable GC patients, MSI-H patients had longer five-year OS and disease-free survival (DFS) compared to patients with microsatellite stable tumors (OS, 77.5% vs. 59.3%; DFS, 71.8% vs. 52.3%) [14,39]. Evidence suggests that dMMR is more likely to activate an immune response and lead to the increased presence of TILs, and PD-L1 upregulation in GC [40–43]. In particular, PD-L1 is expressed on the surface of neoplastic cells in 15–70% of GC [37], with increased expression being associated with non-metastatic cancer tissue [44], well differentiated tumors [44] and improved OS (median OS not reached vs. 40 months; $p = 0.008$) [45] although its association with a favorable OS has not always been consistent [37,46]. The immunohistochemical expression of PD-L1 protein can be scored using the combined positive score (CPS), where CPS > 1 is considered positive [47]. There appears to be an association between PD-L1+ GC and MSI-H or EBV positive tumors [48]. The evaluation of PD-L1 CPS on formalin-fixed paraffin-embedded tumor tissue samples has been proposed as a method to select patients for immune-checkpoint inhibition [49]. High PD-L1 CPS score has been associated with a high density of CD3+/CD8+ TILs. Interestingly, PD-L1 negative tumors with high-density CD3+ and CD8+ cells had a good prognosis [46]. A meta-analysis on various TIL subtypes in GC has shown that high levels of CD8+, CD3+, and CD4+ T cell infiltration is associated with better OS. Additionally, a high density of forkhead box P3 (FOXP3) positive cells within the tumor does not appear to be a negative prognostic indicator [50]. TILs are gathering increasing importance as a prognostic biomarker in GC [51]. Regarding TIL assessment in GC, only the stromal count (= % area occupied by mononuclear inflammatory cells over the total stromal area)—stained by hematoxylin and eosin—has been suggested for evaluation, due to a lack of prognostic significance for intra-tumoral TILs [52]. However, this finding requires further validation [52,53].

In the KEYNOTE 059 study, PD-L1 expression as a potential biomarker of response to pembrolizumab in advanced and refractory GC patients was evaluated and demonstrated a higher overall response rate (ORR) in PD-L1+ compared to the PD-L1 negative tumors (15.5%, CPS $\geq$1 vs. 6.4%, CPS < 1). However, PD-L1 negative tumors displayed greater complete response rate (CR) (2.8% vs. 2.0%) [39,54]. Such findings prompted the need for defining and utilizing further biomarkers of response to immunotherapy. Tumor mutational burden (TMB), dMMR/MSI, TILs and EBV have been broadly explored as the main molecular determinants of immunotherapy response in GC. Of note, TMB (i.e., the number of somatic mutations derived from next-generation sequencing techniques) has been correlated with higher levels of neoantigen expression, and subsequently increased immune responses [55]. High TMB has been suggested in 3% and 5% of patients with esophageal and stomach cancer, respectively (>20 mut/Mb) [30]. Recently, the food and drug administration (FDA) approved the FoundationOneCDx assay (Foundation Medicine, Inc., Cambridge, MA, USA) as a companion diagnostic (CDx) for treatment with pembrolizumab in unresectable or metastatic TMB-high solid tumors ($\geq$10 mut/Mb) [56]. Findings in GC also show an improved OS in TMB-High tumors treated with immunotherapy, compared to those with lower TMB levels: 80% 2-year survival for TMB-high vs. 12% for TMB-low, $p = 0.03$ [57] and median OS = 16.8 vs. 6.62 months, $p = 0.058$ [58]. Yet, TMB as a potential biomarker of response to immunotherapy is challenged by the lack of harmonized sequencing panels as well as lack of clearly defined cut-offs for implementation in clinical practice [36].

MSI-H tumors have also been associated with a good response to immunotherapy [15,59,60]. Based on these findings, the FDA approved pembrolizumab for the treatment of MSI-H tumors that had progressed following prior treatment, irrespective of tumor site [61]. In GC, studies have also demonstrated that dMMR and MSI-H tumors generally have a favorable response to immune-checkpoint blockade [36,59]. A multi cohort study of pembrolizumab monotherapy in advanced GC showed that MSI-H tumors had greater ORR (57.1%) compared to MSS patients (9%) and also a significant disease control rate (DCR) of 71.4% was achieved [30,36]. These results were supported by findings from the phase III, KEYNOTE-062 clinical trial which are discussed in the clinical trial section of this review [62]. MMR status is commonly assessed by immunohistochemistry although the lack of CDx tests and tumor-specific guidelines is seen as a disadvantage [35]. However, unlike in other types of tumors, a high correlation between MMR immunohistochemistry and MSI testing in gastro-esophageal cancer is generally observed [36]. Hence, the PCR-based Bethesda panel, consisting of two mononucleotide repeats and three dinucleotide repeats, and NGS are employed in MSI evaluation [63].

EBV+ tumors are associated with a response to immunotherapy and this appears to be independent of TMB and MSI status [64]. According to a multi-factorial genomic biomarker analysis in GC patients administered pembrolizumab, EBV positivity, MSI and PD-L1 expression are associated with improved ORR (100%, 85.7%, and 50%, respectively) [65]. EBV+ GC appears to be relatively immunogenic. This results in increased infiltration with immune cells and also increased PD-L1 and PD-L2 gene expression [65]. Further investigation into biomarkers of response to immunotherapy in advanced GC/gastro-esophageal cancer is warranted. A summary of the most commonly studied biomarkers along with their strengths and limitations is provided in Table 1.

Table 1. Biomarkers for immunotherapy: detection methods, strengths and limitations.

Biomarker	Method and Interpretation	Clinical Value	Clinical Setting	Strengths	Limitations
PD-L1	IHC 22C3 (CDx): positive if CPS ≥ 1	Predictive (pembrolizumab); prognostic (poor OS)	FDA: advanced or metastatic GC/GEJC treated with ≥2 lines of therapy	Standardized (CDx), reliable	Relatively expensive if CDx, poor inter-observer reproducibility, high intra-tumor heterogeneity
MMR	IHC for MLH1, MSH2, MSH6, and PMS2: deficient if lack of expression in ≥1 biomarker	Predictive (pembrolizumab); prognostic (improved OS)	Tissue/site-agnostic: unresectable or metastatic dMMR GC/GEJC progressed following prior treatment	Reliable, cost-effective, short turn-around times	No CDx and interpretation guidelines, no data on intra-tumor heterogeneity
MSI	FoundationOne (CDx) or NGS: MSI-H by PCR or NGS: hyper-variability ≥2 Bethesda (BAT-25, BAT-26, D2S123, D5S346 and D17S250) or Promega (BAT-25, BAT-26, MONO-27, NR-21 and NR-24) loci	Predictive (pembrolizumab and other ICI) prognostic (improved OS). Validated with tumor specific guidelines	Tissue/site-agnostic: unresectable or metastatic MSI-H GC/GEJC progressed following prior treatment	CDx available, cost-effective (PCR or NGS if high volume)	Expensive (CDx or NGS if low volume), externalized analysis (CDx), no tumor-specific guidelines
TILs	sTILs on HE-stained sections; modified from International TILs Working Group guidelines for breast carcinoma (% of the tumor stromal area containing infiltrating mononuclear inflammatory cells)	Predictive for immunotherapies (emerging); Prognostic (improved RFS).	Not performed in clinical practice	Cost-effective	Controversial clinical value
TMB	FoundationOne (CDx); NGS: TMB-H if >17 mut/MB; SNVs counting by Oncomine Tumor Mutation Load Assay	Predictive for ICB; Prognostic (enhanced ORR and PFS); associated with clinical response to ICI	Not performed in clinical practice	CDx available	Expensive, externalized analysis (CDx), no guidelines, controversial clinical value
EBV	cobas EBV (CDx); EBV-encoded RNA ISH	Prognostic (improved OS and decrease of metastases recurrence); associated with amplification and/or overexpression of PD-L1 and PD-L2 in GC; high density of immune cell infiltration; alterations in the PIK3CA gene	Diagnostic/subtyping	Standardized and cost-effective	Not available in all centers

Legend: CDx: companion diagnostic, CPS:combined positive score, EBV: Ebstein-Barr virus, GC: gastric cancer, GEJC: gastro-esophageal junctional cancer, HE: hematoxylin and eosin, ICB: immune checkpoint blockade, ICI: immune checkpoint inhibitor, IHC: immunohistochemistry, ISH: in situ hybridization, MMR: mismatch repair, MSI: microsatellite instability, OS: overall survival, PCR: polymerase chain reaction, PFS: progression-free survival, RFS: relapse-free survival, SNVs: single nucleotide variants, TILs: tumor infiltrating lymphocytes, TMB: tumor mutational burden, TMB-H: tumor mutational burden-high.

2.2. Circulating Biomarkers

Circulating molecules and their role in predicting response to immunotherapy is a topic of great interest and is an area that still has not been studied in depth. These soluble factors can be released from both tumor cells and immune cells and may provide a simple method to evaluate the dynamic behavior of the immune system in cancer patients during treatment and avoid the need for invasive procedures [66]. Much effort is being spent on identifying primary responders to immunotherapy at a relatively early treatment timepoint. Circulating biomarkers, some of which are currently used in clinical practice, such as pepsinogen, carcinoembryonic antigen (CEA), carbohydrate antigen 19-9 (CA19-9) and soluble IL-2, are not accurate enough to predict prognosis in GC [67–69].

Recent evidence has shown that patients with GC have higher serum soluble PD-L1 (sPD-L1) concentrations than healthy controls. Moreover, both elevated tissue PD-L1 and serum sPD-L1 were independent prognostic factors for poor OS and poor DFS in GC patients who underwent surgery [70–72]. Lymphocyte activation gene 3 (LAG3) is a checkpoint receptor localized on activated T cell surfaces and NK cells. The soluble variant, in turn, can have a regulatory function on immune cells [73,74]. Its role has been investigated in GC patients. High sLAG-3 expression is associated with a better prognosis in GC and its expression was positively correlated with IL-12 and IFN-γ production in GC patients. In a recent in vivo experiment sLAG3 was shown to be able to promote the activation of CD8 T cells and the production of INF and IL-12, resulting in tumor growth inhibition [75].

While the prognostic value of soluble checkpoints is under investigation in several solid tumors, the question that remains to be answered is whether soluble checkpoints can predict response to treatment. Given that the immune system is a key factor involved in the response to treatments such as immunotherapy and CT, there is a clear rationale to suggest that such soluble markers could be biomarkers of response to treatment [76]. A study including 11 patients with NSCLC and 9 patients with GC treated with an anti-PD1 agent showed that pre-treatment levels of sPD-L1 were not associated with OS in these patients. However, reduction in plasma sPD-L1 levels was significantly associated with tumor response after four cycles of treatment [77]. A study including 68 patients with metastatic GC eligible for first line CT analyzed baseline level of sPDL1 and the dynamic changes during therapy. Patients with low levels of sPD-L1 at diagnosis showed a better OS and PFS than patients with a high sPDL1. Patients whose sPDL1 increased after the first cycle of CT showed worse PFS and OS. This result suggests that soluble checkpoints may be the ideal method of studying the immune system as an extremely dynamic entity allowing real-time, non-invasive monitoring during cancer treatment [78]. Takahashi et al. confirmed in their study that high serum levels of sPD-L1 correlated with worse OS in patients with metastatic GC treated with first-line CT [79]. These data suggest the possibility of individualizing the therapeutic choice based on the immunological profile, thereby leading to promising new combination strategies in the near future.

Immunotherapeutics in solid tumors is constantly evolving due to the introduction of new technologies to manipulate the patient's immune system to attack cancer cells. Tumor antigen vaccines are currently being studied in several solid tumors. They are created from cancer cells' pure tumor antigens [80]. The antitumor activity of tumor peptide vaccines, such as G17DT, vascular endothelial growth factor receptor (VEGFR) and OTSGC-A24, have been investigated in GC patients. G17DT is a vaccine able to promote an immune response against gastrin, a hormone involved in carcinogenesis and progression in GC [81–83]. A phase II/III study (NCT00042510) reported that G17DT is able to induce efficient anti-gastrin antibody production and is able to inhibit tumor proliferation and progression [84]. A multi-center study showed that the combination of G17DT and platinum-5FU CT prolonged the median time-to-progression and median survival time for patients with unresectable cancer of the stomach or gastroesophageal junction, compared to platinum-5FU CT alone. Therefore, the FDA approved the fast track designation for the vaccine G17DT in February 2003 [85]. Another peptide vaccine involving the use of VEGFR 1 and 2, receptors of the VEGF angiogenic factor, has been investigated. In a phase I/II study, the administration of the VEGFR1/2 peptide vaccine in combination with CT induced a cytotoxic T cell response. In the 82% of patients with a cytotoxic T lymphocyte response to VEGFR2-169 peptide, time to progression and OS were significantly prolonged compared to those without such a response [86]. Such findings are encouraging, although it should be noted that only 22 patients were included. A phase I/Ib study (NCT01227772) evaluated OTSGC-A24, which is thought to be able to target several specific tumor antigens, such as forkhead box M1, DEP domain containing 1, kinesin family member 20A, URLC10 and VEGFR1. Although the treatment was well tolerated, no radiological responses were observed [83].

An innovative immunotherapeutic strategy uses adoptive T cell therapy to overcome the immune-evasion mechanisms mediated by cancer cells. T lymphocytes are removed from patients and modified in vitro in order to activate specific immune cells. Then, the modified activated T cells are administered to patients, thereby eliciting a tumor response against cancer [87]. Chimeric antigen receptor-T (CAR-T) cell therapy was shown to be effective in hematologic disease and it is actually under investigation in several solid tumors [88,89].

In GC, several antigens, including human epidermal growth factor receptor 2 (HER2), carcinoembryonic antigen (CEA), mucin 1 (MUC1) and epithelial cell adhesion molecule (EpCAM), have been used as targets for CAR-T. The anti-HER2 CAR-modified T cell was evaluated in many pre-clinical studies [90]. Clinical studies are now evaluating it in GC patients (NCT02713984, NCT01935843, NCT00889954). CEA-specific CAR-T cells were confirmed to be active in pre-clinical studies in mice with GC. Since then, a clinical trial is ongoing (NCT02349724) to define the correct dose and safety profile [91,92]. MUC1 and Ep-CAM are transmembrane glycoproteins expressed in different solid tumors, but in GC they are markers of aggressive disease. Clinical Phase I/II trials (NCT02617134, NCT02725125) are evaluating EpCAM and MUC1 modified CAR-T in solid tumors expressing these targets [93].

3. Immunotherapy: From Landmark Trials to Clinical Practice and Future Perspectives

Over the last decade, the safety and efficacy of immunotherapy has been investigated in clinical trials in GC patients, initially in the advanced disease setting and more recently in the earlier disease setting.

3.1. Non-Metastatic Disease

Most immune checkpoint inhibitor trials in the earlier disease setting are ongoing (Table 2). The use of immune checkpoint inhibitors- alone or in association with CT is not currently considered standard of care [94].

In the context of neoadjuvant and perioperative treatments, the phase III Keynote 585 trial (NCT03221426) is evaluating the efficacy of pembrolizumab plus CT versus CT alone [95]. The CT arm was initially cisplatin plus capecitabine or cisplatin plus fluorouracil. Following the favorable results of the FLOT-4 study, the trial protocol was amended to enable the inclusion of the FLOT CT regimen comprising fluorouracil, docetaxel and oxaliplatin as a safety cohort [96]. The primary endpoints are OS, event free survival (EFS) and the rate of pathological complete response (pCR). It is important to note that PD-L1 status is not being used for patient selection, although an exploratory endpoint assessing efficacy by PD-L1 expression is planned.

Table 2. List of major ongoing phase I-III trials with immune checkpoint inhibitors in gastric cancer.

Study Name (NCT Number)	Country	Phase	Line	N	Drugs (Target)	Selected Population	Study Intervention I Experimental Arm/Control Arm or II Experimental Arm	Primary Endpoint
Non-metastatic gastric cancer								
Keynote-585 (NCT03221426)	Global	III	Perioperative	NA	Pembrolizumab (PD-1)	All comers	fluorouracil/capecitabine plus cisplatin or FLOT +/- pembrolizumab	OS EFS pCR
IMAGINE (NCT04062656)	Western	rII	Perioperative	NA	Nivolumab (PD-1) Ipilimumab (CTLA-4) Relatlimab (LAG-3)	All comers	FLOT Nivolumab Nivolumab + ipilimumab Nivolumab + relatlimab	pCR
NCT04354662	Asian	II	Perioperative	NA	Toripalimab (PD-1)	All comers	FLOT + toripalimab	DFS
ICONIC (NCT03399071)	Western	II	Perioperative	NA	Avelumab (PD-L1)	All comers	FLOT + avelumab	pCR
NCT03878472	Asian	II	Neoadjuvant	NA	SHR1210 (PD-1)	All comers	SHR1210 SHR1210 + Apatinib SHR1210 + Apatinib + S-1 SHR1210 + Apatinib + S-1 + oxaliplatin	pRR
Checkmate-577 (NCT02743494)	Global	III	Adjuvant	794	Nivolumab (PD-1)	All comers	Nivolumab versus placebo after neoadjuvant chemoradiotherapy and surgery	DFS
EORTC VESTIGE (NCT03443856)	Western	rII	Adjuvant	NA	Nivolumab (PD-1) Ipilimumab (CTLA-4)	All comers	Nivolumab + ipilimumab versus FLOT after neoadjuvant FLOT and surgery	DFS
Metastatic gastric cancer								
Keynote-859 (NCT03675737)	Global	III	1°	NA	Pembrolizumab (PD-1)	HER-2 negative	cisplatin plus 5-fluorouracil/Xelox +/- pembrolizumab	OS PFS
Keynote-811 (NCT03615326)	Global	III	1°	NA	Pembrolizumab (PD-1)	HER-2 positive	cisplatin plus 5-fluorouracil/Xelox/Folfox/S-1 oxaliplatin + trastuzumab +/- pembrolizumab	PFS OS
APICAL-GE (NCT04278222)	Asian	II	1°	NA	Toripalimab (PD-1)	MSS	Anlotinib Plus Toripalimab	ORR
NCT04202484	Asian	II	1°	NA	Toripalimab (PD-1)	HER-2 negative	Toripalimab combined with oxaliplatin and Tegafur, Gimeracil and Oteracil Porassium Capsules	ORR
SHR-1210-III-316 (NCT04342910)	China	III	2°	550	Camrelizumab (PD-1) Apatinib (VEGFR2)	All comers	Camrelizumab + apatinib paclitaxel or irinotecan	OS
NCT04435652	Asia	II-III	2°	492	QL1604 (PD-1)	HER-2 negative	QL1604 + nab-paclitaxel followed by QL1604 maintenance paclitaxel alone	ORR, safety, OS

Table 2. Cont.

Study Name (NCT Number)	Country	Phase	Line	N	Drugs (Target)	Selected Population	Study Intervention I Experimental Arm/Control Arm or II Experimental Arm	Primary Endpoint
SEQUEL (NCT04069273)	USA	rII	≥2°	58	Pembrolizumab (PD-1) Ramucirumab (VEGFR2)	All comers	Paclitaxel + ramucirumab + pembrolizumab (patient-tailored algorithm) Paclitaxel + ramucirumab + pembrolizumab	ORR
DURIGAST (PRODIGE59-FFCD1707) (NCT03959293)	France	rII	2°	105	Durvalumab (PD-L1) Tremelimumab (CTLA-4)	All comers	FOLFIRI + durvalumab + tremelimumab FOLFIRI + durvalumab	PFS
ESR-15-11655 (NCT03579784)	Korea	II	2°	40	Durvalumab (PD-1) Olaparib (PARP)	All comers	Paclitaxel + olaparib + durvalumab	DCR
NCC2070 (NCT04140318)	China	II	2°	60	Sintilimab (PD-1)	All comers	Nab-paclitaxel + sintilimab	ORR
ASGARD (NCT04089657)	China	II	≥3°	40	Sintilimab (PD-1) Apatinib (VEGFR2)	All comers	Apatinib + sintilimab	DCR
RiME (NCT03995017)	USA	II	2°–3°	61	Nivolumab (PD-1) Rucaparib (PARP) Ramucirumab (VEGFR2)	All comers	Rucaparib + ramucirumab + nivolumab Rucaparib + ramucirumab	ORR
RAP (AIO-STO-0218) (NCT03966118)	Germany	II	2°	59	Avelumab (PD-1) Ramucirumab (VEGFR2)	All comers	Paclitaxel + ramucirumab + avelumab	OS
WaKING (NCT04166721)	UK	II	≥2°	52	Atezolizumab (PD-L1) DKN-01 (DKK1)	MSS/pMMR	Atezolizumab + DKN-01	Safety, ORR
NCT03694977	Korea	II	>2°	30	Lacnotuzumab (CSF-1) Spartalizumab (PD-1)	All comers	Lacnotuzumab + Spartalizumab	Biomarker analysis
NCT04592211	Korea	I-II	2°	71	Pembrolizumab (PD-1) Olaparib (PARP)	HRR/MSS	Pembrolizumab + olaparib + paclitaxel	PFS DLT
NCT04209686	Australia, USA	II	2°	36	Pembrolizumab (PD-1) Olaparib (PARP)	All comers	Pembrolizumab + olaparib + paclitaxel	OS
da VINci (NCT03784040)	Asia	Ib	>2°	40	OTSGC-A24 (cancer vaccine) Nivolumab (PD-1) Ipilimumab (CTLA-4)	All comers	OTSGC-A24 + nivolumab OTSGC-A24 + nivolumab + ipilimumab	Safety, ORR

Legend: N: patient number; r: randomized; CPS: combined positive score for PD-L1 status; MSS/pMMR: microsatellite stable/mismatch repair proficient; DLT: dose-limiting toxicity; DCR: disease control rate; DOR: duration of response; ORR: objective response rate; OS: overall survival; EFS: event free survival; pCR: pathological complete response; PFS: progression-free survival; NA: not applicable; pRR: pathological remission rate.

In the adjuvant setting, the initial results from the phase III Checkmate 577 trial were recently presented [97]. This trial (NCT02743494) assessed the safety and efficacy of nivolumab versus placebo as adjuvant treatment in 794 patients with stage II and III esophageal (squamous tumors and adenocarcinomas) and esophagogastric junctional adenocarcinoma (GEJA) who had received neoadjuvant treatment followed by surgery. Patients were not selected for PD-L1 status. Nivolumab significantly prolonged DFS (22.4 versus 11 months, Hazard Ratio (HR): 0.69; $p = 0.0003$) with a good safety profile (grade 3–4 adverse events: 13% versus 6% in the placebo arm). Whilst these initial results are promising, the full publication is awaited in order to analyze the data in more detail. Additionally, it should be noted that the trial included both esophageal and GEJ cancers as well as squamous tumors and adenocarcinomas. Therefore, it could be argued that these tumor types should be assessed separately in dedicated clinical trials to better understand clinical applicability. For additional details regarding ongoing trials in these settings, see Table 2.

3.2. Metastatic Disease: 1st Line Treatment

Evidence for the role of immune checkpoint inhibitors in first-line treatment of metastatic GC is very recent, arising during the last few months. In this regard, pembrolizumab, nivolumab and avelumab are the main agents that have been investigated (Table 3).

The phase III Keynote 062 trial was a study with a complex design, including both superiority and non-inferiority comparisons. In fact, in the superiority part, the trial evaluated the safety and efficacy of pembrolizumab plus standard CT (cisplatin plus 5-fluorouracil/capecitabine) versus CT alone in first-line treatment of metastatic GC/GEJA patients with epidermal growth factor receptor 2 (HER-2) negative status. Additionally, the trial included a third arm, evaluating the non-inferiority of pembrolizumab as a single agent treatment and compared it to standard CT [62]. Therefore, 763 patients (Asian and non-Asian) were randomized 1:1:1 to one of the three arms. The central assessment of PD-L1 was mandatory at screening and only patients with a PD-L1 $\geq$ 1 tumor according to the CPS score were randomized. After a median follow up of 29.4 months, single agent pembrolizumab was found to be non-inferior to the control arm (median OS: 10.6 versus 11 months; HR: 0.91; 99.2% Confidence Interval (CI): 0.69–1.18; non-inferiority margin: 1.2) with a trend of superiority for patients with PD-L1 CPS $\geq$ 10 (median OS: 17.4 versus 10.8 months, HR: 0.69). However, this last analysis was not planned. The survival rates at 12 and 24 months were 46.9% and 26.5% in the experimental single agent arm versus 45.6% and 19.2% in the control arm. Nevertheless, the trial did not improve OS in the combination arm, both for patients with PD-L1 CPS $\geq$ 1 (median OS: 12.5 versus 11.1 months; HR: 0.85, 95% CI: 0.70–1.03, p: 0.05) and PD-L1 CPS $\geq$ 10 (median OS: 12.3 versus 10.8 months; HR: 0.85; 95%CI: 0.62–1.17; p: 0.16). Likewise, the superiority in PFS was not met for the experimental arm (median PFS: 6.9 versus 6.4 months; HR: 0.84; 95%CI: 0.70–1.02; p: 0.04). Of note, patients with MSI-H benefited the most from pembrolizumab both for patients with PDL-1 CPS $\geq$1 (median OS: not reached (NR) versus 8.5 months in the control arm, HR: 0.29) and PDL-1 CPS $\geq$ 10 (median OS: NR versus 13.6 months). The survival benefit was maintained in this subgroup also in the combination arm (pembrolizumab plus CT: HR: 0.37).

Table 3. List of major completed phase II-III trials with immune checkpoint inhibitors in metastatic gastric cancer.

Study Name [Reference]	Agents (Target)	Country	Phase	Line	PD-L1 Status	Treatment Arms	N	Primary Endpoints	OS	PFS	RR (%)
Keynote-062 [62]	Pembrolizumab (PD-1)	Global	III	1°	CPS ≥ 1%	cisplatin + 5-fluorouracil/capecitabine (CT)	250	OS, PFS	Non-inferiority: 10.6 (I) vs. 11 (CT) Superiority: 12.5 (CT+I) vs. 11.1 (CT)	Superiority: 6.9 (CT+I) vs. 6.4 (CT)	48.6 (CT+I) 37.2 (CT)
						cisplatin + 5-fluorouracil /capecitabine + pembrolizumab (CT + I)	257				
						pembrolizumab (I)	256				
Checkmate-649 (preliminary results) [68]	Nivolumab (PD-1) Ipilimumab (CTLA-4)	Global	III	1°	Unselected	nivolumab + ipilimumab		OS, PFS		CPS ≥ 5%:	NR
						Xelox/Folfox	482		14	7.7	
						Xelox/Folfox + nivolumab	473		11.3	6.1	
Attraction-4 (preliminary results) [94]	Nivolumab (PD-1)	Asian	III	1°	Unselected	Nivolumab + S-1 oxaliplatin/Xelox	362	PFS, OS	17.5	10.5	NR
						S-1 oxaliplatin/Xelox	362		17.2	8.3	
Janjigian et al. [100]	Pembrolizumab (PD-1)	Global	II	1°	Unselected	Xelox/Folfox/cisplatin plus 5-fluorouracil+ trastuzumab+ pembrolizumab	37	PFS at 6 months	27.3	13	100
Javelin Gastric 100 [101]	Avelumab (PD-L1)	Global	III	1° mantainance	Unselected	Avelumab	249	OS	10.4	3.2	13.3
						Folfox/Xelox	250		10.9	4.4	14.4
Keynote-061 [102]	Pembrolizumab (PD-1)	Global	III	2°	CPS ≥ 1%	Pembrolizumab	196	PFS, OS	9.1	1.5	16
						Paclitaxel	199		8.3	4.1	14
Keynote-059 (cohort 1) [54]	Pembrolizumab (PD-1)	Global	II	≥3°	Unselected (57.1% CPS ≥ 1%)	Pembrolizumab	259	RR	5.6	2	11.6
Attraction-02 (ONO-4538-12) [103]	Nivolumab (PD-1)	Asian	III	≥3°	Unselected	Nivolumab	330	OS	7.5	1.6	11
						Placebo	163		5.1	1.5	20
Checkmate-032 [104]	Nivolumab (PD-1) Ipilimumab (CTLA-4)	Western	I-II	≥3°	Unselected	Nivolumab	59	RR	6.2	1.4	12
						Nivolumab1/Ipilimumab3 *	49		6.9	1.6	24
						Nivolumab3/Ipilimumab1 **	52		4.8	1.6	8
Javelin Gastric 300 [105]	Avelumab (PD-L1)	Global	III	3°	TPS ≥ 1%	Avelumab	272	OS	4.6	1.4	4.6
						Physician's choice ‡	133		5	2.7	5

* Nivolumab 1 mg/kg plus ipilimumab 3 mg/kg every 3 weeks. ** Nivolumab 3 mg/kg plus ipilimumab 1 mg/kg every 3 weeks. *** Nivolumab 1 mg/kg plus ipilimumab 1 mg/kg every 3 weeks. ‡ Paclitaxel 80 mg/m² on days 1, 8 and 15 or irinotecan 150 mg/m² on days 1 and 15, each of a 4-week treatment cycle. Legend: N: patient number; NR: not reported; CPS: PD-L1 combined positive score; TPS: PD-L1 tumor proportion score; PD-1: programmed cell death protein-1; CTLA-4: Cytotoxic T-Lymphocyte Antigen 4; PD-L1: programmed cell death protein-ligand 1; OS: overall survival (months); PFS: progression-free survival (months); RR: response rate; NR: not reported.

Recently, the preliminary results of the phase III Checkmate 649 [98] and ATTRACTION-4 trial [99] were presented at the ESMO Congress 2020. The Checkmate 649 trial (NCT02872116) randomized untreated metastatic GC patients to three arms: nivolumab plus ipilimumab, standard CT (Folfox or Xelox), standard CT plus nivolumab [98]. Patients were enrolled regardless of PD-L1 status and HER-2 testing was not mandatory, although patients with known HER-2 positive tumors were excluded. The preliminary results only reported the analysis for the combination arms (1581 patients) and, among those patients, the data focused on those with PDL-1 CPS $\geq$ 5 (955 patients, 60%). In this population, the experimental arm (nivolumab plus CT) was associated with improved survival benefit when compared to CT alone (median OS: 14.4 versus 11.1 months, respectively, HR: 0.71, $p < 0.0001$; median PFS: 7.7 versus 6.1 months, HR: 0.68; p: < 0.0001). However, the benefit was also confirmed in the entire population- including PD-L1 negative tumors- (median OS: 13.8 versus 11.6 months, respectively, HR: 0.8, p: 0.0002) as well as in the PD-L1 CPS $\geq$ 1 subgroup (median OS: 14 versus 11.3 months, respectively, HR: 0.77, p: 0.0001). The safety profile was acceptable and the rate of grade 3–4 adverse events for the experimental versus control arm was 59% versus 44%, respectively. Of note, the trial included 75% non-Asian patients. Therefore, the combination of Folfox/Xelox plus nivolumab seems to be very promising in first-line treatment of metastatic disease in GC. However, the full publication is awaited in order to better understand the biological mechanisms that underpin the positive results and to understand how this combination could be used in clinical practice.

The phase III ATTRACTION-4 trial (NCT02746796) randomized 724 Asian patients to receive CT alone (Xelox or oxaliplatin plus S-1) or with nivolumab as first-line treatment for HER-2 negative metastatic GC, regardless of PDL-1 status [99]. After a follow up of 11.6 months, the addition of nivolumab improved PFS when compared with the control arm (median PFS: 10.5 versus 8.3 months, respectively; HR: 0.68, p: 0.0007). However, with a median follow-up of 26.6 months, OS was not significantly different in the two arms (median OS: 17.5 versus 17.2 months, HR 0.90; 95% CI: 0.75–1.08; p: 0.257), whereas the benefit in PFS and overall response rate (ORR) were confirmed (ORR: 57.5 versus 47.8%; p: 0.0088). Therefore, the Checkmate 649 and ATTRACTION-4 trials provide the first evidence for the efficacy of nivolumab in this setting, even if in different populations. However, the final results and publication from the ATTRACTION-4 trial, are also awaited.

The phase III Keynote-859 [106] and Keynote-811 [107] are currently ongoing in this setting (Table 2). Keynote-859 (NCT03675737) is randomizing untreated metastatic HER-2 negative GC patients to receive standard CT (cisplatin plus 5-fluorouracil/Xelox, investigator choice) alone or with pembrolizumab as first-line treatment [106]. The trial includes patients regardless of PD-L1 status; however, assessment of PD-L1 status is mandatory. The Keynote-811 trial (NCT03615326) is investigating the role of pembrolizumab in first-line treatment for HER-2 positive metastatic GC [107]. The trial was based on the promising results of the phase Ib/II trial PANACEA trial [108] in breast cancer and in the following phase II study in esophageal/GEJA/GC [100]. This latter phase II study was an open-label, non-randomized, single-arm trial that showed promising activity and a good safety profile by using pembrolizumab in addition to standard CT (Folfox/Xelox plus trastuzumab or cisplatin plus 5-fluorouracil/capecitabine plus trastuzumab- according to investigator's choice) in 37 HER-2 positive tumors (5% Asian patients), regardless of PD-L1 status. Of the patients, 70% were alive at six-months and free from relapse (primary endpoint), median PFS and median OS were 13 and 27.3 months, respectively. Of note, ORR was 100%, 17% had a complete response and 74% a partial response. These initial results are of significant interest as they show the potential for a new treatment option in patients with HER-2 positive tumors if confirmed in a larger phase III study. The results of the randomized phase III Keynote-811 trial which includes patients with the same characteristics are therefore eagerly awaited.

Maintenance treatment with immunotherapy after first-line therapy has also been investigated. The phase III Javelin 100 trial assessed the efficacy and safety of using an immune checkpoint inhibitor (avelumab) in this setting [101]. The trial randomized

805 metastatic HER-2 negative GC/GEJA patients who demonstrated a response to first line CT (Folfox/Xelox) to receive either CT (continuation of the ongoing treatment) or avelumab. The trial included Asian patients (20%); patients were not selected by PD-L1 status, although a subgroup analysis for PD-L1 CPS ≥ 1 was pre-planned. The trial failed to show an improvement in OS with avelumab in this setting (median OS: 10.4 versus 10.9 months, HR: 0.91, 95% CI: 0.74–1.11; p: 0.1779). These results were also confirmed in the PD-L1 positive population (median OS: 16.2 versus 17.7 months, HR: 1.13; 95% CI: 0.57–2.23, p: 0.6352). However, in this trial, the small MSI-H subgroup of patients appeared to benefit from immunotherapy (HR: 0.27; 95% CI: 0.06–1.25).

The results from studies using immune checkpoint inhibitors in first-line treatment for metastatic GC are promising. However, it is not yet entirely clear which patients benefit the most from immunotherapy due to the lack of reliable, validated predictive biomarkers to guide the treatment choice for patients with GC [109]. Therefore, the search for new biomarkers as well as a better understanding of the molecular mechanisms underlying the response to immunotherapy is urgently needed. Immunotherapy does not currently represent standard of care in the first line metastatic setting in GC and its use is restricted by local authorities.

3.3. Metastatic Disease: Second Line Treatment and Beyond

Following progression with a first-line platinum- and fluoropyrimidine-based CT regimen [110], the VEGFR2 human monoclonal antibody (mAb) ramucirumab is a standard of care in the second-line setting. Ramucirumab monotherapy improved OS when compared to best supportive care (BSC) (5.2 vs. 3.8 months, HR = 0.77, p = 0.047) and also in association with paclitaxel when compared to paclitaxel alone (9.6 vs. 7.4 months, HR = 0.80, p = 0.017) in two randomized phase III trials (REGARD and RAINBOW, respectively) [111,112]. While efficacy and safety of ramucirumab were confirmed in "real-life" populations [113–115], the randomized phase III TAGS trial confirmed the OS benefit of the cytotoxic oral drug trifluridine/tipiracil over placebo (5.7 vs. 3.6 months, HR = 0.69, p = 0.0005) as a third-line regimen in a global population [116].

The role of immunotherapy was first demonstrated when monotherapy with PD-1 inhibitors (nivolumab and pembrolizumab) showed significant efficacy in later lines of treatment [54,103,117] (Table 3). In the phase III ATTRACTION-02 trial, nivolumab significantly prolonged OS compared to placebo (5.2 vs. 4.1 months, HR = 0.63, p < 0.0001) in patients progressed or intolerant to at least two previous lines of treatment, with a 3-year OS rate of 5.6% and 1.9%, respectively. Therefore, only a small proportion of patients achieved durable clinical benefit from nivolumab. Notably, PD-L1 status did not identify patients likely to benefit from nivolumab. Toxicity profile included mild to moderate diarrhea, fatigue, pruritus, and rash. However, longer OS was observed in patients experiencing immune checkpoint inhibitor (ICI)-related AEs compared to those who did not (2-year OS of 20% and 0%, respectively). These findings resulted in the approval of nivolumab in third- or later-line in Japan, Taiwan and South Korea [103]. Similar data were obtained in Western populations [117] even if phase III data are lacking.

The human anti-PD1 pembrolizumab was first tested in the phase II KEYNOTE-059 trial and obtained higher ORR (15.5% vs. 6.4%) and longer duration of response (DOR, 16.3 vs. 6.9 months) in PD-L1-positive (CPS ≥ 1%) rather than in PD-L1-negative mGC as a third- or later-line treatment. These results led to FDA approval of pembrolizumab as a third- or later line of treatment for CPS ≥ 1% mGC patients in the USA [54].

The positive results of the ATTRACTION-02 trial were not replicated in two phase III trials testing the efficacy of PD1/PD-L1 inhibitors compared to CT. In the JAVELIN Gastric 300 trial, the PD-L1 inhibitor avelumab did not improve survival over standard CT (mOS: 4.6 vs. 5.0 months, p = 0.81, respectively) in third-line treatment, irrespective of PD-L1 status (TPS ≥ 1%) [105].

In the KEYNOTE-061 trial, 592 mGC patients progressed on a first-line platinum- and fluoropyrimidine-based CT were randomized to receive pembrolizumab or paclitaxel as second-line. Primary endpoints were OS and PFS in patients with PD-L1 CPS $\geq$ 1, with significance threshold for OS set at p = 0.0135 (one-sided). Pembrolizumab failed to improve outcome in terms of OS (mOS: 9.1 vs. 8.3 months, HR = 0.82, p = 0.042) and PFS (mPFS: 1.5 vs. 4.1 months) when compared to paclitaxel alone [102]. One of the main limitations of this trial was the control arm of paclitaxel without ramucirumab, which is considered standard of care in the second-line setting of mGC. In an updated 2-year analysis of the KEYNOTE-061 trial, a trend towards improved OS in PD-L1 CPS $\geq$ 1 patients in favor of pembrolizumab was shown. Moreover, a higher benefit from pembrolizumab over paclitaxel in terms of OS, ORR and DOR was described in subgroups of patients with performance status 0, CPS $\geq$ 10% and MSI-high [118].

As multiple immune checkpoint pathways modulate antitumor response, combining PD1/PD-L1 inhibitors with other ICIs is a potential strategy to overcome resistance. For example, the immune checkpoint molecule CTLA-4 suppresses T-cell proliferation early in the immune response, whereas PD-1 acts in a later phase of T-cell suppression [119].

The phase I-II CheckMate-032 trial tested nivolumab alone or in combination with the inhibitor of cytotoxic T-lymphocyte associated protein-4 (CTLA-4) ipilimumab in 160 pretreated Western mGC patients, reaching an ORR of 12% and 24% and G3–4 AEs of 17 and 47%, respectively. These results were obtained regardless of PD-L1 status [104].

The tumor microenvironment (TME) is an integral part of cancer and includes a variety of immune and non-immune cell types and factors playing a pivotal role in driving an inflammatory, immunosuppressive and pro-angiogenic intra-tumoral environment [120]. Tumor-associated macrophages (TAMs) play a role in cancer microenvironment, they can affect inhibitory and growth cancer cell processes depending on stage, tissue type, and host microbiota [121]. Furthermore, TAMs can impact on the antitumor effects of CT and radiotherapy and contribute to intrinsic/acquired resistance to PD-1 inhibitors [122]. Interestingly, these cells can be reduced by inhibiting the colony-stimulating factor-1 (CSF-1)/receptor pathway. The association of the CSF-1 inhibitor lacnotuzumab and the PD-1 inhibitor spartalizumab is under investigation in a phase II trial enrolling pre-treated patients (Table 2). Within the TME, tumor neo-vascularization promoted by tumor-induced angiogenic factors can lead to an imbalance between immunosuppressive cells such as regulatory T cells (Treg) and TAMs, and anti-tumor CD8+ cytotoxic T-lymphocytes (CTLs), causing tumor progression, invasion and angiogenesis [120]. Anti-angiogenic agents may restore the anti-tumor immune activity by disrupting the VEGF/VEGFR axis in the TME [122]. On the other hand, the association of immunotherapy and CT might be of benefit by improving immunogenicity and restoring balance within the TME [120]. This strategy is currently under investigation, safety and activity data from combinations treatments such as paclitaxel and ramucirumab with avelumab (RAP: NCT03966118) or pembrolizumab (SEQUEL: NCT04069273) (Table 2) are awaited.

The multi-targeted tyrosine kinase inhibitor (TKI) regorafenib enhances antitumor immunity through macrophage modulation [123]. In the Japanese EPOC1603 phase Ib trial, the combination of regorafenib and nivolumab showed anti-tumor activity (ORR 44%, mPFS 5.8 months) [124]. The multi-targeted TKI lenvatinib was evaluated together with pembrolizumab in the Japanese EPOC1706 phase II trial, showing promising activity (ORR 69%) [125].

Genomic instability derives from deficient DNA damage response. Poly (ADP-ribose) polymerase (PARP) inhibitors (PARPi) alter the ability to repair DNA damage; their effect is more pronounced in tumors with pre-existing defects in DNA repair (such as MSI/dMMR tumors). Unrepaired DNA damage secondary to PARPi treatment was reported to activate immune pathways and PD-L1 expression on tumor cells, which could in turn increase sensitivity to ICIs [126]. Phase II trials combining ICIs and PARPi with or without VEGFR inhibitors or CT are ongoing (Table 2).

The HER-2 inhibitor trastuzumab has immune mechanisms of action involving innate and adaptive immunity through antibody-dependent cellular cytotoxicity, upregulation of PD-L1 and promotion of immune infiltration [127,128]. In the global phase I-II

CP-MGAH22-05 trial, the association of the novel anti-HER2 mAb margetuximab and pembrolizumab provided positive results in terms of safety and efficacy (ORR 18%, DCR 53%) in 95 pre-treated HER2-positive mGC patients [129].

The composition of the gut microbiome has emerged as a key factor affecting the peripheral immune system in the context of cancer. Moreover, gut microbiota might affect the efficacy of immune checkpoint inhibitors in various cancers [127]. The DELIVER trial (JACCRO GC-08, UMIN000030850) aims to investigate the role of immune-related biomarkers (gut microbiome, genetic polymorphisms, gene expression, and the metabolome in plasma) in patients treated with nivolumab.

4. Discussion

In recent years, immunotherapy has revolutionized cancer care. Due to its efficacy, its long-lasting effect and its relative favorable safety profile, this innovative approach has changed the natural history of different types of tumors, such as lung cancer, head and neck and urological malignancies. For patients with mGC the prognosis disappointingly remains dismal. The standard therapies (chemotherapy, trastuzumab or ramucirumab) have limited impact on patient outcomes, and median survival ranges from four months with BSC only, to 12 months with chemotherapy [22]. Therefore, improving the knowledge of the GC molecular landscape as well as developing targeted therapies may serve as a promising approach in the treatment of GC patients. To date, several studies have been carried out and many are ongoing, aimed to define the magnitude of benefit and the role for immunotherapy, as monotherapy and combined with chemotherapy, targeted agents, and other immunotherapies, in GC. In this context, a huge variety of biomarkers have shown promising results, particularly MSI, PD-L1 and TMB, as well as soluble biomarkers, including sPD-L1, sLAG-3, circulating tumor DNA (ctDNA), exosomes, cytokines, cancer-testis antigens (CTA) [130] and metal chelators, and finally the microbiome [131]. Unfortunately, none of these biomarkers has been validated for use in clinical practice, so far.

Therefore, discovering reliable predictive biomarkers of response to immunotherapy in GC represents a critical unmet need to personalize treatment and improve survival. Despite the success achieved with ICIs for the treatment of other solid tumors, the results in the treatment of GC are uncertain, although the benefit appears to be more pronounced in patients with PD-L1+ expression, MSI-H or dMMR tumors [132]. Consequently, nowadays, the approved indications for immunotherapy in mGC are limited to second or subsequent lines of therapy. However, surgery remains the only curative option in GC and immunotherapy may play an important role even in the neoadjuvant and adjuvant setting. Most trials of immune checkpoint blockade in the earlier disease are ongoing, such as the phase III Keynote 585 trial in the neoadjuvant setting [95] and the Checkmate 577 trial in adjuvant [97]. Combining immunotherapy and chemotherapy might lead to improved tumor immunogenicity, and, in this way, improve immunotherapy efficacy. The rationale to combine an immunosuppressive drug, such as chemotherapy, with agents that act to modulate immune regulatory mechanisms to boost the immune response against cancer cells, is potentially challenging. In mGC the addition of chemotherapy to immunotherapy by increasing TMB with platinum agents could be especially interesting [133].

Several trials are further investigating the activity of the association between ICIs and different chemotherapy agents, as first- or second-line treatment for mGC. Of these, the results of combining paclitaxel and ramucirumab with avelumab (RAP: NCT03966118) or pembrolizumab (SEQUEL: NCT04069273) are eagerly awaited.

Additionally, numerous clinical trials evaluating the combination of immunotherapy with targeted agents (anti-angiogenic agents, PARPi and anti-HER2 mAb) are generating much excitement. In this context, there is a strong rationale to combine ICIs with anti-angiogenic drugs. Preclinical evidence has demonstrated that normalizing the tumor vasculature enhances immunotherapy activity. Notably, evidence suggests that enhanced immune stimulation improves tumor vascular normalization [134]. In mGC encouraging results have been observed for this strategy (i.e., combining nivolumab plus ramucirumab [135] or regorafenib) [124]. However, the level of evidence for these combinations is still limited, thereby hampering their approval for clinical use.

5. Conclusions

In conclusion, despite the efforts made, GC remains a highly lethal cancer and the magnitude of benefit from immunotherapy for these patients is still under debate. A critical open question regarding patient selection for treatment with immunotherapy and the optimal sequence of where it should be used in the treatment paradigm remains. Nowadays, a plethora of potentially useful predictive biomarkers has been investigated, but unfortunately their clinical use is still limited. Additionally, the results achieved with immunotherapy in the metastatic setting are encouraging, but not completely satisfactory. Further studies are urgently needed to deepen the molecular knowledge of the GC milieu. It is hoped that this will eventually lead to a more clearly defined algorithm of key criteria to select candidates likely to obtain the most benefit from immunotherapy.

Author Contributions: Conceptualization, M.G. and A.P. (Angelica Petrillo); methodology, M.G.; software, N.F.; validation, S.K.; formal analysis, M.G.; investigation, A.L.S.; resources, M.G.; data curation, R.P. and E.S.; writing—original draft preparation, A.B., D.T., A.P. (Angelica Petrillo), A.P. (Alessandro Parisi), A.L.S.; writing—review and editing, S.K. and M.G.; visualization, S.K.; supervision, S.K.; project administration, M.G.; funding acquisition, M.G. All authors have read and agreed to the published version of the manuscript.

Funding: This research received no external funding.

Institutional Review Board Statement: Not applicable.

Informed Consent Statement: Not applicable.

Data Availability Statement: Not applicable.

Conflicts of Interest: The authors declare no conflict of interest.

References

1. Bray, F.; Ferlay, J.; Soerjomataram, I.; Siegel, R.L.; Torre, L.A.; Jemal, A. Global cancer statistics 2018: GLOBOCAN estimates of incidence and mortality worldwide for 36 cancers in 185 countries. *CA Cancer J. Clin.* **2018**, *68*, 394–424. [CrossRef] [PubMed]
2. Global Cancer Observatory: Gastric Cancer. Available online: https://gco.iarc.fr/ (accessed on 23 December 2020).
3. Laurén, P. The two histological main types of gastric carcinoma: Diffuse and so-called intestinal-type carcinoma. *Acta Pathol. Microbiol. Scand.* **1965**, *64*, 31–49. [CrossRef]
4. Marqués-Lespier, J.M.; González-Pons, M.; Cruz-Correa, M. Current Perspectives on Gastric Cancer. *Gastroenterol. Clin. North Am.* **2016**, *45*, 413–428. [CrossRef]
5. Ma, J.; Shen, H.; Kapesa, L.; Zeng, S. Lauren classification and individualized chemotherapy in gastric cancer. *Oncol. Lett.* **2016**, *11*, 2959–2964. [CrossRef]
6. Blair, V.R.; McLeod, M.; Carneiro, F.; Coit, D.G.; D'Addario, J.L.; van Dieren, J.M.; Harris, K.L.; Hoogerbrugge, N.; Oliveira, C.; van der Post, R.S.; et al. Hereditary diffuse gastric cancer: Updated clinical practice guidelines. *Lancet Oncol.* **2020**, *21*, e386–e397. [CrossRef]
7. Berlth, F. Pathohistological classification systems in gastric cancer: Diagnostic relevance and prognostic value. *World. J. Gastroenterol.* **2014**, *20*, 5679. [CrossRef] [PubMed]
8. Bosman, F.T.; Carneiro, F.; Hruban, R.H.; Theise, N.D. *WHO Classification of Tumours of the Digestive System*; World Health Organization: Geneva, Switzerland, 2010; ISBN 9789283224327.
9. Cancer Genome Atlas Research Network. Comprehensive molecular characterization of gastric adenocarcinoma. *Nature* **2014**, *513*, 202–209. [CrossRef]
10. Ling, Y.; Watanabe, Y.; Nagahashi, M.; Shimada, Y.; Ichikawa, H.; Wakai, T.; Okuda, S. Genetic profiling for diffuse type and genomically stable subtypes in gastric cancer. *Comput. Struct. Biotechnol. J.* **2020**, *18*, 3301–3308. [CrossRef]
11. Rodriquenz, M.G.; Roviello, G.; D'Angelo, A.; Lavacchi, D.; Roviello, F.; Polom, K. MSI and EBV Positive Gastric Cancer's Subgroups and Their Link with Novel Immunotherapy. *J. Clin. Med.* **2020**, *9*, 1427. [CrossRef]
12. Li, X.; Wu, W.K.K.; Xing, R.; Wong, S.H.; Liu, Y.; Fang, X.; Zhang, Y.; Wang, M.; Wang, J.; Li, L.; et al. Distinct Subtypes of Gastric Cancer Defined by Molecular Characterization Include Novel Mutational Signatures with Prognostic Capability. *Cancer Res.* **2016**, *76*, 1724–1732. [CrossRef]

13. Leung, S.Y.; Yuen, S.T.; Chung, L.P.; Chu, K.M.; Chan, A.S.Y.; Ho, J.C.I. hMLH1 Promoter Methylation and Lack of hMLH1 Expression in Sporadic Gastric Carcinomas with High-Frequency Microsatellite Instability. *Cancer Res.* 1999, 59, 159–164.
14. Pietrantonio, F.; Miceli, R.; Raimondi, A.; Kim, Y.W.; Kang, W.K.; Langley, R.E.; Choi, Y.Y.; Kim, K.-M.; Nankivell, M.G.; Morano, F.; et al. Individual Patient Data Meta-Analysis of the Value of Microsatellite Instability As a Biomarker in Gastric Cancer. *J. Clin. Oncol.* 2019, 37, 3392–3400. [CrossRef]
15. Le, D.T.; Durham, J.N.; Smith, K.N.; Wang, H.; Bartlett, B.R.; Aulakh, L.K.; Lu, S.; Kemberling, H.; Wilt, C.; Luber, B.S.; et al. Mismatch repair deficiency predicts response of solid tumors to PD-1 blockade. *Science* 2017, 357, 409–413. [CrossRef]
16. Le, D.T.; Uram, J.N.; Wang, H.; Bartlett, B.R.; Kemberling, H.; Eyring, A.D.; Skora, A.D.; Luber, B.S.; Azad, N.S.; Laheru, D.; et al. PD-1 Blockade in Tumors with Mismatch-Repair Deficiency. *N. Engl. J. Med.* 2015, 372, 2509–2520. [CrossRef]
17. Eichelberg, M.R.; Welch, R.; Guidry, J.T.; Ali, A.; Ohashi, M.; Makielski, K.R.; McChesney, K.; Van Sciver, N.; Lambert, P.F.; Keleş, S.; et al. Epstein-Barr Virus Infection Promotes Epithelial Cell Growth by Attenuating Differentiation-Dependent Exit from the Cell Cycle. *MBio* 2019, 10. [CrossRef]
18. Jung, H.; Kim, H.S.; Kim, J.Y.; Sun, J.-M.; Ahn, J.S.; Ahn, M.-J.; Park, K.; Esteller, M.; Lee, S.-H.; Choi, J.K. DNA methylation loss promotes immune evasion of tumours with high mutation and copy number load. *Nat. Commun.* 2019, 10, 4278. [CrossRef] [PubMed]
19. Geddert, H.; Zur Hausen, A.; Gabbert, H.E.; Sarbia, M. EBV-infection in cardiac and non-cardiac gastric adenocarcinomas is associated with promoter methylation of p16, p14 and APC, but not hMLH1. *Anal. Cell. Pathol. (Amst.)* 2010, 33, 143–149. [CrossRef]
20. Xin Yu, J.; Hubbard-Lucey, V.M.; Tang, J. Immuno-oncology drug development goes global. *Nat. Rev. Drug Discov.* 2019, 18, 899–900. [CrossRef] [PubMed]
21. Yang, L.; Wang, Y.; Wang, H. Use of immunotherapy in the treatment of gastric cancer (Review). *Oncol. Lett.* 2019, 18, 5681–5690. [CrossRef]
22. Zhao, L.; Li, J.; Bai, C.; Nie, Y.; Lin, G. Multi-Modality Treatment for Patients With Metastatic Gastric Cancer: A Real-World Study in China. *Front. Oncol.* 2019, 9, 1155. [CrossRef]
23. Ebinger, S.M.; Warschkow, R.; Tarantino, I.; Schmied, B.M.; Güller, U.; Schiesser, M. Modest overall survival improvements from 1998 to 2009 in metastatic gastric cancer patients: A population-based SEER analysis. *Gastric Cancer* 2016, 19, 723–734. [CrossRef] [PubMed]
24. Robert, C. A decade of immune-checkpoint inhibitors in cancer therapy. *Nat. Commun.* 2020, 11, 3801. [CrossRef] [PubMed]
25. Schumacher, T.N.; Scheper, W.; Kvistborg, P. Cancer Neoantigens. *Annu. Rev. Immunol.* 2019, 37, 173–200. [CrossRef] [PubMed]
26. Hendrickx, W.; Simeone, I.; Anjum, S.; Mokrab, Y.; Bertucci, F.; Finetti, P.; Curigliano, G.; Seliger, B.; Cerulo, L.; Tomei, S.; et al. Identification of genetic determinants of breast cancer immune phenotypes by integrative genome-scale analysis. *Oncoimmunology* 2017, 6, e1253654. [CrossRef]
27. Wagner, J.; Wickman, E.; DeRenzo, C.; Gottschalk, S. CAR T Cell Therapy for Solid Tumors: Bright Future or Dark Reality? *Mol. Ther.* 2020, 28, 2320–2339. [CrossRef] [PubMed]
28. Huang, J.; Rong, L.; Wang, E.; Fang, Y. Pseudoprogression of extramedullary disease in relapsed acute lymphoblastic leukemia after CAR T-cell therapy. *Immunotherapy* 2021, 13, 5–10. [CrossRef] [PubMed]
29. Ou, Z. PCN198 Global regulatory challenges of CAR T-Cell therapies: Approval, pricing, and access. *Value Health* 2019, 22, S93. [CrossRef]
30. Lin, E.M.; Gong, J.; Klempner, S.J.; Chao, J. Advances in immuno-oncology biomarkers for gastroesophageal cancer: Programmed death ligand 1, microsatellite instability, and beyond. *World J. Gastroenterol.* 2018, 24, 2686–2697. [CrossRef] [PubMed]
31. Ratti, M.; Lampis, A.; Hahne, J.C.; Passalacqua, R.; Valeri, N. Microsatellite instability in gastric cancer: Molecular bases, clinical perspectives, and new treatment approaches. *Cell. Mol. Life Sci.* 2018, 75, 4151–4162. [CrossRef] [PubMed]
32. Kim, J.-Y.; Shin, N.R.; Kim, A.; Lee, H.-J.; Park, W.; Kim, J.-Y.; Lee, C.-H.; Huh, G.-Y.; Park, D.Y. Microsatellite Instability Status in Gastric Cancer: A Reappraisal of Its Clinical Significance and Relationship with Mucin Phenotypes. *Korean J. Pathol.* 2013, 47, 28. [CrossRef] [PubMed]
33. Trenner, A.; Sartori, A.A. Harnessing DNA Double-Strand Break Repair for Cancer Treatment. *Front. Oncol.* 2019, 9, 1388. [CrossRef] [PubMed]
34. Motegi, A.; Masutani, M.; Yoshioka, K.; Bessho, T. Aberrations in DNA repair pathways in cancer and therapeutic significances. *Semin. Cancer Biol.* 2019, 58, 29–46. [CrossRef] [PubMed]
35. Corti, C.; Sajjadi, E.; Fusco, N. Determination of Mismatch Repair Status in Human Cancer and Its Clinical Significance. *Adv. Anat. Pathol.* 2019, 26, 270–279. [CrossRef] [PubMed]
36. Lopez, G.; Venetis, K.; Sajjadi, E.; Fusco, N. Mismatch Repair System Genomic Scars in Gastroesophageal Cancers: Biology and Clinical Testing. *Gastrointest. Disord.* 2020, 2, 341–352. [CrossRef]
37. Matsuoka, T.; Yashiro, M. Biomarkers of gastric cancer: Current topics and future perspective. *World J. Gastroenterol.* 2018, 24, 2818–2832. [CrossRef] [PubMed]
38. Dhakras, P.; Uboha, N.; Horner, V.; Reinig, E.; Matkowskyj, K.A. Gastrointestinal cancers: Current biomarkers in esophageal and gastric adenocarcinoma. *Transl. Gastroenterol. Hepatol.* 2020, 5, 55. [CrossRef] [PubMed]

39. Pagni, F.; Guerini-Rocco, E.; Schultheis, A.M.; Grazia, G.; Rijavec, E.; Ghidini, M.; Lopez, G.; Venetis, K.; Croci, G.A.; Malapelle, U.; et al. Targeting Immune-Related Biological Processes in Solid Tumors: We do Need Biomarkers. *Int. J. Mol. Sci.* **2019**, *20*, 5452. [CrossRef] [PubMed]
40. Sajjadi, E.; Venetis, K.; Scatena, C.; Fusco, N. Biomarkers for precision immunotherapy in the metastatic setting: Hope or reality? *Ecancermedicalscience* **2020**, *14*. [CrossRef]
41. Polom, K.; Marano, L.; Marrelli, D.; De Luca, R.; Roviello, G.; Savelli, V.; Tan, P.; Roviello, F. Meta-analysis of microsatellite instability in relation to clinicopathological characteristics and overall survival in gastric cancer. *Br. J. Surg.* **2018**, *105*, 159–167. [CrossRef]
42. Giampieri, R.; Maccaroni, E.; Mandolesi, A.; Del Prete, M.; Andrikou, K.; Faloppi, L.; Bittoni, A.; Bianconi, M.; Scarpelli, M.; Bracci, R.; et al. Mismatch repair deficiency may affect clinical outcome through immune response activation in metastatic gastric cancer patients receiving first-line chemotherapy. *Gastric Cancer* **2017**, *20*, 156–163. [CrossRef]
43. Yuza, K.; Nagahashi, M.; Watanabe, S.; Takabe, K.; Wakai, T. Hypermutation and microsatellite instability in gastrointestinal cancers. *Oncotarget* **2017**, *8*, 112103–112115. [CrossRef] [PubMed]
44. He, P.; Ma, Z.; Han, H.; Zhang, X.; Niu, S.; Du, L.; Zheng, Y.; Liu, H. Expression of programmed death ligand 1 (PD-L1) is associated with metastasis and differentiation in gastric cancer. *Life Sci.* **2020**, *242*, 117247. [CrossRef]
45. Liu, X.; Choi, M.G.; Kim, K.; Kim, K.-M.; Kim, S.T.; Park, S.H.; Cristescu, R.; Peter, S.; Lee, J. High PD-L1 expression in gastric cancer (GC) patients and correlation with molecular features. *Pathol. Res. Pract.* **2020**, *216*, 152881. [CrossRef] [PubMed]
46. Ju, X.; Shen, R.; Huang, P.; Zhai, J.; Qian, X.; Wang, Q.; Chen, M. Predictive relevance of PD-L1 expression with pre-existing TILs in gastric cancer. *Oncotarget* **2017**, *8*, 99372–99381. [CrossRef]
47. Fassan, M.; Brignola, S.; Pennelli, G.; Alberti, G.; Angerilli, V.; Bressan, A.; Pellino, A.; Lanza, C.; Salmaso, R.; Lonardi, S.; et al. PD-L1 expression in gastroesophageal dysplastic lesions. *Virchows Arch.* **2020**, *477*, 151–156. [CrossRef] [PubMed]
48. Ma, C.; Patel, K.; Singhi, A.D.; Ren, B.; Zhu, B.; Shaikh, F.; Sun, W. Programmed Death-Ligand 1 Expression Is Common in Gastric Cancer Associated With Epstein-Barr Virus or Microsatellite Instability. *Am. J. Surg. Pathol.* **2016**, *40*, 1496–1506. [CrossRef]
49. Ye, D.; Xu, G.; Ma, W.; Li, Y.; Luo, W.; Xiao, Y.; Liu, Y.; Zhang, Z. Significant function and research progress of biomarkers in gastric cancer (Review). *Oncol. Lett.* **2019**, *19*, 17–29. [CrossRef]
50. Zhang, N.; Cao, M.; Duan, Y.; Bai, H.; Li, X.; Wang, Y. Prognostic role of tumor-infiltrating lymphocytes in gastric cancer: A meta-analysis and experimental validation. *Arch. Med. Sci.* **2020**, *16*, 1092–1103. [CrossRef]
51. Lee, J.S.; Won, H.S.; Sun, D.S.; Hong, J.H.; Ko, Y.H. Prognostic role of tumor-infiltrating lymphocytes in gastric cancer. *Medicine (Baltimore)* **2018**, *97*, e11769. [CrossRef]
52. Hendry, S.; Salgado, R.; Gevaert, T.; Russell, P.A.; John, T.; Thapa, B.; Christie, M.; van de Vijver, K.; Estrada, M.V.; Gonzalez-Ericsson, P.I.; et al. Assessing Tumor-Infiltrating Lymphocytes in Solid Tumors. *Adv. Anat. Pathol.* **2017**, *24*, 311–335. [CrossRef]
53. Liu, J.; Xu, Y.; Yu, M.; Liu, Z.; Xu, Y.; Ma, G.; Zhou, W.; Kong, P.; Ling, L.; Wang, S.; et al. Increased Stromal Infiltrating Lymphocytes are Associated with Circulating Tumor Cells and Metastatic Relapse in Breast Cancer Patients After Neoadjuvant Chemotherapy. *Cancer Manag. Res.* **2019**, *11*, 10791–10800. [CrossRef]
54. Fuchs, C.S.; Doi, T.; Jang, R.W.; Muro, K.; Satoh, T.; Machado, M.; Sun, W.; Jalal, S.I.; Shah, M.A.; Metges, J.-P.; et al. Safety and Efficacy of Pembrolizumab Monotherapy in Patients With Previously Treated Advanced Gastric and Gastroesophageal Junction Cancer. *JAMA Oncol.* **2018**, *4*, e180013. [CrossRef]
55. Sholl, L.M.; Hirsch, F.R.; Hwang, D.; Botling, J.; Lopez-Rios, F.; Bubendorf, L.; Mino-Kenudson, M.; Roden, A.C.; Beasley, M.B.; Borczuk, A.; et al. The Promises and Challenges of Tumor Mutation Burden as an Immunotherapy Biomarker: A Perspective from the International Association for the Study of Lung Cancer Pathology Committee. *J. Thorac. Oncol.* **2020**, *15*, 1409–1424. [CrossRef] [PubMed]
56. U.S. Food and Drug Administration. FDA Approves Pembrolizumab for Adults and Children with TMB-H Solid Tumors. Available online: https://www.fda.gov/drugs/drug-approvals-and-databases/fda-approves-pembrolizumab-adults-and-children-tmb-h-solid-tumors (accessed on 19 December 2020).
57. Ku, G.Y.; Sanchez-Vega, F.; Chatila, W.; Margolis, M.; Fein, C.; Ilson, D.H.; Hechtman, J.F.; Tuvy, Y.; Bouvier, N.; Kundra, R.; et al. Correlation of benefit from immune checkpoint inhibitors with next gen sequencing (NGS) profiles in esophagogastric cancer (EGC) patients. *J. Clin. Oncol.* **2017**, *35*, 4025. [CrossRef]
58. Janjigian, Y.Y.; Sanchez-Vega, F.; Jonsson, P.; Chatila, W.K.; Hechtman, J.F.; Ku, G.Y.; Riches, J.C.; Tuvy, Y.; Kundra, R.; Bouvier, N.; et al. Genetic Predictors of Response to Systemic Therapy in Esophagogastric Cancer. *Cancer Discov.* **2018**, *8*, 49–58. [CrossRef] [PubMed]
59. Sundar, R.; Smyth, E.C.; Peng, S.; Yeong, J.P.S.; Tan, P. Predictive Biomarkers of Immune Checkpoint Inhibition in Gastroesophageal Cancers. *Front. Oncol.* **2020**, *10*, 763. [CrossRef] [PubMed]
60. Zhao, P.; Li, L.; Jiang, X.; Li, Q. Mismatch repair deficiency/microsatellite instability-high as a predictor for anti-PD-1/PD-L1 immunotherapy efficacy. *J. Hematol. Oncol.* **2019**, *12*, 54. [CrossRef] [PubMed]
61. Marcus, L.; Lemery, S.J.; Keegan, P.; Pazdur, R. FDA Approval Summary: Pembrolizumab for the Treatment of Microsatellite Instability-High Solid Tumors. *Clin. Cancer Res.* **2019**, *25*, 3753–3758. [CrossRef]
62. Shitara, K.; Van Cutsem, E.; Bang, Y.-J.; Fuchs, C.; Wyrwicz, L.; Lee, K.-W.; Kudaba, I.; Garrido, M.; Chung, H.C.; Lee, J.; et al. Efficacy and Safety of Pembrolizumab or Pembrolizumab Plus Chemotherapy vs Chemotherapy Alone for Patients With First-line, Advanced Gastric Cancer. *JAMA Oncol.* **2020**, *6*, 1571. [CrossRef]

63. Cho, J.; Kang, S.Y.; Kim, K.-M. MMR protein immunohistochemistry and microsatellite instability in gastric cancers. *Pathology* **2019**, *51*, 110–113. [CrossRef]
64. Luchini, C.; Bibeau, F.; Ligtenberg, M.J.L.; Singh, N.; Nottegar, A.; Bosse, T.; Miller, R.; Riaz, N.; Douillard, J.-Y.; Andre, F.; et al. ESMO recommendations on microsatellite instability testing for immunotherapy in cancer, and its relationship with PD-1/PD-L1 expression and tumour mutational burden: A systematic review-based approach. *Ann. Oncol.* **2019**, *30*, 1232–1243. [CrossRef] [PubMed]
65. Kim, S.T.; Cristescu, R.; Bass, A.J.; Kim, K.-M.; Odegaard, J.I.; Kim, K.; Liu, X.Q.; Sher, X.; Jung, H.; Lee, M.; et al. Comprehensive molecular characterization of clinical responses to PD-1 inhibition in metastatic gastric cancer. *Nat. Med.* **2018**, *24*, 1449–1458. [CrossRef]
66. Chen, Y.; Wang, Q.; Shi, B.; Xu, P.; Hu, Z.; Bai, L.; Zhang, X. Development of a sandwich ELISA for evaluating soluble PD-L1 (CD274) in human sera of different ages as well as supernatants of PD-L1+ cell lines. *Cytokine* **2011**, *56*, 231–238. [CrossRef] [PubMed]
67. Duraker, N.; Naci Çelik, A.; Gençler, N. The prognostic significance of gastric juice CA 19-9 and CEA levels in gastric carcinoma patients. *Eur. J. Surg. Oncol.* **2002**, *28*, 844–849. [CrossRef] [PubMed]
68. Miki, K.; Morita, M.; Sasajima, M.; Hoshina, R.; Kanda, E.; Urita, Y. Usefulness of gastric cancer screening using the serum pepsinogen test method. *Am. J. Gastroenterol.* **2003**, *98*, 735–739. [CrossRef]
69. Miki, K. Gastric cancer screening using the serum pepsinogen test method. *Gastric Cancer* **2006**, *9*, 245–253. [CrossRef]
70. Zheng, Z.; Bu, Z.; Liu, X.; Zhang, L.; Li, Z.; Wu, A.; Wu, X.; Cheng, X.; Xing, X.; Du, H.; et al. Level of circulating PD-L1 expression in patients with advanced gastric cancer and its clinical implications. *Chin. J. Cancer Res.* **2014**, *26*, 104–111.
71. Shigemori, T.; Toiyama, Y.; Okugawa, Y.; Yamamoto, A.; Yin, C.; Narumi, A.; Ichikawa, T.; Ide, S.; Shimura, T.; Fujikawa, H.; et al. Soluble PD-L1 Expression in Circulation as a Predictive Marker for Recurrence and Prognosis in Gastric Cancer: Direct Comparison of the Clinical Burden Between Tissue and Serum PD-L1 Expression. *Ann. Surg. Oncol.* **2019**, *26*, 876–883. [CrossRef]
72. Gershtein, E.S.; Ognerubov, N.A.; Chang, V.L.; Delektorskaya, V.V.; Korotkova, E.A.; Sokolov, N.Y.; Polikarpova, S.B.; Stilidi, I.S.; Kushlinskii, N.E. [The content of the soluble forms PD-1 and PD-L1 in blood serum of patients with gastric cancer and their relationship with clinical and morphological characteristics of the disease.]. *Klin. Lab. Diagn.* **2020**, *65*, 347–352. [CrossRef]
73. Shapiro, M.; Herishanu, Y.; Katz, B.-Z.; Dezorella, N.; Sun, C.; Kay, S.; Polliack, A.; Avivi, I.; Wiestner, A.; Perry, C. Lymphocyte activation gene 3: A novel therapeutic target in chronic lymphocytic leukemia. *Haematologica* **2017**, *102*, 874–882. [CrossRef]
74. Okamura, T.; Fujio, K.; Sumitomo, S.; Yamamoto, K. Roles of LAG3 and EGR2 in regulatory T cells. *Ann. Rheum. Dis.* **2012**, *71*, i96–i100. [CrossRef]
75. Li, N.; Jilisihan, B.; Wang, W.; Tang, Y.; Keyoumu, S. Soluble LAG3 acts as a potential prognostic marker of gastric cancer and its positive correlation with CD8+T cell frequency and secretion of IL-12 and INF-γ in peripheral blood. *Cancer Biomarkers* **2018**, *23*, 341–351. [CrossRef] [PubMed]
76. Botticelli, A.; Mezi, S.; Pomati, G.; Cerbelli, B.; Di Rocco, C.; Amirhassankhani, S.; Sirgiovanni, G.; Occhipinti, M.; Napoli, V.; Emiliani, A.; et al. The 5-Ws of immunotherapy in head and neck cancer. *Crit. Rev. Oncol. Hematol.* **2020**, *153*, 103041. [CrossRef] [PubMed]
77. Ando, K.; Hamada, K.; Watanabe, M.; Ohkuma, R.; Shida, M.; Onoue, R.; Kubota, Y.; Matsui, H.; Ishiguro, T.; Hirasawa, Y.; et al. Plasma Levels of Soluble PD-L1 Correlate With Tumor Regression in Patients With Lung and Gastric Cancer Treated With Immune Checkpoint Inhibitors. *Anticancer Res.* **2019**, *39*, 5195–5201. [CrossRef] [PubMed]
78. Park, W.; Bang, J.-H.; Nam, A.-R.; Jin, M.H.; Seo, H.; Kim, J.-M.; Oh, K.S.; Kim, T.-Y.; Oh, D.-Y. Prognostic Value of Serum Soluble Programmed Death-Ligand 1 and Dynamics During Chemotherapy in Advanced Gastric Cancer Patients. *Cancer Res. Treat.* **2021**, *53*, 199–206. [CrossRef]
79. Takahashi, N.; Iwasa, S.; Sasaki, Y.; Shoji, H.; Honma, Y.; Takashima, A.; Okita, N.T.; Kato, K.; Hamaguchi, T.; Yamada, Y. Serum levels of soluble programmed cell death ligand 1 as a prognostic factor on the first-line treatment of metastatic or recurrent gastric cancer. *J. Cancer Res. Clin. Oncol.* **2016**, *142*, 1727–1738. [CrossRef] [PubMed]
80. Ribas, A.; Butterfield, L.H.; Glaspy, J.A.; Economou, J.S. Current developments in cancer vaccines and cellular immunotherapy. *J. Clin. Oncol.* **2003**, *21*, 2415–2432. [CrossRef] [PubMed]
81. Gilliam, A.D.; Watson, S.A. G17DT: An antigastrin immunogen for the treatment of gastrointestinal malignancy. *Expert Opin. Biol. Ther.* **2007**, *7*, 397–404. [CrossRef]
82. Park, D.J.; Thomas, N.J.; Yoon, C.; Yoon, S.S. Vascular Endothelial Growth Factor A Inhibition in Gastric Cancer. *Gastric Cancer* **2015**, *18*, 33–42. [CrossRef]
83. Sundar, R.; Rha, S.Y.; Yamaue, H.; Katsuda, M.; Kono, K.; Kim, H.S.; Kim, C.; Mimura, K.; Kua, L.-F.; Yong, W.P. A phase I/Ib study of OTSGC-A24 combined peptide vaccine in advanced gastric cancer. *BMC Cancer* **2018**, *18*, 332. [CrossRef] [PubMed]
84. Gilliam, A.D.; Watson, S.; Henwood, M.; McKenzie, A.; Humphreys, J.; Elder, J.; Iftikhar, S.; Welch, N.; Fielding, J.; Broome, P.; et al. A phase II study of G17DT in gastric carcinoma. *Eur. J. Surg. Oncol.* **2004**, *30*, 536–543. [CrossRef]
85. Ajani, J.A.; Randolph Hecht, J.; Ho, L.; Baker, J.; Oortgiesen, M.; Eduljee, A.; Michaeli, D. An open-label, multinational, multicenter study of G17DT vaccination combined with cisplatin and 5-fluorouracil in patients with untreated, advanced gastric or gastroesophageal cancer: The GC4 study. *Cancer* **2006**, *106*, 1908–1916. [CrossRef] [PubMed]

86. Masuzawa, T.; Yoshiyuki, F.; Okada, K.; Nakamura, A.; Takiguchi, S.; Nakajima, K.; Miyata, H.; Yamasaki, M.; Kurokawa, Y.; Osawa, R.; et al. Phase I/II study of S-1 plus cisplatin combined with peptide vaccines for human vascular endothelial growth factor receptor 1 and 2 in patients with advanced gastric cancer. *Int. J. Oncol.* **2012**, *41*, 1297–1304. [CrossRef] [PubMed]
87. Stauss, H.J.; Morris, E.C.; Abken, H. Cancer gene therapy with T cell receptors and chimeric antigen receptors. *Curr. Opin. Pharmacol.* **2015**, *24*, 113–118. [CrossRef]
88. Li, J.; Li, W.; Huang, K.; Zhang, Y.; Kupfer, G.; Zhao, Q. Chimeric antigen receptor T cell (CAR-T) immunotherapy for solid tumors: Lessons learned and strategies for moving forward. *J. Hematol. Oncol.* **2018**, *11*, 22. [CrossRef] [PubMed]
89. Gill, S.; Maus, M.V.; Porter, D.L. Chimeric antigen receptor T cell therapy: 25years in the making. *Blood Rev.* **2016**, *30*, 157–167. [CrossRef]
90. Whilding, L.M.; Maher, J. ErbB-targeted CAR T-cell immunotherapy of cancer. *Immunotherapy* **2015**, *7*, 229–241. [CrossRef]
91. Wang, L.; Ma, N.; Okamoto, S.; Amaishi, Y.; Sato, E.; Seo, N.; Mineno, J.; Takesako, K.; Kato, T.; Shiku, H. Efficient tumor regression by adoptively transferred CEA-specific CAR-T cells associated with symptoms of mild cytokine release syndrome. *Oncoimmunology* **2016**, *5*, e1211218. [CrossRef]
92. Guest, R.D.; Kirillova, N.; Mowbray, S.; Gornall, H.; Rothwell, D.G.; Cheadle, E.J.; Austin, E.; Smith, K.; Watt, S.M.; Kühlcke, K.; et al. Definition and application of good manufacturing process-compliant production of CEA-specific chimeric antigen receptor expressing T-cells for phase I/II clinical trial. *Cancer Immunol. Immunother.* **2014**, *63*, 133–145. [CrossRef]
93. Warneke, V.S.; Behrens, H.-M.; Haag, J.; Krüger, S.; Simon, E.; Mathiak, M.; Ebert, M.P.A.; Röcken, C. Members of the EpCAM signalling pathway are expressed in gastric cancer tissue and are correlated with patient prognosis. *Br. J. Cancer* **2013**, *109*, 2217–2227. [CrossRef]
94. Smyth, E.C.; Verheij, M.; Allum, W.; Cunningham, D.; Cervantes, A.; Arnold, D. Gastric cancer: ESMO Clinical Practice Guidelines for diagnosis, treatment and follow-up. *Ann. Oncol.* **2016**, *27*, v38–v49. [CrossRef] [PubMed]
95. Bang, Y.-J.; Van Cutsem, E.; Fuchs, C.S.; Ohtsu, A.; Tabernero, J.; Ilson, D.H.; Hyung, W.J.; Strong, V.E.; Goetze, T.O.; Yoshikawa, T.; et al. KEYNOTE-585: Phase III study of perioperative chemotherapy with or without pembrolizumab for gastric cancer. *Future Oncol.* **2019**, *15*, 943–952. [CrossRef]
96. Al-Batran, S.-E.; Homann, N.; Pauligk, C.; Goetze, T.O.; Meiler, J.; Kasper, S.; Kopp, H.-G.; Mayer, F.; Haag, G.M.; Luley, K.; et al. Perioperative chemotherapy with fluorouracil plus leucovorin, oxaliplatin, and docetaxel versus fluorouracil or capecitabine plus cisplatin and epirubicin for locally advanced, resectable gastric or gastro-oesophageal junction adenocarcinoma (FLOT4): A randomised, phase 2/3 trial. *Lancet* **2019**, *393*, 1948–1957.
97. Kelly, R.J.; Ajani, J.A.; Kuzdzal, J.; Zander, T.; Van Cutsem, E.; Piessen, G.; Mendez, G.; Feliciano, J.L.; Motoyama, S.; Lièvre, A.; et al. LBA9_PR Adjuvant nivolumab in resected esophageal or gastroesophageal junction cancer (EC/GEJC) following neoadjuvant chemoradiation therapy (CRT): First results of the CheckMate 577 study. *Ann. Oncol.* **2020**, *31*, S1193–S1194. [CrossRef]
98. Moehler, M.; Shitara, K.; Garrido, M.; Salman, P.; Shen, L.; Wyrwicz, L.; Yamaguchi, K.; Skoczylas, T.; Campos Bragagnoli, A.; Liu, T.; et al. LBA6_PR Nivolumab (nivo) plus chemotherapy (chemo) versus chemo as first-line (1L) treatment for advanced gastric cancer/gastroesophageal junction cancer (GC/GEJC)/esophageal adenocarcinoma (EAC): First results of the CheckMate 649 study. *Ann. Oncol.* **2020**, *31*, S1191. [CrossRef]
99. Boku, N.; Ryu, M.H.; Oh, D.-Y.; Oh, S.C.; Chung, H.C.; Lee, K.-W.; Omori, T.; Shitara, K.; Sakuramoto, S.; Chung, I.J.; et al. LBA7_PR Nivolumab plus chemotherapy versus chemotherapy alone in patients with previously untreated advanced or recurrent gastric/gastroesophageal junction (G/GEJ) cancer: ATTRACTION-4 (ONO-4538–37) study. *Ann. Oncol.* **2020**, *31*, S1192. [CrossRef]
100. Janjigian, Y.Y.; Maron, S.B.; Chatila, W.K.; Millang, B.; Chavan, S.S.; Alterman, C.; Chou, J.F.; Segal, M.F.; Simmons, M.Z.; Momtaz, P.; et al. First-line pembrolizumab and trastuzumab in HER2-positive oesophageal, gastric, or gastro-oesophageal junction cancer: An open-label, single-arm, phase 2 trial. *Lancet Oncol.* **2020**, *21*, 821–831. [CrossRef]
101. Moehler, M.; Dvorkin, M.; Boku, N.; Özgüroğlu, M.; Ryu, M.-H.; Muntean, A.S.; Lonardi, S.; Nechaeva, M.; Bragagnoli, A.C.; Coşkun, H.S.; et al. Phase III Trial of Avelumab Maintenance After First-Line Induction Chemotherapy Versus Continuation of Chemotherapy in Patients With Gastric Cancers: Results From JAVELIN Gastric 100. *J. Clin. Oncol.* **2020**, *39*, 966–977. [CrossRef]
102. Shitara, K.; Özgüroğlu, M.; Bang, Y.-J.; Di Bartolomeo, M.; Mandalà, M.; Ryu, M.-H.; Fornaro, L.; Olesiński, T.; Caglevic, C.; Chung, H.C.; et al. Pembrolizumab versus paclitaxel for previously treated, advanced gastric or gastro-oesophageal junction cancer (KEYNOTE-061): A randomised, open-label, controlled, phase 3 trial. *Lancet* **2018**, *392*, 123–133. [CrossRef]
103. Kang, Y.-K.; Boku, N.; Satoh, T.; Ryu, M.-H.; Chao, Y.; Kato, K.; Chung, H.C.; Chen, J.-S.; Muro, K.; Kang, W.K.; et al. Nivolumab in patients with advanced gastric or gastro-oesophageal junction cancer refractory to, or intolerant of, at least two previous chemotherapy regimens (ONO-4538–12, ATTRACTION-2): A randomised, double-blind, placebo-controlled, phase 3 trial. *Lancet (Lond. Engl.)* **2017**, *390*, 2461–2471. [CrossRef]
104. Janjigian, Y.Y.; Bendell, J.; Calvo, E.; Kim, J.W.; Ascierto, P.A.; Sharma, P.; Ott, P.A.; Peltola, K.; Jaeger, D.; Evans, J.; et al. CheckMate-032 Study: Efficacy and Safety of Nivolumab and Nivolumab Plus Ipilimumab in Patients With Metastatic Esophagogastric Cancer. *J. Clin. Oncol.* **2018**, *36*, 2836–2844. [CrossRef] [PubMed]

105. Bang, Y.-J.; Ruiz, E.Y.; Van Cutsem, E.; Lee, K.-W.; Wyrwicz, L.; Schenker, M.; Alsina, M.; Ryu, M.-H.; Chung, H.-C.; Evesque, L.; et al. Phase III, randomised trial of avelumab versus physician's choice of chemotherapy as third-line treatment of patients with advanced gastric or gastro-oesophageal junction cancer: Primary analysis of JAVELIN Gastric 300. *Ann. Oncol.* **2018**, *29*, 2052–2060. [CrossRef] [PubMed]
106. Tabernero, J.; Bang, Y.; Van Cutsem, E.; Fuchs, C.; Janjigian, Y.; Bhagia, P.; Li, K.; Adelberg, D.; Qin, S. P-38 KEYNOTE-859: A randomized, double-blind, placebo-controlled phase 3 trial of first-line pembrolizumab plus chemotherapy in patients with advanced gastric or gastroesophageal junction adenocarcinoma. *Ann. Oncol.* **2020**, *31*, S101–S102. [CrossRef]
107. Chung, H.C.; Bang, Y.-J.; Fuchs, C.S.; Qin, S.-K.; Satoh, T.; Shitara, K.; Tabernero, J.; van Cutsem, E.; Alsina, M.; Cao, Z.A.; et al. First-line pembrolizumab/placebo plus trastuzumab and chemotherapy in HER2-positive advanced gastric cancer: KEYNOTE-811. *Futur. Oncol.* **2020**, *17*, 491–501. [CrossRef]
108. Loi, S.; Giobbie-Hurder, A.; Gombos, A.; Bachelot, T.; Hui, R.; Curigliano, G.; Campone, M.; Biganzoli, L.; Bonnefoi, H.; Jerusalem, G.; et al. Pembrolizumab plus trastuzumab in trastuzumab-resistant, advanced, HER2-positive breast cancer (PANACEA): A single-arm, multicentre, phase 1b–2 trial. *Lancet Oncol.* **2019**, *20*, 371–382. [CrossRef]
109. Petrillo, A.; Smyth, E.C. Biomarkers for Precision Treatment in Gastric Cancer. *Visc. Med.* **2020**, *36*, 364–372. [CrossRef]
110. Parisi, A.; Porzio, G.; Ficorella, C. Multimodality Treatment in Metastatic Gastric Cancer: From Past to Next Future. *Cancers (Basel)* **2020**, *12*, 2598. [CrossRef] [PubMed]
111. Wilke, H.; Muro, K.; Van Cutsem, E.; Oh, S.-C.; Bodoky, G.; Shimada, Y.; Hironaka, S.; Sugimoto, N.; Lipatov, O.; Kim, T.-Y.; et al. Ramucirumab plus paclitaxel versus placebo plus paclitaxel in patients with previously treated advanced gastric or gastro-oesophageal junction adenocarcinoma (RAINBOW): A double-blind, randomised phase 3 trial. *Lancet Oncol.* **2014**, *15*, 1224–1235. [CrossRef]
112. Fuchs, C.S.; Tomasek, J.; Yong, C.J.; Dumitru, F.; Passalacqua, R.; Goswami, C.; Safran, H.; dos Santos, L.V.; Aprile, G.; Ferry, D.R.; et al. Ramucirumab monotherapy for previously treated advanced gastric or gastro-oesophageal junction adenocarcinoma (REGARD): An international, randomised, multicentre, placebo-controlled, phase 3 trial. *Lancet* **2014**, *383*, 31–39. [CrossRef]
113. Parisi, A.; Cortellini, A.; Roberto, M.; Venditti, O.; Santini, D.; Dell'Aquila, E.; Stellato, M.; Marchetti, P.; Occhipinti, M.A.; Zoratto, F.; et al. Weight loss and body mass index in advanced gastric cancer patients treated with second-line ramucirumab: A real-life multicentre study. *J. Cancer Res. Clin. Oncol.* **2019**, *145*, 2365–2373. [CrossRef]
114. Di Bartolomeo, M.; Niger, M.; Tirino, G.; Petrillo, A.; Berenato, R.; Laterza, M.M.; Pietrantonio, F.; Morano, F.; Antista, M.; Lonardi, S.; et al. Ramucirumab as Second-Line Therapy in Metastatic Gastric Cancer: Real-World Data from the RAMoss Study. *Target. Oncol.* **2018**, *13*, 227–234. [CrossRef]
115. Paulson, A.S.; Hess, L.M.; Liepa, A.M.; Cui, Z.L.; Aguilar, K.M.; Clark, J.; Schelman, W. Ramucirumab for the treatment of patients with gastric or gastroesophageal junction cancer in community oncology practices. *Gastric Cancer* **2018**, *21*, 831–844. [CrossRef]
116. Shitara, K.; Doi, T.; Dvorkin, M.; Mansoor, W.; Arkenau, H.-T.; Prokharau, A.; Alsina, M.; Ghidini, M.; Faustino, C.; Gorbunova, V.; et al. Trifluridine/tipiracil versus placebo in patients with heavily pretreated metastatic gastric cancer (TAGS): A randomised, double-blind, placebo-controlled, phase 3 trial. *Lancet. Oncol.* **2018**, *19*, 1437–1448. [CrossRef]
117. Petrillo, A.; Tirino, G.; Zito Marino, F.; Pompella, L.; Sabetta, R.; Panarese, I.; Pappalardo, A.; Caterino, M.; Ventriglia, A.; Laterza, M.M.; et al. Nivolumab in Heavily Pretreated Metastatic Gastric Cancer Patients: Real-Life Data from a Western Population. *Onco. Targets. Ther.* **2020**, *13*, 867–876. [CrossRef]
118. Fuchs, C.S.; Özgüroğlu, M.; Bang, Y.-J.; Di Bartolomeo, M.; Mandalà, M.; Ryu, M.; Fornaro, L.; Olesinski, T.; Caglevic, C.; Chung, H.C.; et al. Pembrolizumab versus paclitaxel for previously treated patients with PD-L1–positive advanced gastric or gastroesophageal junction cancer (GC): Update from the phase III KEYNOTE-061 trial. *J. Clin. Oncol.* **2020**, *38*, 4503. [CrossRef]
119. Buchbinder, E.I.; Desai, A. CTLA-4 and PD-1 Pathways. *Am. J. Clin. Oncol.* **2016**, *39*, 98–106. [CrossRef] [PubMed]
120. Pitt, J.M.; Marabelle, A.; Eggermont, A.; Soria, J.-C.; Kroemer, G.; Zitvogel, L. Targeting the tumor microenvironment: Removing obstruction to anticancer immune responses and immunotherapy. *Ann. Oncol.* **2016**, *27*, 1482–1492. [CrossRef]
121. Gambardella, V.; Castillo, J.; Tarazona, N.; Gimeno-Valiente, F.; Martínez-Ciarpaglini, C.; Cabeza-Segura, M.; Roselló, S.; Roda, D.; Huerta, M.; Cervantes, A.; et al. The role of tumor-associated macrophages in gastric cancer development and their potential as a therapeutic target. *Cancer Treat. Rev.* **2020**, *86*, 102015. [CrossRef] [PubMed]
122. Mantovani, A.; Marchesi, F.; Malesci, A.; Laghi, L.; Allavena, P. Tumour-associated macrophages as treatment targets in oncology. *Nat. Rev. Clin. Oncol.* **2017**, *14*, 399–416. [CrossRef]
123. Arai, H.; Battaglin, F.; Wang, J.; Lo, J.H.; Soni, S.; Zhang, W.; Lenz, H.-J. Molecular insight of regorafenib treatment for colorectal cancer. *Cancer Treat. Rev.* **2019**, *81*, 101912. [CrossRef]
124. Fukuoka, S.; Hara, H.; Takahashi, N.; Kojima, T.; Kawazoe, A.; Asayama, M.; Yoshii, T.; Kotani, D.; Tamura, H.; Mikamoto, Y.; et al. Regorafenib Plus Nivolumab in Patients With Advanced Gastric or Colorectal Cancer: An Open-Label, Dose-Escalation, and Dose-Expansion Phase Ib Trial (REGONIVO, EPOC1603). *J. Clin. Oncol.* **2020**, *38*, 2053–2061. [CrossRef]
125. Kawazoe, A.; Fukuoka, S.; Nakamura, Y.; Kuboki, Y.; Mikamoto, Y.; Shima, H.; Fujishiro, N.; Higuchi, T.; Wakabayashi, M.; Nomura, S.; et al. An open-label phase II study of lenvatinib plus pembrolizumab in patients with advanced gastric cancer (EPOC1706). *J. Clin. Oncol.* **2020**, *38*, 374. [CrossRef]
126. Peyraud, F.; Italiano, A. Combined PARP Inhibition and Immune Checkpoint Therapy in Solid Tumors. *Cancers (Basel)* **2020**, *12*, 1502. [CrossRef] [PubMed]

127. Zitvogel, L.; Ma, Y.; Raoult, D.; Kroemer, G.; Gajewski, T.F. The microbiome in cancer immunotherapy: Diagnostic tools and therapeutic strategies. *Science* **2018**, *359*, 1366–1370. [CrossRef] [PubMed]
128. Park, S.; Jiang, Z.; Mortenson, E.D.; Deng, L.; Radkevich-Brown, O.; Yang, X.; Sattar, H.; Wang, Y.; Brown, N.K.; Greene, M.; et al. The Therapeutic Effect of Anti-HER2/neu Antibody Depends on Both Innate and Adaptive Immunity. *Cancer Cell* **2010**, *18*, 160–170. [CrossRef] [PubMed]
129. Catenacci, D.V.T.; Kang, Y.-K.; Park, H.; Uronis, H.E.; Lee, K.-W.; Ng, M.C.H.; Enzinger, P.C.; Park, S.H.; Gold, P.J.; Lacy, J.; et al. Margetuximab plus pembrolizumab in patients with previously treated, HER2-positive gastro-oesophageal adenocarcinoma (CP-MGAH22–05): A single-arm, phase 1b–2 trial. *Lancet Oncol.* **2020**, *21*, 1066–1076. [CrossRef]
130. Li, X.-F.; Ren, P.; Shen, W.-Z.; Jin, X.; Zhang, J. The expression, modulation and use of cancer-testis antigens as potential biomarkers for cancer immunotherapy. *Am. J. Transl. Res.* **2020**, *12*, 7002–7019. [PubMed]
131. Nasr, R.; Shamseddine, A.; Mukherji, D.; Nassar, F.; Temraz, S. The Crosstalk between Microbiome and Immune Response in Gastric Cancer. *Int. J. Mol. Sci.* **2020**, *21*, 6586. [CrossRef] [PubMed]
132. Pietrantonio, F.; Randon, G.; Di Bartolomeo, M.; Luciani, A.; Chao, J.; Smyth, E.C.; Petrelli, F. Predictive role of microsatellite instability for of PD-1 blockade in patients with advanced gastric cancer: A meta-analysis of randomized clinical trials. *ESMO Open* **2021**, *6*, 100036. [CrossRef]
133. Murugaesu, N.; Wilson, G.A.; Birkbak, N.J.; Watkins, T.B.K.; McGranahan, N.; Kumar, S.; Abbassi-Ghadi, N.; Salm, M.; Mitter, R.; Horswell, S.; et al. Tracking the Genomic Evolution of Esophageal Adenocarcinoma through Neoadjuvant Chemotherapy. *Cancer Discov.* **2015**, *5*, 821–831. [CrossRef]
134. Liu, Z.; Wang, Y.; Huang, Y.; Kim, B.Y.S.; Shan, H.; Wu, D.; Jiang, W. Tumor Vasculatures: A New Target for Cancer Immunotherapy. *Trends Pharmacol. Sci.* **2019**, *40*, 613–623. [CrossRef]
135. Hara, H.; Shoji, H.; Takahari, D.; Esaki, T.; Machida, N.; Nagashima, K.; Aoki, K.; Honda, K.; Miyamoto, T.; Boku, N.; et al. Phase I/II study of ramucirumab plus nivolumab in patients in second-line treatment for advanced gastric adenocarcinoma (NivoRam study). *J. Clin. Oncol.* **2019**, *37*, 129. [CrossRef]

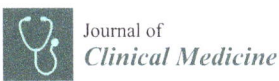

Review

The Emerging Role of Liquid Biopsy in Gastric Cancer

Csongor György Lengyel [1,*], Sadaqat Hussain [2], Dario Trapani [3], Khalid El Bairi [4], Sara Cecilia Altuna [5], Andreas Seeber [6], Andrew Odhiambo [7], Baker Shalal Habeeb [8] and Fahmi Seid [9]

1. Head and Neck Surgery, National Institute of Oncology Hungary, 1122 Budapest, Hungary
2. North West Cancer Center, Altnagelvin Hospital, Londonderry BT47 6SB, UK; oncologysh@gmail.com
3. European Institute of Oncology, IRCCS, 20141 Milan, Italy; dario.trapani@ieo.it
4. Cancer Biomarkers Working Group, Oujda 60000, Morocco; k.elbairi@ump.ac.ma
5. Oncomédica C.A., Medical Oncology Department, Caracas 1010, Venezuela; altunamujica.md@gmail.com
6. Department of Hematology and Oncology, Comprehensive Cancer Center Innsbruck, Medical University of Innsbruck, 6020 Innsbruck, Austria; andreas.seeber@tirol-kliniken.at
7. Unit of Medical Oncology, Department of Clinical Medicine, University of Nairobi, Nairobi 30197, Kenya; andrewodhiambo@gmail.com
8. Department of Medical Oncology, Shaqlawa Teaching Hospital, Shaqlawa, Erbil 44005, Iraq; bakershalal@gmail.com
9. School of Medicine and Health Sciences, Hawassa University, Hawassa 1560, Ethiopia; fahmizeek@gmail.com
* Correspondence: lengyel.csongor@gmail.com

Abstract: (1) Background: Liquid biopsy (LB) is a novel diagnostic method with the potential of revolutionizing the prevention, diagnosis, and treatment of several solid tumors. The present paper aims to summarize the current knowledge and explore future possibilities of LB in the management of metastatic gastric cancer. (2) Methods: This narrative review examined the most recent literature on the use of LB-based techniques in metastatic gastric cancer and the current LB-related clinical trial landscape. (3) Results: In gastric cancer, the detection of circulating cancer cells (CTCs) has been recognized to have a prognostic role in all the disease stages. In the setting of localized disease, cell-free DNA (cfDNA) and circulating tumor DNA (ctDNA) qualitative and quantitative detection have the potential to inform on the risk of cancer recurrence and metastatic dissemination. In addition, gastric cancer-released exosomes may play an essential part in metastasis formation. In the metastatic setting, the levels of cfDNA show a positive correlation with tumor burden. There is evidence that circulating tumor microemboli (CTM) in the blood of metastatic patients is an independent prognostic factor for shorter overall survival. Gastric cancer-derived exosomal microRNAs or clonal mutations and copy number variations detectable in ctDNA may contribute resistance to chemotherapy or targeted therapies, respectively. There is conflicting and limited data on CTC-based PD-L1 verification and cfDNA-based Epstein–Barr virus detection to predict or monitor immunotherapy responses. (4) Conclusions: Although preliminary studies analyzing LBs in patients with advanced gastric cancer appear promising, more research is required to obtain better insights into the molecular mechanisms underlying resistance to systemic therapies. Moreover, validation and standardization of LB methods are crucial before introducing them in clinical practice. The feasibility of repeatable, minimally invasive sampling opens up the possibility of selecting or dynamically changing therapies based on prognostic risk or predictive biomarkers, such as resistance markers. Research is warranted to exploit a possible transforming area of cancer care.

Keywords: liquid biopsy; circulating tumor cell; cfDNA; ctDNA; metastatic gastric cancer; epithelial–mesenchymal transition; resistance to treatment; HER2-inhibition; VEGFR-inhibition; immunotherapy; response monitoring

1. Introduction

The term liquid biopsy simultaneously encompasses a group of significantly different techniques, emerging as a tool that clinical practitioners can use to diagnose cancer, assess prognosis, identify targetable alterations, predict the effectiveness of treatments, and monitor tumor burden and therapeutic resistance. Among solid tumors, the potential for liquid biopsy has been most thoroughly studied in colorectal cancer, non-small cell lung cancer, and breast cancer and less explored in gastric cancer [1–3]. In our introduction, following a brief description of gastric cancer's prognostic and predictive biomarkers, we provide a brief overview of the history and applications of liquid biopsy. It is not the purpose of this article to describe the technical and procedural background and limitations of liquid biopsy, which would go beyond the scope of this review. Readers may also refer to some of the excellent recent reviews on this topic [1–3].

1.1. Overview of the Prognostic and Predictive Tissue Biomarkers in Gastric Cancer

Stomach cancer is the fifth most prevalent tumor globally, with a worldwide incidence in increasing trend of growth [4]. According to the Global Cancer Observatory of the World Health Organization, from the 1.09 million cases diagnosed in 2020, the incidence will rise to 1.77 million by 2040 [5].

Histologically, around 90% of gastroesophageal junction cancer (GEJC) and gastric cancer cases are adenocarcinomas [6,7]. Gastric adenocarcinomas can be further divided into four categories based on The Cancer Genome Atlas (TCGA) Research Network's molecular classification. The classification differentiated (i) chromosomally unstable, (ii) Epstein–Barr virus-induced, (iii) genomically stable, and (iv) microsatellite unstable groups [8].

Several biomarkers have prognostic or predictive value in gastric cancer, and their prevalence may vary depending on the disease stage. Both Programmed cell death ligand 1 (PD-L1) and Human epidermal growth factor receptor 2 (HER2)-positive tumors have been linked to aggressive disease and reduced survival, although some conflicting evidence still exists [9–12]. A decreased risk of lymph node metastasis, tumor invasion, and mortality has been correlated with microsatellite instability (MSI) in stomach cancer. However, the connection with improved prognosis remains unclear in light of conflicting evidence [13]. Several publications have questioned the role of neoadjuvant chemotherapy in microsatellite-instable tumors and supported a surgery-only approach. The predictive value of microsatellite instability in the clinical decision of providing perioperative chemotherapy may be prospectively confirmed by subgroup analyses of the FLOT-4 and JACCRO GC-07 studies [14–17]. In EBV-positive gastric cancers, subsequent studies have also demonstrated that PD-L1 expression is increased and associated with a decrease in survival [18,19].

The clinical benefit of immunotherapy has been reported in two subgroups of gastric cancer, in tumors with elevated PD-L1 expression and in tumors with microsatellite instability [20–22]. Correlation between HER2 positive status and clinical response to trastuzumab has also been observed [11]. Therefore, according to the National Comprehensive Cancer Network (NCCN)'s newest guidelines in the USA, MSI testing is suggested in all newly diagnosed patients, and HER2 and PD-L1 testing are recommended in all metastatic cases [23]. High tumor mutational burden and positive EBV status are emerging predictive biomarkers for gastric cancer immunotherapy [24–26].

1.2. A Brief Introduction to Liquid Biopsy

In 1948, Mandel and Métais published the results of discovering extracellular nucleic acids (DNA and RNA) in the blood [27]. In 1966, Leon et al. measured circulating free DNA (cfDNA) levels in 173 oncology patients and 55 healthy controls by using radioimmunoassay. The authors observed that 50% of cancer patients had normal cfDNA levels. However, they reported substantially higher levels of cfDNA in the serum of metastatic patients. In some patients, dynamic changes in cfDNA have been observed after radiation therapy by using serial sampling [28]. Nearly thirty years later, evidence has been provided that tumor cells release their DNA into the bloodstream. By parallel testing of the primary tumor and the plasma, characteristic mutations of selected genes like RAS or gene alterations in the genes involved in DNA mismatch repair (MMR) (i.e., present in the primary tumors) could also be detected in the matching plasma. This phenomenon was reported across the indications by several groups [29–31]. In 2008, Diehl et al. demonstrated that it is possible to molecularly detect tumor relapse in colorectal cancer by tracking individually selected tumor-specific mutations in the plasma. The authors summed this approach's benefits in its high specificity, and the downside was to create a unique mutation-specific probe marker for each subject [32]. Simultaneously, it was recognized that tumor DNA could be isolated from many other body fluids, such as cerebrospinal fluid, saliva, pleural fluid, urine, and fecal samples [33–36]. Nowadays, liquid biopsy is composed of different biological sources such as circulating tumor microemboli (CTM), circulating tumor cells (CTC), cell-free nucleic acids, exosomes, or tumor-educated platelets (TEP) [37,38]. Additional information can be obtained by molecular characterization in addition to detecting these specific circulating factors' presence or concentration.

The aim of this narrative review, based on this context, is to study the current landscape and the future application of liquid biopsy in metastatic gastric cancer. Therefore, we present an outline of its potential role in the diagnosis of metastatic disease and monitoring of clonal dynamics during systemic therapies together with possible future applications.

2. The Role of Liquid Biopsy in Gastric Cancer in the Early Detection of Metastatic Disease

Circulating free DNA (cfDNA) in the blood is mainly derived from apoptotic cells, mostly from leukocytes [39]. Invasive primary tumors, circulating tumor cells, and metastatic sites may also be the source of circulating free DNA passively or actively releasing tumor DNA into the circulation [40]. In a case-control study, enrolling 30 gastric cancer patients and 34 healthy individuals, Kim et al. demonstrated that mean plasma cfDNA levels were the lowest among healthy subjects and highest in patients with advanced gastric cancer [41]. In a larger trial, among the subset of 18 gastric cancer patients, an association has been observed between the higher level of postoperative cfDNA and recurrence [42]. One study followed the dynamics of total circulating cell-free DNA (cfDNA) levels in 73 gastric cancer patients in the postoperative period. The authors reported that plasma cfDNA levels might increase for three months after surgery, then decrease [43]. Circulating tumor DNA (ctDNA) is usually only a small portion of circulating free DNA and has recently emerged to predict recurrence or relapse in several cancer types. For example, in breast cancer, serial ctDNA sampling is reliable in identifying tumor progression or distant metastatic disease. Circulating tumor DNA may be detected from the plasma up to 1 year before radiologically detectable disease progression [44]. Other similar studies have found that liquid biopsies can also be used for surveillance of other gastrointestinal malignancies. In addition to detecting relapsed or recurrent disease, the presence of ctDNA may influence the choice of adjuvant chemotherapy [45,46].

In gastric cancer patients undergoing gastrectomy, a Japanese study has monitored somatic mutations of the TP53 (tumor protein P53) gene in plasma that were initially present in (matched) tumor samples and ctDNA (detected in 3/42 patients). Elevated TP53-mutant ctDNA levels were associated with a higher risk of disease progression; however, the number of patients that the authors could track (n = 3) was relatively small [47]. The hypothesis of detecting molecular residual disease (MRD) by ctDNA has been prospectively investigated in 46 patients with stage I–III gastric cancer resected with curative purpose. Baseline ctDNA was positive in 45 percent of the plasma samples and independently associated with the primary tumor's extent (p = 0.006). Patients with early tumors with no gastric *muscularis propria* infiltration had no detectable pre-operative ctDNA (p = 0.024), irrespective of the involvement of the regional lymph nodes. Postoperative ctDNA detection was associated with disease recurrence in all patients in this study. The ctDNA positivity preceded radiological recurrence by a median of 6 months, and its positivity at any time postoperatively associated with worse disease-free and overall survival [48]. Another study analyzed the personalized cancer-specific rearrangements of 25 gastric cancer patients in the postoperative period for one year. While no correlation was found between ctDNA positivity preoperatively and cancer recurrence, the detection of ctDNA postoperatively was significantly associated with cancer recurrence in the first year ($p = 0.029$), and the median time observed between ctDNA detection and radiologic cancer recurrence was 4.05 months [49]. The Japanese MONSTAR-SCREEN study performed a serial ctDNA assay involving 540 patients with advanced solid tumors, of whom 133 had gastrointestinal (GI) tumors (48 patients had gastric tumors). Published results showed that ctDNA levels in GI tumors were significantly higher compared to non-GI tumors. One-third of the alterations detected in tumors were detected only in ctDNA, not in the tissue sample [50]. The SCRUM-Japan GOZILA (UMIN000016343) study examined the role of ctDNA-based comprehensive genomic profiling in facilitating the recruitment of patients for clinical trials compared to tissue-based detection. The use of liquid biopsy, according to the authors, reduced the lead time of testing to its one-third (11 vs. 33 days) and doubled the rate of patient enrolment into studies (9.5 vs. 4.1%). When detectable target alterations in tumors were determined using ct-DNA, the efficacy of the treatment was not inferior to that associated with tissue-based determination [51].

In gastric cancer, the detection of circulating tumor cells (CTCs) in peripheral blood may have clinical utility in monitoring tumor recurrence and metastatic spread [52]. According to a meta-analysis encompassing 2566 patients from 26 trials, the detection of CTCs was correlated with a substantial inferior effect on the patients' overall survival in all stages [53].

In a prospective trial that has enrolled 93 patients with resectable gastric cancer, patients with CTCs $\geq 5/7.5$ mL detected in postoperative blood samples had significantly inferior disease-free survival (DFS) and overall survival (OS) than those with a smaller number of CTCs. The increased number of CTCs after treatment correlated with early recurrence as well [54]. In addition to the detection and concentration of CTCs, additional methods can be used to characterize CTCs, including chromosomal abnormalities, cell surface markers, and receptors. One example of this is the CD44 positivity of the CTCs, which may have a negative prognostic significance in epithelial tumors. A prospective trial that enrolled 228 patients with resectable gastric cancer found that during the long-term follow-up, among the 99 cytokeratin-positive tumors, distant metastases were observed in half of the CD44-positive patients, compared with 19% of patients in the CD44-negative group [55]. CTCs often contain more than two copies of chromosome 8. Based on this feature, they can be identified by specific methods (e.g., SET-iFISH). According to Li et al., monitoring the therapeutic response in metastatic gastric cancer by tracking chromosome eight aneuploidy may be a useful tool [56,57]. Cancerous stem cell features, tumor cell invasiveness, and chemoresistance properties are all gained during the epithelial–mesenchymal transformation (EMT). The emergence of mesenchymal markers and a decline in epithelial markers accompany this transformation. As a result, epithelial markers are unable to identify CTCs undergoing EMT (EpCAM-based enrichment methods) [58–60].

The development of peritoneal metastases is relatively common, affecting one in two patients with gastric cancer. Predisposing factors for the development of peritoneal metastases are less well known. Tumor implantation, hematogenous spread, or exosomes have all been described as possible mechanisms for developing peritoneal metastasis [61]. Several authors have questioned the practical utility of using CTC identification for the early detection of peritoneal metastases. According to a prospective study involving 136 patients with advanced gastric cancer, the presence of peritoneal metastases did not correlate with the number of CTCs [57]. In contrast to CTCs, gastric cancer-released exosomes may play an essential part during the process of peritoneal metastatic spread in the transformation of the premetastatic microenvironment. Exosomes may weaken the mesothelial barrier by inducing apoptosis of the peritoneal cells and fibrosis [62]. The content of exosomes consists of proteins, lipids, and RNA (miRNA and mRNA) that are characteristic of the original cell secreting them, thus allowing further segmentation [63]. The composition of microRNA (miRNA) contained in exosomes may induce proliferation and has been reported to determine the site of metastasis formation (organotropism) [64,65]. In a bioinformatics study of exosomal miRNAs, three candidates were suggested as biomarkers for gastric cancer metastasis, namely miR-10b-5p for nodal metastasis, miR-101-3p for ovarian metastasis, and miR-143-5p for liver metastasis [66]. Another study described gastric cancer exosomes enriched with miR-106a being able to induce the formation of peritoneal metastases [67]. Among serosa-involved gastric cancer patients, reduced exosomal miR 29 levels in peritoneal lavage fluid or ascites are correlated with the enhanced risk of developing peritoneal metastases and worse OS [68]. In addition to exosomal information transfer from tumor cells, there is also crosstalk between healthy tissues and tumor cells. A proteomic study confirmed the role of omental exosomes in the growth of gastric cancer and the development of peritoneal metastases [69]. In the circulation, microRNAs can not only be found in exosomes or microvesicles, but also in a protein-bound state. MicroRNAs primarily bind to Argonaute2 (Ago2) protein or to High-density lipoprotein (HDL). As described in colon cancer, monitoring of Ago2 as well as Ago2-miRNA levels in the blood of gastric cancer patients may be a possible marker of tumor progression and response to chemotherapy [70–72].

3. The Role of Liquid Biopsy in Disease Monitoring

Circulating tumor microemboli (CTM) are clusters of CTCs in the blood, which are not only entirely composed of tumor cells. Non-cancerous cell types found in CTMs are white blood cells, fibroblasts, endothelial cells, pericytes, and platelets [73]. Several authors have described that tumor cells in CTM have specific phenotypic and molecular characteristics. In contrast to CTCs, no apoptotic signals are observed in CTMs, suggesting that the CTM clusters are not developing within the blood, but tumor cells are cleaved together from their site of origin, retaining their cell–cell connections [74]. In a study that enrolled 41 patients with treatment-naive metastatic gastric cancer, Zheng et al. examined the prognostic significance of CTM in peripheral blood samples. In a multivariate analysis, detectable CTM in the blood was an independent prognostic factor for shorter overall survival [58].

In the next section, we detail the role of liquid biopsy in the therapy follow-up and treatment resistance.

3.1. Liquid Biopsy in Response Monitoring or Detection of Resistance Mechanisms to Chemotherapy or Targeted Therapy

In recent years, monitoring the response to anti-cancer treatment has undergone a rapid change. Liquid biopsy has proven to be helpful in different solid malignancies for detecting new resistance mechanisms to chemotherapy and targeted therapy. However, data available for molecular mechanisms of resistance to gastric cancer treatment in this clinical setting is still scarce. Liquid biopsies may also help diagnose resistance to treatment before radiological progression and are gaining more relevance as a tool for optimizing patient care. The serum exosome proteome of metastatic gastric cancer patients was defined recently in detail by Ding et al. [75]. A study showed that, in gastric cell lines, exosomal Ribosomal Protein S3 (RPS3) secreted by cisplatin-resistant tumor cells could be taken up by cisplatin-sensitive cells and thus become chemoresistant (through activation of the PI3K-Akt-cofilin-1 signaling pathway) [76]. Another gastric cell-line experiment has identified the microRNA-501-5p (miR-501) as an inductor of doxorubicin resistance [77]. Overexpressed long noncoding RNAs (lncRNAs) may regulate chemotherapy resistance indirectly through a variety of mechanisms [78].

Two main targeted therapy groups are approved for their use in metastatic gastric cancer, namely anti-angiogenics and HER2 inhibitors. The retrospective biomarker analysis of the phase III REGARD trial examined the role of VEGFR2 (vascular endothelial growth factor receptor 2) expression on survival and the response to ramucirumab. This analysis ruled out any predictive value of the VEGFR2 expression levels and suggested a non-significant prognostic trend of shorter PFS among the high expressors. The analysis proved no relationship between the baseline concentration of serum circulating VEGF-C, VEGF-D, VEGFR1, VEGFR3 proteins, and the efficacy of ramucirumab treatment [79]. In the phase III AVAGAST trial, resistance to treatment with bevacizumab was seen among patients with lower baseline VEGF-A plasma levels and a trend towards lower survival rates. Another examined biomarker was baseline neuropilin-1 expression. Low initial neuropilin-1 expression was not only prognostic (indicating poor survival), but was predictive of the response to bevacizumab [80]. The novel VEGFR2 inhibitor apatinib appeared to antagonize the chemotherapy resistance by inhibiting the transport function of the multi-drug resistance proteins MDR1 and BCRP and could be considered in combination with platinum compounds or fluoropyrimidines. However, the clinical benefit of such strategies is still to be determined [81]. The anti-HER2 monoclonal antibody trastuzumab is a standard-of-care in treating HER-2 positive metastatic gastric cancer. Interestingly, according to a report, the examination of the HER2 status of circulating tumor cells (CTCs) reported higher positivity in CTCs (43%) compared to primary tumors (11%) [82].

Several resistance mechanisms against HER-2 inhibition have already been described [83]. One such mechanism is downregulation of the ERBB2 at a transcriptional level, leading to lower HER2 expression and failure of HER-2 inhibition strategies [84,85]. In vitro and in vivo models with gastric cancer cell lines show that the activation of several alternative pathways is an alternative mechanism for developing resistance to HER2 inhibition. The HER4–YAP1 axis is activated after chronic exposure to trastuzumab in cell cultures and translates into a higher rate of EMT and resistance to therapy. Blocking HER4 phosphorylation lowers the activity of YAP1, a downstream transcription factor directly involved in regulating the expression of HER2 and E-Cadherin [86]. Other alternative activations in resistant gastric cancer include another downstream effector of HER2, FGF3, and RAS/PI3K, and MAPK/ERK signaling pathways, mainly through the activation of other members of the ERBB family, such as EGFR or HER3. In another experimental model, simultaneous inhibition of these three receptors potentially overcame trastuzumab resistance [87]. The activation of the PI3K pathway also upregulates the factor known as metastasis-associated in colon cancer 1 (MACC1), which promotes the Warburg effect in cancer cells, resulting in a poor prognosis [88]. A clinical trial that investigated the utility of ctDNA for the detection of biomarkers of resistance to trastuzumab therapy was conducted on 39 patients with advanced gastric cancer. The authors showed a consistent correlation of clonal mutations between tumor and peripheral blood samples, identifying 32 mutations potentially related to trastuzumab resistance, and defined another valuable biomarker to monitor response to chemotherapy, the molecular Tumor Burden Index (mTBI), as an independent prognostic factor for progression-free survival [89]. The concept of serial plasma sampling for response monitoring has been proven by Wang et al. CtDNA reliably predicted antitumor response or tumor growth in 24 trastuzumab-treated patients. By tracking HER2 copy numbers' changes, the leading mechanism of primary or acquired resistance could be differentiated (in the case of acquired resistance, HER2 copy numbers decreased during progression, compared to baseline) [90].

3.2. Liquid Biopsy in Response Monitoring or Detection of Resistance Mechanisms to Immunotherapy

Immunotherapy treatment of gastric cancer has shown promising activity and recently demonstrated improved survival in selected patients with metastatic disease. In the first-line setting, the use of the anti-PD1 pembrolizumab was shown to be non-inferior to the platinum-based chemotherapy in patients with HER2-negative, PD-L1 positive tumors (i.e., Combined Positive Score [CPS] equal or higher than 1, intended as the PD-L1 positive fraction of tumor and/or immune-cell), in the KEYNOTE-062 trial [91]. Such an effect seemed driven by the subset of patients with highly immune-sensitive tumors for the presence of DNA microsatellite instability (MSI). The CheckMate 649 study has tested the combination of the anti-PD1 nivolumab and chemotherapy and demonstrated a consistent benefit in the patients with CPS > 5%, establishing a role in the first-line setting [92].

Among patients failing on first-line therapy, the use of the anti-PD1 pembrolizumab also showed to be superior to paclitaxel (CPS ≥ 1 subset) for the OS in the KEYNOTE-061 trial [25]. However, the PD-L1 expression in gastric cancer has not been demonstrated to be a reproducible or univocal marker, and many concerns have been reported in confirming a predictive role of the PD-L1 CPS in selecting patients for immunotherapy [93,94]. Therefore, identifying predictive biomarkers for cancer immunotherapy is highly desirable, including less invasive diagnostic procedures and dynamic monitoring assays. The informative potential of the ctDNA in gastric tumors has been proposed for the upfront selection of patients or disease-course monitoring, either for qualitative (e.g., molecular typization) and quantitative (e.g., ctDNA change) measurements [95]. This concept is relatively new and only recently implemented in clinical research.

An emerging biomarker for tumor-agnostic utilization is the tumor mutational burden (TMB) [96]. TMB has been identified as a marker of improved survival in patients with gastric cancer receiving immune-checkpoint inhibitors [97,98].

While tissue-assessed TMB has been broadly implemented in clinical practice and research, blood-based assays (bTMB) are technically more challenging, representing an essential barrier for their validation and clinical uptake [99]. In addition, the predictive role of TMB seems partially overlapping and less significant than microsatellite instability (MSI), positivity to Epstein–Barr virus (EBV), and PD-L1 CPS [100]. These three markers are established prognostic and predictive indicators in gastric cancer [26,101–103]. First, the initial attempts to test circulating cancer cells for PD-L1 expression revealed challenges to differentiate them from macrophages, which might express this biomarker and be misinterpreted. Accordingly, the patient selection based on non-tissue PD-L1 assessments seems not ready for clinical utilization and requires technology improvements [104]. Exosomal PD-L1 in metastatic gastric cancer has been discovered to be an independent predictor for OS and was negatively correlated with CD4+ or CD8+ T-cell count and granzyme B levels [105,106]. Ishiba et al. examined the possibility of detecting ctRNA in the blood of 760 patients with solid tumors, including 44 cases of gastric cancer. Their study showed that it is possible to determine the mRNA of the PD-L1 gene, and quantification of PD-L1 gene expression is feasible. The authors suggest that ctRNA isolated from blood may be a potential alternative to tissue PD-L1 assay [107]. Second, applications of liquid biopsy have also been reported across several tumor types to evaluate the status of the microsatellites [108]. The ctDNA sequencing technologies have demonstrated a good concordance with the tissue-MSI assessment: 99.5% (95% CI, 98.7–99.8) and 87% (95% CI, 77–93) for low- and high-MSI, respectively [109]. Third, for the EBV status ascertainment via liquid biopsy, the evidence is less robust. Viral ctDNA can be detected in patients with EBV-positive gastric cancer by quantitative real-time polymerase chain reaction (PCR), with reasonable specificity (97%) and modest sensitivity (71%)—and mostly in patients with larger primary tumors [110]. Essentially, PCR assay detects EBV viremia in the context of EBV infection and gastric cancer, but this is not always the case for EBV-immortalized cancer cells. However, the demonstration of latent EBV in ctDNA from cancer cells is more challenging, as these cells are commonly apoptotic or necrotic, and the EBV cannot be consistently demonstrated, often not preserved and destroyed [111]. However, methylation genome markers that are recurrently present in EBV-positive tumors have been identified as surrogate indicators of EBV and may help predict the immune response [112].

Recently, the first analysis of the phase II clinical INSPIRE trial (NCT02644369; drug: pembrolizumab) has been provided. This study assesses changes between genomic and immune biomarkers with tissue- and liquid biopsy-based assays at baseline, during treatment and at progression. In the first analysis, the investigators identified tumor-specific mutations at baseline from tissue and developed a tumor-informed personalized ctDNA assay for the on-treatment monitoring [113]. The investigators confirmed a baseline prognostic significance of the ctDNA with immunotherapy, as reported in other studies, including gastric cancer cohorts [114,115]. More interestingly, the study demonstrated an informative role of the ctDNA changes to discriminate between actual disease progression and radiological pseudo-progression: when ctDNA was rising, patients were unlikely to derive a benefit from immunotherapy and, vice versa, ctDNA decline was associated with a shrinkage of the actual tumor burden [113]. This observation seems to suggest the role of liquid biopsy to confirm the disease progression and initiate immediate treatment changes in patients more unlikely to derive a clinical benefit [116]. Interestingly, ctDNA clearance was associated with sustained and durable responses to pembrolizumab, although this occurred in only a subset of patients. The radiographic response was also preceded by ctDNA clearance. Although Bratman et al. provided the first evidence for the clinical utility of ctDNA in patients receiving immunotherapy, unfortunately, it is not clear whether the study has included gastric cancer patients [113].

4. Ongoing Clinical Trials Using Liquid Biopsy Approaches for Gastric Cancer

Although the impact of liquid biopsy in gastric cancer is thought to be immature, significant progress is ongoing in almost all areas of gastric cancer (Table 1). The Danish CURE study is a continuous prospective cohort (NCT04576858) designed to examine the relevance of ctDNA determination in the plasma of patients with gastroesophageal cancer in different clinical cohorts: (1) Scheduled for surgical resection and perioperative chemotherapy; (2) Neoadjuvant chemoradiotherapy followed by surgical resection; (3) Definitive chemoradiotherapy with curative intent; (4) Systemic treatment to extend the patient's life; and (5) Palliative treatment without the use of chemotherapy. A Chinese prospective cohort study (NCT04000425) uses serial sampling to evaluate the clinical use of ctDNA as a potential indicator of minimal residual disease (MRD) after radical gastrectomy. One primary endpoint of the trial is ctDNA clearance among patients with positive postoperative ctDNA; in these patient segments, the clearance of ctDNA could reflect a response to adjuvant chemotherapy. The other primary endpoint of the trial would validate the use of ctDNA for the detection of recurrent disease, measuring the time between the first ctDNA positivity and the occurrence of clinically detectable disease recurrence.

Several clinical studies from China investigate whether serial ctDNA mutation profiling may support the early diagnosis of the disease (NCT04665687) or predict recurrence in the postoperative setting (NCT02887612). Since the KEYNOTE-012 study investigated the efficacy of pembrolizumab in patients with advanced PD-L1 positive gastric cancer, a study is being performed to predict the efficacy of ctDNA for the immune-checkpoint blockade in advanced gastric cancer (NCT04053725). Three phase II trials are in progress, including one study investigating adjuvant doublet pembrolizumab and trastuzumab versus trastuzumab alone in patients with HER2+ esophagogastric cancer with persistent ctDNA following curative surgery (NCT04510285). Moreover, another phase II trial will explore the clinical value of dynamic detection of circulating tumor cells (CTCs), ctDNA, and cell-free DNA (cfDNA) in neoadjuvant chemotherapy and surgery for resectable or locally advanced gastric or gastroesophageal junction cancer settings (NCT03957564). Promisingly, GAS-THER2 is another phase II trial evaluating the efficacy of adding trastuzumab to standard chemotherapy in patients with advanced HER2-negative gastric cancer and HER2-positive expression in CTCs (NCT04168931). The role of ctDNA and CTCs as a biomarker for cytoreductive surgery combined with hyperthermic intraperitoneal chemotherapy and systemic chemotherapy in gastric cancer with regional peritoneal metastasis is also being investigated in a multicenter and single-arm and phase III study (NCT03023436).

Table 1. Ongoing clinical trials using liquid biopsy approaches for gastric cancer.

Study Setting	Study Type (NCT Number and Trial Name)	Liquid Biopsy Approach	Estimated Enrollment	Primary Objectives	Estimated Primary Completion Date [1]
Early stage	Prospective cohort (NCT04665687)	ctDNA	1730	To differentiate early gastric cancer and precancerous adenoma and predict recurrence by finding biomarkers through molecular profiling	December 2022
Neoadjuvant	Phase II (NCT03957564)	ctDNA, CTCs, and cfDNA	40	To evaluate CTC numbers/types, ctDNA mutation rate, cfDNA concentration and tumor response to neoadjuvant chemotherapy and surgery for resectable or locally advanced gastric or gastro-esophageal junction cancer patients	May 2024
Adjuvant	Phase II trial (NCT04510285)	ctDNA	48	To evaluate differences in 6-month ctDNA clearance rate in HER2+ esophagogastric cancer with persistent ctDNA following curative surgery when treated with "second adjuvant" trastuzumab with or without pembrolizumab	August 2022
Adjuvant and recurrence detection	Prospective cohort (NCT04000425)	ctDNA	55	To evaluate the role of ctDNA clearance during adjuvant chemotherapy (among patients with detectable ctDNA), and to define risk of recurrence in patients with newly detected positive ctDNA after radical gastrectomy	May 2021
Recurrence detection	Prospective cohort (NCT02887612)	ctDNA	200	To evaluate the positive predictive value of serum ctDNA positivity in the prediction of relapse after surgery in early and intermediate stage gastric cancer	June 2020
Advanced	Phase III trial (NCT03023436)	ctDNA and CTCs	220	To assess of ctDNA and CTC alterations as potential biomarkers for debulking surgery combined with hyperthermic intraperitoneal chemotherapy and systemic chemotherapy in patients with gastric cancer and peritoneal dissemination (as a secondary outcome measure)	June 2022
Advanced	Phase II (NCT04168931 GASTHER2)	CTCs	85	To investigate whether HER2-expressing CTCs may be suitable for prediction of response in patients with relapsed or metastatic gastric cancer who are histologically HER2-negative and treated with trastuzumab combination chemotherapy	January 2025
Advanced	Prospective cohort (NCT04053725)	ctDNA	200	To investigate the predictive dynamics of ctDNA mutation changes during immune-checkpoint blockade of gastric cancer patients	November 2021
All settings (from neoadjuvant to advanced)	Prospective cohort (NCT04576858 CURE)	ctDNA	1950	Prediction of prognosis and therapy response	July 2025

[1] per ClinicalTrials.gov. (Accessed 24 March 2021).

5. Discussion

There is a clear need for novel non-invasive diagnostic methods in both non-metastatic and metastatic gastric cancer settings, which may also capture tumor heterogeneity [117–120]. A real challenge in the early detection of gastric cancer is that its diagnosis requires an invasive procedure, and most patients are asymptomatic at an early stage [121]. Liquid biopsy may play a prominent role in early diagnosis in the future. Two studies show that elevated postoperative cfDNA may be associated with a higher risk of recurrence [42,43]. Several reports have described that ctDNA may be used as a marker of MRD and may influence the choice of adjuvant chemotherapy, and may allow personalized monitoring of progression [45–47]. A strong relationship between the detectability of CTCs and a substantial inferior effect on the patients' overall survival in all stages has been reported in the literature. CTCs may also help identify high-risk patients by detecting minimal residual disease (MRD) may provide an option for risk stratifying and identifying the patients at the highest risk of recurrence [53,122]. In summary, in the nonmetastatic setting, several data show that liquid biopsy may provide valuable biomarkers to diagnose cancer early, estimate tumor volume, determine the completeness of the tumor resection and prognosis. Identification and detailed analysis of cancer-derived exosomes may be useful in identifying tumor-preferred metastatic sites, outlining the potential for a more active, organ-focused follow-up. Accurate knowledge of exosomal data transfer may open new perspectives in tumor diagnosis, monitoring of therapy, and non-invasive follow-up of the patient and may hold new therapeutic options in the future.

In the metastatic setting, the levels of cfDNA show a positive correlation with tumor burden [41]. There is evidence that detectable CTM in the blood among metastatic patients was an independent prognostic factor for shorter overall survival [58]. Gastric cancer-derived exosomal microRNAs and clonal mutations or CNVs detectable in ctDNA may contribute resistance to chemotherapy or HER2 inhibition, respectively [76–78,89,90,123]. Although there are limitations to CTC-based PD-L1 verification, there are other ways to determine PD-L1: from exosomal PD-L1 or to detect and quantify PD-L1 mRNA from ctRNA [104,105,107]. Data are conflicting and limited around cfDNA-based EBV detection and epigenomic applications [110,111]. If gastric cancer patients were also included in the phase II INSPIRE clinical trial, an analysis of the study may provide valuable information on tumor-based, personalized monitoring of the disease by ctDNA. Monitoring of cfDNA provided valuable information to differentiate between actual disease progression and radiological pseudo-progression, thus opening a window for immediate treatment changes in non-responders [113,116].

Most ongoing clinical trials address the pre- and post- surgical interval; two trials focus on the metastatic setting. The phase II GASTHER2 NCT04168931 trial examines the HER2 status of CTCs as a predictor of response to standard therapy combined with trastuzumab. The NCT04053725 trial investigates the predictive dynamics of serial ctDNA sampling during the immune-checkpoint blockade.

6. Conclusions

Recent revolutionary advancements in technology and the incorporation of genetic tumor characterization have significantly improved the possibilities of forecasting the prognosis of patients with metastatic gastric cancer, but the future holds even more excitement. Integrating broad tumor genomic characterization, dynamic monitoring of responses by the techniques of liquid biopsy will allow the implementation of adaptive, real-time treatment modifications in precision oncology. Clinical validation and standardization of novel liquid biopsy procedures are also necessary before being widely used in everyday practice. Although initial experiments analyzing liquid biopsies look very promising in patients with advanced gastric cancer, more prospective studies are needed to understand the molecular mechanisms behind resistance to targeted therapies. Applications of liquid biopsy to select and monitor patients receiving immunotherapy seem promising for identifying established and innovative qualitative–quantitative biomarkers in the 'circulome' and prompt treatment change in the primary- and secondary-resistant tumors. It seems that if the liquid biopsy and the immunotherapy revolution in cancer treatment eventually meet, they can facilitate patient compliance and improve overall outcomes.

Author Contributions: D.T. gathered data about immunotherapy, S.C.A. and A.S. collected data with targeted therapy, A.O., F.S. and B.S.H. accumulated data with chemotherapy, S.H. and K.E.B. reviewed clinical trial data, B.S.H. provided further help with references, C.G.L. wrote the paper. All authors have read and agreed to the published version of the manuscript.

Funding: This research received no external funding

Data Availability Statement: No new data were created or analyzed in this study. Data sharing is not applicable to this article.

Conflicts of Interest: C.G.L. reports employment by Bristol Myers Squibb. Other authors declare no conflict of interest.

References

1. Dasari, A.; Morris, V.K.; Allegra, C.J.; Atreya, C.; Benson, A.B., 3rd; Boland, P.; Chung, K.; Copur, M.S.; Corcoran, R.B.; Deming, D.A.; et al. ctDNA applications and integration in colorectal cancer: An NCI Colon and Rectal-Anal Task Forces whitepaper. *Nat. Rev. Clin. Oncol.* **2020**, *17*, 757–770. [CrossRef] [PubMed]
2. Ignatiadis, M.; Sledge, G.W.; Jeffrey, S.S. Liquid biopsy enters the clinic—Implementation issues and future challenges. *Nat. Rev. Clin. Oncol.* **2021**. [CrossRef] [PubMed]
3. Rodríguez, J.; Avila, J.; Rolfo, C.; Ruíz-Patiño, A.; Russo, A.; Ricaurte, L.; Ordóñez-Reyes, C.; Arrieta, O.; Zatarain-Barrón, Z.L.; Recondo, G.; et al. When Tissue is an Issue the Liquid Biopsy is Nonissue: A Review. *Oncol. Ther.* **2021**. [CrossRef]
4. Bray, F.; Ferlay, J.; Soerjomataram, I.; Siegel, R.L.; Torre, L.A.; Jemal, A. Global cancer statistics 2018: GLOBOCAN estimates of incidence and mortality worldwide for 36 cancers in 185 countries. *CA Cancer J. Clin.* **2018**, *68*, 394–424. [CrossRef] [PubMed]
5. World Health Organization. Global Cancer Observatory. Available online: https://gco.iarc.fr/tomorrow/en/dataviz/isotype?cancers=7&single_unit=50000 (accessed on 14 February 2021).
6. Gobbi, P.G.; Bergonzi, M.; Pozzoli, D.; Villano, L.; Vanoli, A.; Corbella, F.; Dionigi, P.; Corazza, G.R. Tumors of the gastroesophageal junction have intermediate prognosis compared to tumors of the esophagus and stomach, but share the same clinical determinants. *Oncol. Lett.* **2011**, *2*, 503–507. [CrossRef] [PubMed]
7. Cellini, F.; Morganti, A.G.; Di Matteo, F.M.; Mattiucci, G.C.; Valentini, V. Clinical management of gastroesophageal junction tumors: Past and recent evidences for the role of radiotherapy in the multidisciplinary approach. *Radiat. Oncol.* **2014**, *9*, 45. [CrossRef] [PubMed]
8. Cancer Genome Atlas Research Network; Analysis Working Group: Asan University; BC Cancer Agency; Brigham and Women's Hospital; Broad Institute; Brown University; Case Western Reserve University; Dana-Farber Cancer Institute; Duke University; Greater Poland Cancer Centre; et al. Integrated genomic characterization of oesophageal carcinoma. *Nature* **2017**, *541*, 169–175. [CrossRef] [PubMed]
9. Kim, J.W.; Nam, K.H.; Ahn, S.H.; Park, D.J.; Kim, H.H.; Kim, S.H.; Chang, H.; Lee, J.O.; Kim, Y.J.; Lee, H.S.; et al. Prognostic implications of immunosuppressive protein expression in tumors as well as immune cell infiltration within the tumor microenvironment in gastric cancer. *Gastric Cancer* **2016**, *19*, 42–52. [CrossRef] [PubMed]
10. Zhang, L.; Qiu, M.; Jin, Y.; Ji, J.; Li, B.; Wang, X.; Yan, S.; Xu, R.; Yang, D. Programmed cell death ligand 1 (PD-L1) expression on gastric cancer and its relationship with clinicopathologic factors. *Int. J. Clin. Exp. Pathol.* **2015**, *8*, 11084–11091. [PubMed]
11. Bang, Y.J.; Van Cutsem, E.; Feyereislova, A.; Chung, H.C.; Shen, L.; Sawaki, A.; Lordick, F.; Ohtsu, A.; Omuro, Y.; Satoh, T.; et al. Trastuzumab in combination with chemotherapy versus chemotherapy alone for treatment of HER2-positive advanced gastric or gastro-oesophageal junction cancer (ToGA): A phase 3, open-label, randomised controlled trial. *Lancet* **2010**, *376*, 687–697. [CrossRef]
12. Boku, N. HER2-positive gastric cancer. *Gastric Cancer* **2014**, *17*, 1–12. [CrossRef] [PubMed]
13. Zhu, L.; Li, Z.; Wang, Y.; Zhang, C.; Liu, Y.; Qu, X. Microsatellite instability and survival in gastric cancer: A systematic review and meta-analysis. *Mol. Clin. Oncol.* **2015**, *3*, 699–705. [CrossRef] [PubMed]
14. Smyth, E.C.; Wotherspoon, A.; Peckitt, C.; Gonzalez, D.; Hulkki-Wilson, S.; Eltahir, Z.; Fassan, M.; Rugge, M.; Valeri, N.; Okines, A.; et al. Mismatch Repair Deficiency, Microsatellite Instability, and Survival: An Exploratory Analysis of the Medical Research Council Adjuvant Gastric Infusional Chemotherapy (MAGIC) Trial. *JAMA Oncol.* **2017**, *3*, 1197–1203. [CrossRef] [PubMed]
15. Kohlruss, M.; Grosser, B.; Krenauer, M.; Slotta-Huspenina, J.; Jesinghaus, M.; Blank, S.; Novotny, A.; Reiche, M.; Schmidt, T.; Ismani, L.; et al. Prognostic implication of molecular subtypes and response to neoadjuvant chemotherapy in 760 gastric carcinomas: Role of Epstein-Barr virus infection and high- and low-microsatellite instability. *J. Pathol. Clin. Res.* **2019**, *5*, 227–239. [CrossRef] [PubMed]

16. Polom, K.; Marano, L.; Marrelli, D.; De Luca, R.; Roviello, G.; Savelli, V.; Tan, P.; Roviello, F. Meta-analysis of microsatellite instability in relation to clinicopathological characteristics and overall survival in gastric cancer. *Br. J. Surg.* **2018**, *105*, 159–167. [CrossRef] [PubMed]
17. Puliga, E.; Corso, S.; Pietrantonio, F.; Giordano, S. Microsatellite instability in Gastric Cancer: Between lights and shadows. *Cancer Treat. Rev.* **2021**, *95*, 102175. [CrossRef]
18. Ma, C.; Patel, K.; Singhi, A.D.; Ren, B.; Zhu, B.; Shaikh, F.; Sun, W. Programmed Death-Ligand 1 Expression Is Common in Gastric Cancer Associated With Epstein-Barr Virus or Microsatellite Instability. *Am. J. Surg. Pathol.* **2016**, *40*, 1496–1506. [CrossRef] [PubMed]
19. Derks, S.; Liao, X.; Chiaravalli, A.M.; Xu, X.; Camargo, M.C.; Solcia, E.; Sessa, F.; Fleitas, T.; Freeman, G.J.; Rodig, S.J.; et al. Abundant PD-L1 expression in Epstein-Barr Virus-infected gastric cancers. *Oncotarget* **2016**, *7*, 32925–32932. [CrossRef]
20. Fuchs, C.S.; Doi, T.; Jang, R.W.; Muro, K.; Satoh, T.; Machado, M.; Sun, W.; Jalal, S.I.; Shah, M.A.; Metges, J.P.; et al. Safety and Efficacy of Pembrolizumab Monotherapy in Patients With Previously Treated Advanced Gastric and Gastroesophageal Junction Cancer: Phase 2 Clinical KEYNOTE-059 Trial. *JAMA Oncol.* **2018**, *4*, e180013. [CrossRef]
21. Shitara, K.; Özgüroğlu, M.; Bang, Y.J.; Di Bartolomeo, M.; Mandalà, M.; Ryu, M.H.; Fornaro, L.; Olesiński, T.; Caglevic, C.; Chung, H.C.; et al. Pembrolizumab versus paclitaxel for previously treated, advanced gastric or gastro-oesophageal junction cancer (KEYNOTE-061): A randomised, open-label, controlled, phase 3 trial. *Lancet* **2018**, *392*, 123–133. [CrossRef]
22. Tabernero, J.; Cutsem, E.V.; Bang, Y.-J.; Fuchs, C.S.; Wyrwicz, L.; Lee, K.W.; Kudaba, I.; Garrido, M.; Chung, H.C.; Salguero, H.R.C.; et al. Pembrolizumab with or without chemotherapy versus chemotherapy for advanced gastric or gastroesophageal junction (G/GEJ) adenocarcinoma: The phase III KEYNOTE-062 study. *J. Clin. Oncol.* **2019**, *37*, LBA4007. [CrossRef]
23. National Comprehensive Cancer Network. Gastric Cancer (Version 1.2021). Available online: https://www.nccn.org/professionals/physician_gls/default.aspx#gastric (accessed on 21 February 2021).
24. Shitara, K.; Özgüroğlu, M.; Bang, Y.-J.; Bartolomeo, M.D.; Mandalà, M.; Ryu, M.-h.; Vivaldi, C.; Olesinski, T.; Chung, H.C.; Muro, K.; et al. The association of tissue tumor mutational burden (tTMB) using the Foundation Medicine genomic platform with efficacy of pembrolizumab versus paclitaxel in patients (pts) with gastric cancer (GC) from KEYNOTE-061. *J. Clin. Oncol.* **2020**, *38*, 4537. [CrossRef]
25. Fuchs, C.S.; Özgüroğlu, M.; Bang, Y.-J.; Bartolomeo, M.D.; Mandalà, M.; Ryu, M.-h.; Fornaro, L.; Olesinski, T.; Caglevic, C.; Chung, H.C.; et al. Pembrolizumab versus paclitaxel for previously treated patients with PD-L1–positive advanced gastric or gastroesophageal junction cancer (GC): Update from the phase III KEYNOTE-061 trial. *J. Clin. Oncol.* **2020**, *38*, 4503. [CrossRef]
26. Kim, S.T.; Cristescu, R.; Bass, A.J.; Kim, K.M.; Odegaard, J.I.; Kim, K.; Liu, X.Q.; Sher, X.; Jung, H.; Lee, M.; et al. Comprehensive molecular characterization of clinical responses to PD-1 inhibition in metastatic gastric cancer. *Nat. Med.* **2018**, *24*, 1449–1458. [CrossRef]
27. Mandel, P.; Metais, P. [Nuclear Acids In Human Blood Plasma]. *Comptes Rendus Seances Soc. Biol. Fil.* **1948**, *142*, 241–243.
28. Leon, S.A.; Shapiro, B.; Sklaroff, D.M.; Yaros, M.J. Free DNA in the serum of cancer patients and the effect of therapy. *Cancer Res.* **1977**, *37*, 646–650.
29. Sorenson, G.D.; Pribish, D.M.; Valone, F.H.; Memoli, V.A.; Bzik, D.J.; Yao, S.L. Soluble normal and mutated DNA sequences from single-copy genes in human blood. *Cancer Epidemiol. Biomark. Prev.* **1994**, *3*, 67–71.
30. Vasioukhin, V.; Anker, P.; Maurice, P.; Lyautey, J.; Lederrey, C.; Stroun, M. Point mutations of the N-ras gene in the blood plasma DNA of patients with myelodysplastic syndrome or acute myelogenous leukaemia. *Br. J. Haematol.* **1994**, *86*, 774–779. [CrossRef] [PubMed]
31. Chen, X.Q.; Stroun, M.; Magnenat, J.L.; Nicod, L.P.; Kurt, A.M.; Lyautey, J.; Lederrey, C.; Anker, P. Microsatellite alterations in plasma DNA of small cell lung cancer patients. *Nat. Med.* **1996**, *2*, 1033–1035. [CrossRef]
32. Diehl, F.; Schmidt, K.; Choti, M.A.; Romans, K.; Goodman, S.; Li, M.; Thornton, K.; Agrawal, N.; Sokoll, L.; Szabo, S.A.; et al. Circulating mutant DNA to assess tumor dynamics. *Nat. Med.* **2008**, *14*, 985–990. [CrossRef] [PubMed]
33. Wang, Y.; Springer, S.; Mulvey, C.L.; Silliman, N.; Schaefer, J.; Sausen, M.; James, N.; Rettig, E.M.; Guo, T.; Pickering, C.R.; et al. Detection of somatic mutations and HPV in the saliva and plasma of patients with head and neck squamous cell carcinomas. *Sci. Transl. Med.* **2015**, *7*, 293ra104. [CrossRef] [PubMed]
34. Kimura, H.; Fujiwara, Y.; Sone, T.; Kunitoh, H.; Tamura, T.; Kasahara, K.; Nishio, K. EGFR mutation status in tumour-derived DNA from pleural effusion fluid is a practical basis for predicting the response to gefitinib. *Br. J. Cancer* **2006**, *95*, 1390–1395. [CrossRef] [PubMed]
35. Diehl, F.; Schmidt, K.; Durkee, K.H.; Moore, K.J.; Goodman, S.N.; Shuber, A.P.; Kinzler, K.W.; Vogelstein, B. Analysis of mutations in DNA isolated from plasma and stool of colorectal cancer patients. *Gastroenterology* **2008**, *135*, 489–498. [CrossRef] [PubMed]
36. De Mattos-Arruda, L.; Mayor, R.; Ng, C.K.Y.; Weigelt, B.; Martínez-Ricarte, F.; Torrejon, D.; Oliveira, M.; Arias, A.; Raventos, C.; Tang, J.; et al. Cerebrospinal fluid-derived circulating tumour DNA better represents the genomic alterations of brain tumours than plasma. *Nat. Commun.* **2015**, *6*, 8839. [CrossRef]
37. Poulet, G.; Massias, J.; Taly, V. Liquid Biopsy: General Concepts. *Acta Cytol.* **2019**, *63*, 449–455. [CrossRef]
38. In 't Veld, S.G.J.G.; Wurdinger, T. Tumor-educated platelets. *Blood* **2019**, *133*, 2359–2364. [CrossRef]
39. Heitzer, E.; Auinger, L.; Speicher, M.R. Cell-Free DNA and Apoptosis: How Dead Cells Inform About the Living. *Trends Mol. Med.* **2020**, *26*, 519–528. [CrossRef] [PubMed]

40. Schwarzenbach, H.; Hoon, D.S.; Pantel, K. Cell-free nucleic acids as biomarkers in cancer patients. *Nat. Rev. Cancer* **2011**, *11*, 426–437. [CrossRef] [PubMed]
41. Kim, K.; Shin, D.G.; Park, M.K.; Baik, S.H.; Kim, T.H.; Kim, S.; Lee, S. Circulating cell-free DNA as a promising biomarker in patients with gastric cancer: Diagnostic validity and significant reduction of cfDNA after surgical resection. *Ann. Surg. Treat. Res.* **2014**, *86*, 136–142. [CrossRef]
42. Lan, Y.T.; Chen, M.H.; Fang, W.L.; Hsieh, C.C.; Lin, C.H.; Jhang, F.Y.; Yang, S.H.; Lin, J.K.; Chen, W.S.; Jiang, J.K.; et al. Clinical relevance of cell-free DNA in gastrointestinal tract malignancy. *Oncotarget* **2017**, *8*, 3009–3017. [CrossRef]
43. Pu, W.Y.; Zhang, R.; Xiao, L.; Wu, Y.Y.; Gong, W.; Lv, X.D.; Zhong, F.Y.; Zhuang, Z.X.; Bai, X.M.; Li, K.; et al. Prediction of cancer progression in a group of 73 gastric cancer patients by circulating cell-free DNA. *BMC Cancer* **2016**, *16*, 943. [CrossRef] [PubMed]
44. Olsson, E.; Winter, C.; George, A.; Chen, Y.; Howlin, J.; Tang, M.H.; Dahlgren, M.; Schulz, R.; Grabau, D.; van Westen, D.; et al. Serial monitoring of circulating tumor DNA in patients with primary breast cancer for detection of occult metastatic disease. *EMBO Mol. Med.* **2015**, *7*, 1034–1047. [CrossRef] [PubMed]
45. Reinert, T.; Schøler, L.V.; Thomsen, R.; Tobiasen, H.; Vang, S.; Nordentoft, I.; Lamy, P.; Kannerup, A.S.; Mortensen, F.V.; Stribolt, K.; et al. Analysis of circulating tumour DNA to monitor disease burden following colorectal cancer surgery. *Gut* **2016**, *65*, 625–634. [CrossRef] [PubMed]
46. Tie, J.; Cohen, J.D.; Wang, Y.; Christie, M.; Simons, K.; Lee, M.; Wong, R.; Kosmider, S.; Ananda, S.; McKendrick, J.; et al. Circulating Tumor DNA Analyses as Markers of Recurrence Risk and Benefit of Adjuvant Therapy for Stage III Colon Cancer. *JAMA Oncol.* **2019**, *5*, 1710–1717. [CrossRef] [PubMed]
47. Hamakawa, T.; Kukita, Y.; Kurokawa, Y.; Miyazaki, Y.; Takahashi, T.; Yamasaki, M.; Miyata, H.; Nakajima, K.; Taniguchi, K.; Takiguchi, S.; et al. Monitoring gastric cancer progression with circulating tumour DNA. *Br. J. Cancer* **2015**, *112*, 352–356. [CrossRef]
48. Yang, J.; Gong, Y.; Lam, V.K.; Shi, Y.; Guan, Y.; Zhang, Y.; Ji, L.; Chen, Y.; Zhao, Y.; Qian, F.; et al. Deep sequencing of circulating tumor DNA detects molecular residual disease and predicts recurrence in gastric cancer. *Cell Death Dis.* **2020**, *11*, 346. [CrossRef]
49. Kim, Y.-W.; Kim, Y.-H.; Song, Y.; Kim, H.-S.; Sim, H.W.; Poojan, S.; Eom, B.W.; Kook, M.-C.; Joo, J.; Hong, K.-M. Monitoring circulating tumor DNA by analyzing personalized cancer-specific rearrangements to detect recurrence in gastric cancer. *Exp. Mol. Med.* **2019**, *51*, 1–10. [CrossRef]
50. Nakamura, Y.; Fujisawa, T.; Kadowaki, S.; Takahashi, N.; Goto, M.; Yoshida, K.; Kawakami, T.; Esaki, T.; Oki, E.; Nishida, N.; et al. Characteristics of genomic alterations in circulating tumor DNA (ctDNA) in patients (Pts) with advanced gastrointestinal (GI) cancers in nationwide large-scale ctDNA screening:SCRUM-Japan Monstar-Screen. *J. Clin. Oncol.* **2021**, *39*, 106. [CrossRef]
51. Nakamura, Y.; Taniguchi, H.; Ikeda, M.; Bando, H.; Kato, K.; Morizane, C.; Esaki, T.; Komatsu, Y.; Kawamoto, Y.; Takahashi, N.; et al. Clinical utility of circulating tumor DNA sequencing in advanced gastrointestinal cancer: SCRUM-Japan GI-SCREEN and GOZILA studies. *Nat. Med.* **2020**, *26*, 1859–1864. [CrossRef] [PubMed]
52. Pantel, K.; Alix-Panabières, C. Liquid biopsy in 2016: Circulating tumour cells and cell-free DNA in gastrointestinal cancer. *Nat. Rev. Gastroenterol. Hepatol.* **2017**, *14*, 73–74. [CrossRef] [PubMed]
53. Huang, X.; Gao, P.; Sun, J.; Chen, X.; Song, Y.; Zhao, J.; Xu, H.; Wang, Z. Clinicopathological and prognostic significance of circulating tumor cells in patients with gastric cancer: A meta-analysis. *Int. J. Cancer* **2015**, *136*, 21–33. [CrossRef]
54. Zhang, Q.; Shan, F.; Li, Z.; Gao, J.; Li, Y.; Shen, L.; Ji, J.; Lu, M. A prospective study on the changes and clinical significance of pre-operative and post-operative circulating tumor cells in resectable gastric cancer. *J. Transl. Med.* **2018**, *16*, 171. [CrossRef] [PubMed]
55. Szczepanik, A.; Sierzega, M.; Drabik, G.; Pituch-Noworolska, A.; Kołodziejczyk, P.; Zembala, M. CD44(+) cytokeratin-positive tumor cells in blood and bone marrow are associated with poor prognosis of patients with gastric cancer. *Gastric Cancer* **2019**, *22*, 264–272. [CrossRef] [PubMed]
56. Li, Y.; Zhang, X.; Ge, S.; Gao, J.; Gong, J.; Lu, M.; Zhang, Q.; Cao, Y.; Wang, D.D.; Lin, P.P.; et al. Clinical significance of phenotyping and karyotyping of circulating tumor cells in patients with advanced gastric cancer. *Oncotarget* **2014**, *5*, 6594–6602. [CrossRef] [PubMed]
57. Li, Y.; Gong, J.; Zhang, Q.; Lu, Z.; Gao, J.; Li, Y.; Cao, Y.; Shen, L. Dynamic monitoring of circulating tumour cells to evaluate therapeutic efficacy in advanced gastric cancer. *Br. J. Cancer* **2016**, *114*, 138–145. [CrossRef] [PubMed]
58. Zheng, X.; Fan, L.; Zhou, P.; Ma, H.; Huang, S.; Yu, D.; Zhao, L.; Yang, S.; Liu, J.; Huang, A.; et al. Detection of Circulating Tumor Cells and Circulating Tumor Microemboli in Gastric Cancer. *Transl. Oncol.* **2017**, *10*, 431–441. [CrossRef] [PubMed]
59. Gorges, T.M.; Tinhofer, I.; Drosch, M.; Röse, L.; Zollner, T.M.; Krahn, T.; von Ahsen, O. Circulating tumour cells escape from EpCAM-based detection due to epithelial-to-mesenchymal transition. *BMC Cancer* **2012**, *12*, 178. [CrossRef] [PubMed]
60. Gazzaniga, P.; Naso, G.; Gradilone, A.; Cortesi, E.; Gandini, O.; Gianni, W.; Fabbri, M.A.; Vincenzi, B.; di Silverio, F.; Frati, L.; et al. Chemosensitivity profile assay of circulating cancer cells: Prognostic and predictive value in epithelial tumors. *Int. J. Cancer* **2010**, *126*, 2437–2447. [CrossRef] [PubMed]
61. Wang, Z.; Chen, J.-q.; Liu, J.-l.; Tian, L. Issues on peritoneal metastasis of gastric cancer: An update. *World J. Surg. Oncol.* **2019**, *17*, 215. [CrossRef] [PubMed]
62. Deng, G.; Qu, J.; Zhang, Y.; Che, X.; Cheng, Y.; Fan, Y.; Zhang, S.; Na, D.; Liu, Y.; Qu, X. Gastric cancer-derived exosomes promote peritoneal metastasis by destroying the mesothelial barrier. *FEBS Lett.* **2017**, *591*, 2167–2179. [CrossRef]

63. Keerthikumar, S.; Chisanga, D.; Ariyaratne, D.; Al Saffar, H.; Anand, S.; Zhao, K.; Samuel, M.; Pathan, M.; Jois, M.; Chilamkurti, N.; et al. ExoCarta: A Web-Based Compendium of Exosomal Cargo. *J. Mol. Biol.* **2016**, *428*, 688–692. [CrossRef] [PubMed]
64. Qu, J.L.; Qu, X.J.; Zhao, M.F.; Teng, Y.E.; Zhang, Y.; Hou, K.Z.; Jiang, Y.H.; Yang, X.H.; Liu, Y.P. Gastric cancer exosomes promote tumour cell proliferation through PI3K/Akt and MAPK/ERK activation. *Dig. Liver Dis.* **2009**, *41*, 875–880. [CrossRef] [PubMed]
65. Li, C.; Liu, D.-R.; Li, G.-G.; Wang, H.-H.; Li, X.-W.; Zhang, W.; Wu, Y.-L.; Chen, L. CD97 promotes gastric cancer cell proliferation and invasion through exosome-mediated MAPK signaling pathway. *World J. Gastroenterol.* **2015**, *21*, 6215–6228. [CrossRef] [PubMed]
66. Zhang, Y.; Han, T.; Feng, D.; Li, J.; Wu, M.; Peng, X.; Wang, B.; Zhan, X.; Fu, P. Screening of non-invasive miRNA biomarker candidates for metastasis of gastric cancer by small RNA sequencing of plasma exosomes. *Carcinogenesis* **2020**, *41*, 582–590. [CrossRef] [PubMed]
67. Zhu, M.; Zhang, N.; He, S.; Lu, X. Exosomal miR-106a derived from gastric cancer promotes peritoneal metastasis via direct regulation of Smad7. *Cell Cycle* **2020**, *19*, 1200–1221. [CrossRef] [PubMed]
68. Ohzawa, H.; Saito, A.; Kumagai, Y.; Kimura, Y.; Yamaguchi, H.; Hosoya, Y.; Lefor, A.K.; Sata, N.; Kitayama, J. Reduced expression of exosomal miR-29s in peritoneal fluid is a useful predictor of peritoneal recurrence after curative resection of gastric cancer with serosal involvement. *Oncol. Rep.* **2020**, *43*, 1081–1088. [CrossRef] [PubMed]
69. Kersy, O.; Loewenstein, S.; Lubezky, N.; Sher, O.; Simon, N.B.; Klausner, J.M.; Lahat, G. Omental Tissue-Mediated Tumorigenesis of Gastric Cancer Peritoneal Metastases. *Front. Oncol.* **2019**, *9*, 1267. [CrossRef] [PubMed]
70. Sohel, M.M.H. Circulating microRNAs as biomarkers in cancer diagnosis. *Life Sci.* **2020**, *248*, 117473. [CrossRef]
71. Fuji, T.; Umeda, Y.; Nyuya, A.; Taniguchi, F.; Kawai, T.; Yasui, K.; Toshima, T.; Yoshida, K.; Fujiwara, T.; Goel, A.; et al. Detection of circulating microRNAs with Ago2 complexes to monitor the tumor dynamics of colorectal cancer patients during chemotherapy. *Int. J. Cancer* **2019**, *144*, 2169–2180. [CrossRef] [PubMed]
72. Zhang, J.; Fan, X.S.; Wang, C.X.; Liu, B.; Li, Q.; Zhou, X.J. Up-regulation of Ago2 expression in gastric carcinoma. *Med. Oncol.* **2013**, *30*, 628. [CrossRef] [PubMed]
73. Umer, M.; Vaidyanathan, R.; Nguyen, N.T.; Shiddiky, M.J.A. Circulating tumor microemboli: Progress in molecular understanding and enrichment technologies. *Biotechnol. Adv.* **2018**, *36*, 1367–1389. [CrossRef] [PubMed]
74. Hou, J.M.; Krebs, M.; Ward, T.; Sloane, R.; Priest, L.; Hughes, A.; Clack, G.; Ranson, M.; Blackhall, F.; Dive, C. Circulating tumor cells as a window on metastasis biology in lung cancer. *Am. J. Pathol.* **2011**, *178*, 989–996. [CrossRef] [PubMed]
75. Ding, X.-Q.; Wang, Z.-Y.; Xia, D.; Wang, R.-X.; Pan, X.-R.; Tong, J.-H. Proteomic Profiling of Serum Exosomes From Patients With Metastatic Gastric Cancer. *Front. Oncol.* **2020**, *10*, 1113. [CrossRef] [PubMed]
76. Sun, M.Y.; Xu, B.; Wu, Q.X.; Chen, W.L.; Cai, S.; Zhang, H.; Tang, Q.F. Cisplatin-Resistant Gastric Cancer Cells Promote the Chemoresistance of Cisplatin-Sensitive Cells via the Exosomal RPS3-Mediated PI3K-Akt-Cofilin-1 Signaling Axis. *Front. Cell Dev. Biol.* **2021**, *9*, 618899. [CrossRef] [PubMed]
77. Xu, Y.C.; Liu, X.; Li, M.; Li, Y.; Li, C.Y.; Lu, Y.; Sanches, J.; Wang, L.; Du, Y.; Mao, L.M.; et al. A Novel Mechanism of Doxorubicin Resistance and Tumorigenesis Mediated by MicroRNA-501-5p-Suppressed BLID. *Mol. Ther. Nucleic Acids* **2018**, *12*, 578–590. [CrossRef]
78. Zhao, W.; Shan, B.; He, D.; Cheng, Y.; Li, B.; Zhang, C.; Duan, C. Recent Progress in Characterizing Long Noncoding RNAs in Cancer Drug Resistance. *J. Cancer* **2019**, *10*, 6693–6702. [CrossRef]
79. Fuchs, C.S.; Tabernero, J.; Tomášek, J.; Chau, I.; Melichar, B.; Safran, H.; Tehfe, M.A.; Filip, D.; Topuzov, E.; Schlittler, L.; et al. Biomarker analyses in REGARD gastric/GEJ carcinoma patients treated with VEGFR2-targeted antibody ramucirumab. *Br. J. Cancer* **2016**, *115*, 974–982. [CrossRef]
80. Van Cutsem, E.; de Haas, S.; Kang, Y.K.; Ohtsu, A.; Tebbutt, N.C.; Ming Xu, J.; Peng Yong, W.; Langer, B.; Delmar, P.; Scherer, S.J.; et al. Bevacizumab in combination with chemotherapy as first-line therapy in advanced gastric cancer: A biomarker evaluation from the AVAGAST randomized phase III trial. *J. Clin. Oncol.* **2012**, *30*, 2119–2127. [CrossRef] [PubMed]
81. Zhao, D.; Hou, H.; Zhang, X. Progress in the treatment of solid tumors with apatinib: A systematic review. *OncoTargets Ther.* **2018**, *11*, 4137–4147. [CrossRef]
82. Abdallah, E.A.; Braun, A.C.; Flores, B.; Senda, L.; Urvanegia, A.C.; Calsavara, V.; Fonseca de Jesus, V.H.; Almeida, M.F.A.; Begnami, M.D.; Coimbra, F.J.F.; et al. The Potential Clinical Implications of Circulating Tumor Cells and Circulating Tumor Microemboli in Gastric Cancer. *Oncologist* **2019**, *24*, e854–e863. [CrossRef] [PubMed]
83. Mitani, S.; Kawakami, H. Emerging Targeted Therapies for HER2 Positive Gastric Cancer That Can Overcome Trastuzumab Resistance. *Cancers* **2020**, *12*, 400. [CrossRef] [PubMed]
84. Marin, J.J.G.; Perez-Silva, L.; Macias, R.I.R.; Asensio, M.; Peleteiro-Vigil, A.; Sanchez-Martin, A.; Cives-Losada, C.; Sanchon-Sanchez, P.; Sanchez De Blas, B.; Herraez, E.; et al. Molecular Bases of Mechanisms Accounting for Drug Resistance in Gastric Adenocarcinoma. *Cancers* **2020**, *12*, 2116. [CrossRef] [PubMed]
85. Piro, G.; Carbone, C.; Cataldo, I.; Di Nicolantonio, F.; Giacopuzzi, S.; Aprile, G.; Simionato, F.; Boschi, F.; Zanotto, M.; Mina, M.M.; et al. An FGFR3 Autocrine Loop Sustains Acquired Resistance to Trastuzumab in Gastric Cancer Patients. *Clin. Cancer Res.* **2016**, *22*, 6164. [CrossRef] [PubMed]
86. Shi, J.; Li, F.; Yao, X.; Mou, T.; Xu, Z.; Han, Z.; Chen, S.; Li, W.; Yu, J.; Qi, X.; et al. The HER4-YAP1 axis promotes trastuzumab resistance in HER2-positive gastric cancer by inducing epithelial and mesenchymal transition. *Oncogene* **2018**, *37*, 3022–3038. [CrossRef] [PubMed]

87. Sampera, A.; Sánchez-Martín, F.J.; Arpí, O.; Visa, L.; Iglesias, M.; Menéndez, S.; Gaye, É.; Dalmases, A.; Clavé, S.; Gelabert-Baldrich, M.; et al. HER-Family Ligands Promote Acquired Resistance to Trastuzumab in Gastric Cancer. *Mol. Cancer Ther.* **2019**, *18*, 2135–2145. [CrossRef] [PubMed]
88. Liu, J.; Pan, C.; Guo, L.; Wu, M.; Guo, J.; Peng, S.; Wu, Q.; Zuo, Q. A new mechanism of trastuzumab resistance in gastric cancer: MACC1 promotes the Warburg effect via activation of the PI3K/AKT signaling pathway. *J. Hematol. Oncol.* **2016**, *9*, 76. [CrossRef] [PubMed]
89. Wang, Y.; Zhao, C.; Chang, L.; Jia, R.; Liu, R.; Zhang, Y.; Gao, X.; Li, J.; Chen, R.; Xia, X.; et al. Circulating tumor DNA analyses predict progressive disease and indicate trastuzumab-resistant mechanism in advanced gastric cancer. *EBioMedicine* **2019**, *43*, 261–269. [CrossRef] [PubMed]
90. Wang, D.-S.; Liu, Z.-X.; Lu, Y.-X.; Bao, H.; Wu, X.; Zeng, Z.-L.; Liu, Z.; Zhao, Q.; He, C.-Y.; Lu, J.-H.; et al. Liquid biopsies to track trastuzumab resistance in metastatic HER2-positive gastric cancer. *Gut* **2019**, *68*, 1152. [CrossRef] [PubMed]
91. Shitara, K.; Van Cutsem, E.; Bang, Y.J.; Fuchs, C.; Wyrwicz, L.; Lee, K.W.; Kudaba, I.; Garrido, M.; Chung, H.C.; Lee, J.; et al. Efficacy and Safety of Pembrolizumab or Pembrolizumab Plus Chemotherapy vs Chemotherapy Alone for Patients With First-line, Advanced Gastric Cancer: The KEYNOTE-062 Phase 3 Randomized Clinical Trial. *JAMA Oncol.* **2020**, *6*, 1571–1580. [CrossRef]
92. Moehler, M.; Shitara, K.; Garrido, M.; Salman, P.; Shen, L.; Wyrwicz, L.; Yamaguchi, K.; Skoczylas, T.; Campos Bragagnoli, A.; Liu, T.; et al. LBA6_PR Nivolumab (nivo) plus chemotherapy (chemo) versus chemo as first-line (1L) treatment for advanced gastric cancer/gastroesophageal junction cancer (GC/GEJC)/esophageal adenocarcinoma (EAC): First results of the CheckMate 649 study. *Ann. Oncol.* **2020**, *31* (Suppl. 4). [CrossRef]
93. Sundar, R.; Smyth, E.C.; Peng, S.; Yeong, J.P.S.; Tan, P. Predictive Biomarkers of Immune Checkpoint Inhibition in Gastroesophageal Cancers. *Front. Oncol.* **2020**, *10*, 763. [CrossRef] [PubMed]
94. Folprecht, G. Tumor mutational burden as a new biomarker for PD-1 antibody treatment in gastric cancer. *Cancer Commun.* **2019**, *39*, 74. [CrossRef] [PubMed]
95. Snyder, A.; Morrissey, M.P.; Hellmann, M.D. Use of Circulating Tumor DNA for Cancer Immunotherapy. *Clin. Cancer Res.* **2019**, *25*, 6909–6915. [CrossRef] [PubMed]
96. Marabelle, A.; Fakih, M.; Lopez, J.; Shah, M.; Shapira-Frommer, R.; Nakagawa, K.; Chung, H.C.; Kindler, H.L.; Lopez-Martin, J.A.; Miller, W.H., Jr.; et al. Association of tumour mutational burden with outcomes in patients with advanced solid tumours treated with pembrolizumab: Prospective biomarker analysis of the multicohort, open-label, phase 2 KEYNOTE-158 study. *Lancet Oncol.* **2020**, *21*, 1353–1365. [CrossRef]
97. Wang, F.; Wei, X.L.; Wang, F.H.; Xu, N.; Shen, L.; Dai, G.H.; Yuan, X.L.; Chen, Y.; Yang, S.J.; Shi, J.H.; et al. Safety, efficacy and tumor mutational burden as a biomarker of overall survival benefit in chemo-refractory gastric cancer treated with toripalimab, a PD-1 antibody in phase Ib/II clinical trial NCT02915432. *Ann. Oncol.* **2019**, *30*, 1479–1486. [CrossRef] [PubMed]
98. Cho, J.; Ahn, S.; Son, D.S.; Kim, N.K.; Lee, K.W.; Kim, S.; Lee, J.; Park, S.H.; Park, J.O.; Kang, W.K.; et al. Bridging genomics and phenomics of gastric carcinoma. *Int. J. Cancer* **2019**, *145*, 2407–2417. [CrossRef] [PubMed]
99. Gandara, D.R.; Paul, S.M.; Kowanetz, M.; Schleifman, E.; Zou, W.; Li, Y.; Rittmeyer, A.; Fehrenbacher, L.; Otto, G.; Malboeuf, C.; et al. Blood-based tumor mutational burden as a predictor of clinical benefit in non-small-cell lung cancer patients treated with atezolizumab. *Nat. Med.* **2018**, *24*, 1441–1448. [CrossRef]
100. Kim, J.; Kim, B.; Kang, S.Y.; Heo, Y.J.; Park, S.H.; Kim, S.T.; Kang, W.K.; Lee, J.; Kim, K.M. Tumor Mutational Burden Determined by Panel Sequencing Predicts Survival After Immunotherapy in Patients With Advanced Gastric Cancer. *Front. Oncol.* **2020**, *10*, 314. [CrossRef]
101. Sohn, B.H.; Hwang, J.E.; Jang, H.J.; Lee, H.S.; Oh, S.C.; Shim, J.J.; Lee, K.W.; Kim, E.H.; Yim, S.Y.; Lee, S.H.; et al. Clinical Significance of Four Molecular Subtypes of Gastric Cancer Identified by The Cancer Genome Atlas Project. *Clin. Cancer Res.* **2017**. [CrossRef]
102. Morihiro, T.; Kuroda, S.; Kanaya, N.; Kakiuchi, Y.; Kubota, T.; Aoyama, K.; Tanaka, T.; Kikuchi, S.; Nagasaka, T.; Nishizaki, M.; et al. PD-L1 expression combined with microsatellite instability/CD8+ tumor infiltrating lymphocytes as a useful prognostic biomarker in gastric cancer. *Sci. Rep.* **2019**, *9*, 4633. [CrossRef]
103. Pietrantonio, F.; Miceli, R.; Raimondi, A.; Kim, Y.W.; Kang, W.K.; Langley, R.E.; Choi, Y.Y.; Kim, K.M.; Nankivell, M.G.; Morano, F.; et al. Individual Patient Data Meta-Analysis of the Value of Microsatellite Instability As a Biomarker in Gastric Cancer. *J. Clin. Oncol.* **2019**, *37*, 3392–3400. [CrossRef] [PubMed]
104. Schehr, J.L.; Schultz, Z.D.; Warrick, J.W.; Guckenberger, D.J.; Pezzi, H.M.; Sperger, J.M.; Heninger, E.; Saeed, A.; Leal, T.; Mattox, K.; et al. High Specificity in Circulating Tumor Cell Identification Is Required for Accurate Evaluation of Programmed Death-Ligand 1. *PLoS ONE* **2016**, *11*, e0159397. [CrossRef]
105. Fan, Y.; Che, X.; Qu, J.; Hou, K.; Wen, T.; Li, Z.; Li, C.; Wang, S.; Xu, L.; Liu, Y.; et al. Exosomal PD-L1 Retains Immunosuppressive Activity and is Associated with Gastric Cancer Prognosis. *Ann. Surg. Oncol.* **2019**, *26*, 3745–3755. [CrossRef] [PubMed]
106. Ayala-Mar, S.; Donoso-Quezada, J.; González-Valdez, J. Clinical Implications of Exosomal PD-L1 in Cancer Immunotherapy. *J. Immunol. Res.* **2021**, *2021*, 8839978. [CrossRef] [PubMed]
107. Ishiba, T.; Hoffmann, A.C.; Usher, J.; Elshimali, Y.; Sturdevant, T.; Dang, M.; Jaimes, Y.; Tyagi, R.; Gonzales, R.; Grino, M.; et al. Frequencies and expression levels of programmed death ligand 1 (PD-L1) in circulating tumor RNA (ctRNA) in various cancer types. *Biochem. Biophys. Res. Commun.* **2018**, *500*, 621–625. [CrossRef] [PubMed]

108. Mayrhofer, M.; De Laere, B.; Whitington, T.; Van Oyen, P.; Ghysel, C.; Ampe, J.; Ost, P.; Demey, W.; Hoekx, L.; Schrijvers, D.; et al. Cell-free DNA profiling of metastatic prostate cancer reveals microsatellite instability, structural rearrangements and clonal hematopoiesis. *Genome Med.* **2018**, *10*, 85. [CrossRef] [PubMed]
109. Willis, J.; Lefterova, M.I.; Artyomenko, A.; Kasi, P.M.; Nakamura, Y.; Mody, K.; Catenacci, D.V.T.; Fakih, M.; Barbacioru, C.; Zhao, J.; et al. Validation of Microsatellite Instability Detection Using a Comprehensive Plasma-Based Genotyping Panel. *Clin. Cancer Res.* **2019**, *25*, 7035–7045. [CrossRef]
110. Shoda, K.; Ichikawa, D.; Fujita, Y.; Masuda, K.; Hiramoto, H.; Hamada, J.; Arita, T.; Konishi, H.; Kosuga, T.; Komatsu, S.; et al. Clinical utility of circulating cell-free Epstein-Barr virus DNA in patients with gastric cancer. *Oncotarget* **2017**, *8*, 28796–28804. [CrossRef] [PubMed]
111. Ignatova, E.; Seriak, D.; Fedyanin, M.; Tryakin, A.; Pokataev, I.; Menshikova, S.; Vakhabova, Y.; Smirnova, K.; Tjulandin, S.; Ajani, J.A. Epstein-Barr virus-associated gastric cancer: Disease that requires special approach. *Gastric Cancer* **2020**, *23*, 951–960. [CrossRef] [PubMed]
112. Cao, Y.; Xie, L.; Shi, F.; Tang, M.; Li, Y.; Hu, J.; Zhao, L.; Zhao, L.; Yu, X.; Luo, X.; et al. Targeting the signaling in Epstein-Barr virus-associated diseases: Mechanism, regulation, and clinical study. *Signal Transduct. Target. Ther.* **2021**, *6*, 15. [CrossRef] [PubMed]
113. Bratman, S.V.; Yang, S.Y.C.; Iafolla, M.A.J.; Liu, Z.; Hansen, A.R.; Bedard, P.L.; Lheureux, S.; Spreafico, A.; Razak, A.A.; Shchegrova, S.; et al. Personalized circulating tumor DNA analysis as a predictive biomarker in solid tumor patients treated with pembrolizumab. *Nat. Cancer* **2020**, *1*, 873–881. [CrossRef]
114. Matsusaka, S.; Chìn, K.; Ogura, M.; Suenaga, M.; Shinozaki, E.; Mishima, Y.; Terui, Y.; Mizunuma, N.; Hatake, K. Circulating tumor cells as a surrogate marker for determining response to chemotherapy in patients with advanced gastric cancer. *Cancer Sci.* **2010**, *101*, 1067–1071. [CrossRef] [PubMed]
115. Uenosono, Y.; Arigami, T.; Kozono, T.; Yanagita, S.; Hagihara, T.; Haraguchi, N.; Matsushita, D.; Hirata, M.; Arima, H.; Funasako, Y.; et al. Clinical significance of circulating tumor cells in peripheral blood from patients with gastric cancer. *Cancer* **2013**, *119*, 3984–3991. [CrossRef] [PubMed]
116. Jensen, T.J.; Goodman, A.M.; Kato, S.; Ellison, C.K.; Daniels, G.A.; Kim, L.; Nakashe, P.; McCarthy, E.; Mazloom, A.R.; McLennan, G.; et al. Genome-Wide Sequencing of Cell-Free DNA Identifies Copy-Number Alterations That Can Be Used for Monitoring Response to Immunotherapy in Cancer Patients. *Mol. Cancer Ther.* **2019**, *18*, 448–458. [CrossRef]
117. Ye, M.; Huang, D.; Zhang, Q.; Weng, W.; Tan, C.; Qin, G.; Jiang, W.; Sheng, W.; Wang, L. Heterogeneous programmed death-ligand 1 expression in gastric cancer: Comparison of tissue microarrays and whole sections. *Cancer Cell Int.* **2020**, *20*, 186. [CrossRef] [PubMed]
118. Vogelstein, B.; Papadopoulos, N.; Velculescu, V.E.; Zhou, S.; Diaz, L.A.; Kinzler, K.W. Cancer Genome Landscapes. *Science* **2013**, *339*, 1546. [CrossRef]
119. Uchôa Guimarães, C.T.; Ferreira Martins, N.N.; Cristina da Silva Oliveira, K.; Almeida, C.M.; Pinheiro, T.M.; Gigek, C.O.; Roberto de Araújo Cavallero, S.; Assumpção, P.P.; Cardoso Smith, M.A.; Burbano, R.R.; et al. Liquid biopsy provides new insights into gastric cancer. *Oncotarget* **2018**, *9*, 15144–15156. [CrossRef] [PubMed]
120. Crowley, E.; Di Nicolantonio, F.; Loupakis, F.; Bardelli, A. Liquid biopsy: Monitoring cancer-genetics in the blood. *Nat. Rev. Clin. Oncol.* **2013**, *10*, 472–484. [CrossRef] [PubMed]
121. Necula, L.; Matei, L.; Dragu, D.; Neagu, A.I.; Mambet, C.; Nedeianu, S.; Bleotu, C.; Diaconu, C.C.; Chivu-Economescu, M. Recent advances in gastric cancer early diagnosis. *World J. Gastroenterol.* **2019**, *25*, 2029–2044. [CrossRef] [PubMed]
122. Yang, C.; Chen, F.; Wang, S.; Xiong, B. Circulating Tumor Cells in Gastrointestinal Cancers: Current Status and Future Perspectives. *Front. Oncol.* **2019**, *9*, 1427. [CrossRef]
123. Liu, X.; Lu, Y.; Xu, Y.; Hou, S.; Huang, J.; Wang, B.; Zhao, J.; Xia, S.; Fan, S.; Yu, X.; et al. Exosomal transfer of miR-501 confers doxorubicin resistance and tumorigenesis via targeting of BLID in gastric cancer. *Cancer Lett.* **2019**, *459*, 122–134. [CrossRef] [PubMed]

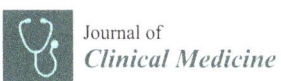

Communication

The Mutational Concordance of Fixed Formalin Paraffin Embedded and Fresh Frozen Gastro-Oesophageal Tumours Using Whole Exome Sequencing

Irene Y. Chong [1,2,*], Naureen Starling [2], Alistair Rust [3], John Alexander [4], Lauren Aronson [1], Marta Llorca-Cardenosa [1], Ritika Chauhan [3], Asif Chaudry [2], Sacheen Kumar [2], Kerry Fenwick [3], Ioannis Assiotis [3], Nik Matthews [3], Ruwaida Begum [2], Andrew Wotherspoon [2], Monica Terlizzo [2], David Watkins [2], Ian Chau [2], Christopher J. Lord [4], Syed Haider [4], Sheela Rao [2] and David Cunningham [2]

[1] The Division of Molecular Pathology, The Institute of Cancer Research, 237 Fulham Road, London SW3 6JB, UK; lauren.aronson@icr.ac.uk (L.A.); marta.llorca@icr.ac.uk (M.L.-C.)

[2] The Royal Marsden Hospital NHS Foundation Trust, 203 Fulham Road, London SW3 6JJ, UK; Naureen.starling@rmh.nhs.uk (N.S.); asif.chaudry@rmh.nhs.uk (A.C.); sacheen.kumar@rmh.nhs.uk (S.K.); ruwaida.begum@rmh.nhs.uk (R.B.); andrew.wotherspoon@rmh.nhs.uk (A.W.); monica.terlizzo@rmh.nhs.uk (M.T.); david.watkins@rmh.nhs.uk (D.W.); ian.chau@rmh.nhs.uk (I.C.); sheela.rao@rmh.nhs.uk (S.R.); david.cunningham@rmh.nhs.uk (D.C.)

[3] The Tissue Profiling Unit, The Institute of Cancer Research, 237 Fulham Road, London SW3 6JB, UK; alistair.rust@icr.ac.uk (A.R.); ritika.chauhan@icr.ac.uk (R.C.); kerry.fenwick@icr.ac.uk (K.F.); ioannis.assiotis@icr.ac.uk (I.A.); nik.matthews@icr.ac.uk (N.M.)

[4] Breast Cancer Now Toby Robins Research Centre, The Institute of Cancer Research, London SW3 6JB, UK; John.Alexander@icr.ac.uk (J.A.); Chris.lord@icr.ac.uk (C.J.L.); Syed.Haider@icr.ac.uk (S.H.)

* Correspondence: irene.chong@icr.ac.uk; Tel.: +44-0207-153-5138

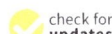

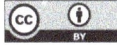

Citation: Chong, I.Y.; Starling, N.; Rust, A.; Alexander, J.; Aronson, L.; Llorca-Cardenosa, M.; Chauhan, R.; Chaudry, A.; Kumar, S.; Fenwick, K.; et al. The Mutational Concordance of Fixed Formalin Paraffin Embedded and Fresh Frozen Gastro-Oesophageal Tumours Using Whole Exome Sequencing. *J. Clin. Med.* **2021**, *10*, 215. https://doi.org/10.3390/jcm10020215

Received: 3 December 2020
Accepted: 4 January 2021
Published: 9 January 2021

Publisher's Note: MDPI stays neutral with regard to jurisdictional claims in published maps and institutional affiliations.

Copyright: © 2021 by the authors. Licensee MDPI, Basel, Switzerland. This article is an open access article distributed under the terms and conditions of the Creative Commons Attribution (CC BY) license (https://creativecommons.org/licenses/by/4.0/).

Abstract: 1. Background: The application of massively parallel sequencing has led to the identification of aberrant druggable pathways and somatic mutations within therapeutically relevant genes in gastro-oesophageal cancer. Given the widespread use of formalin-fixed paraffin-embedded (FFPE) samples in the study of this disease, it would be beneficial, especially for the purposes of biomarker evaluation, to assess the concordance between comprehensive exome-wide sequencing data from archival FFPE samples originating from a prospective clinical study and those derived from fresh-frozen material. 2. Methods: We analysed whole-exome sequencing data to define the mutational concordance of 16 matched fresh-frozen and FFPE gastro-oesophageal tumours (N = 32) from a prospective clinical study. We assessed DNA integrity prior to sequencing and then identified coding mutations in genes that have previously been implicated in other cancers. In addition, we calculated the mutant-allele heterogeneity (MATH) for these samples. 3. Results: Although there was increased degradation of DNA in FFPE samples compared with frozen samples, sequencing data from only two FFPE samples failed to reach an adequate mapping quality threshold. Using a filtering threshold of mutant read counts of at least ten and a minimum of 5% variant allele frequency (VAF) we found that there was a high median mutational concordance of 97% (range 80.1–98.68%) between fresh-frozen and FFPE gastro-oesophageal tumour-derived exomes. However, the majority of FFPE tumours had higher mutant-allele heterogeneity (MATH) scores when compared with corresponding frozen tumours ($p < 0.001$), suggesting that FFPE-based exome sequencing is likely to over-represent tumour heterogeneity in FFPE samples compared to fresh-frozen samples. Furthermore, we identified coding mutations in 120 cancer-related genes, including those associated with chromatin remodelling and Wnt/β-catenin and Receptor Tyrosine Kinase signalling. 4. Conclusions: These data suggest that comprehensive genomic data can be generated from exome sequencing of selected DNA samples extracted from archival FFPE gastro-oesophageal tumour tissues within the context of prospective clinical trials.

Keywords: gastro-oesophageal cancer; mutational concordance; exome sequencing; formalin fixed paraffin embedded; biomarkers

1. Introduction

Gastric and oesophageal cancers are, respectively, the third and seventh leading causes of cancer-related deaths [1–3]. Disease relapse following first-line treatment in patients with advanced disease is frequent, with limited subsequent treatment options. Previously studied targeted therapies in patients with advanced gastro-oesophageal cancer include inhibitors of erythroblastic oncogene B (ERBB2) [4], epidermal growth factor receptor (EGFR) [5,6], vascular endothelial growth factor (VEGF) [7], vascular endothelial growth factor receptor (VEGFR2) [8,9], and poly (ADP-ribose) polymerase (PARP) [10]. However, an improved understanding of individual patient responses is required to identify actionable mechanisms of treatment response and resistance. Genome-wide DNA sequencing studies have confirmed that gastro-oesophageal adenocarcinomas are highly mutated and heterogeneous tumours [11,12]. We and others have identified aberrant druggable pathways and somatic mutations within therapeutically relevant genes in the treatment of naïve frozen gastro-oesophageal tumours using massively parallel sequencing techniques [11,13–15]. For the purposes of biomarker evaluation, it would be beneficial to utilise whole-exome DNA sequencing to generate comprehensive genomic data that could be compared with clinical response and outcome within mature phase III studies. Unfortunately, only formalin-fixed paraffin-embedded (FFPE) tissues are available for genomic evaluation in most of these trials; this could potentially be problematic as the process of tissue immobilisation by the FFPE process can result in cross-linked and fragmented DNA that may not be fit for purpose for massively parallel sequencing [16]. It is, therefore, important to understand the level of mutational concordance between frozen and FFPE tumours to assess the utility of next-generation sequencing of DNA extracted from FFPE tissues. Here, we describe an analysis of whole-exome sequencing data to define the mutational concordance of DNA extracted from matched fresh frozen and FFPE gastro-oesophageal tumours, and to estimate the feasibility of this approach within the context of prospective clinical trials.

2. Experimental Section

2.1. Sample Description and Preparation

Snap frozen and matched FFPE gastro-oesophageal tumour biopsies used for exome sequencing were obtained from patients at the time of endoscopic ultrasound staging, prior to treatment by the same endoscopist at the Royal Marsden Hospital, UK. The biopsies were fixed in neutral buffered formalin for 5–8 h. Oesophageal tumour samples with malignant cell purities of over 70% were selected for DNA extraction and subsequent whole-exome sequencing. Signed written informed consent from each patient was obtained before recruitment to the study according to regulations of the local ethics review board.

2.2. Genomic DNA Extraction and Whole-Exome

Genomic DNA was isolated from tumour biopsies using the DNeasy Blood and Tissue kit (Qiagen, Hilden, Germany) and quantified using Qubit fluorometric quantitation (Invitrogen Life Technologies, Carlsbad, CA, USA). Genomic DNA was fragmented to 200 basepairs (bps) using a Covaris E Series instrument (Covaris Inc., Woburn, MA, USA). The resultant library was subjected to DNA capture using the 50 Mb SureSelect Human All Exon V5 kit (Agilent, Santa Clara, CA, USA). DNA capture was carried out, and Illumina paired-end libraries were prepared from the captured target regions and quantified using a Bioanalyzer DNA chip (Agilent). This process was then followed by sequencing on a HiSeq2500 platform (Illumina, San Diego, CA, USA), acquiring 2 × 100 bps reads. Bcl2fastq software (v1.8.4, Illumina) was used for converting the raw basecalls to fastqs and to further demultiplex the sequencing data. The demultiplexed paired-end fastq files were used for further analysis.

2.3. Read Mapping and Detection of Mutations from Exome Sequencing

BWA-mem (v0.7.5a) was used to align reads to the human reference genome (GRCh37) [17]. Variant calling was carried out using the Broad Best Practice pipeline with standard settings [18]. In summary, GATK (v3.3-0) was used to detect frameshifts and MuTect (v1.1.4) was used to detect point mutations. The effects of single-point mutations were determined by SnpEff (v3.3h). Candidate mutations were selected using the following list of heuristic rules: (1) variants detected at a mutant allele frequency (MAF) of greater than 5% in any of the 1000 Genomes project populations were excluded from analysis, (2) variants called in regions not covered by the exome capture probes were excluded, (3) variants marked as low quality (QUAL below 30) were excluded, and (4) variants not reaching a depth threshold of 10 reads were excluded.

3. Results

3.1. Clinicopathological Features of Patients

All patients were treatment-naïve at the time of biopsy retrieval. The median age was 64 years for the 16 patients included in this study (Table 1). The majority were male (81.2%). The most common disease site was at the gastro-oesophageal junction (GOJ, 68.8%). The GOJ and gastric tumours were adenocarcinomas (93.8%) that were either moderately or poorly differentiated (grade 2 or 3). The remaining cancer was an early, well-differentiated (grade 1) neuroendocrine tumour located in the distal oeosphagus. The majority of tumours were locally advanced (T3 N0/1 M0, 62%). Four patients had early disease (T1/2 N0, M0, 25%), and two patients presented with metastatic disease (T3 N1 M1, 12.5%). The storage period of the tissues ranged from 4 to 10 years, with a median time of 8.5 years.

Table 1. Clinicopathological characteristics of patients.

Characteristic	(N = 16)
Age at diagnosis	
Median—y	64
Range—y	22–82
Sex—No. (%)	
Male	13 (81.2)
Female	3 (18.8)
Site of tumour—No. (%)	
Distal oesophagus	1 (6.3)
GOJ type I	3 (18.7)
GOJ type II	4 (25)
GOJ type III	4 (25)
Stomach	4 (25)
Histology—No. (%)	
Adenocarcinoma	15 (93.8)
Neuroendocrine	1 (6.2)
Grade—No. (%)	
1	1 (6.2)
2	5 (31.3)
3	10 (62.5)
TNM Stage—No. (%)	
T1/2 N0 M0	4 (25)
T3 N0/1 M0	10 (62.5)
T3 N1 M1	2 (12.5)
Time from biopsy to sequencing	
Median—y	8.5
Range—y	4–10

3.2. Assessment of DNA Integrity

We observed that there was a significant difference in the concentration of double-stranded DNA extracted from frozen compared with FFPE oesophageal tumour ($p = 0.0026$, Mann–Whitney U test), suggesting improved integrity of DNA extracted from frozen samples and increased degradation of FFPE biospecimens (Figure 1A) [19]. However, there was no significant difference in either the total quantity of pre-hybridisation PCR product generated or the number of PCR cycles required to generate the pre-hybridisation library prior to exome sequencing (Figure 1B,C). Following exome sequencing, mutation filtering was applied including mapping quality threshold of ≥ 30, depth threshold of ≥ 10 reads, and variant allele frequency (VAF) threshold of ≥ 0.05. Of note, in the absence of matched blood samples, many germline variants are likely to exist in our mutational repertoire. By applying these thresholds, mutation calls detected in frozen tumour samples were considered a gold standard, allowing for the calculation of true positive, false positive, and false negative rates. For each set of thresholds, combined numbers for sensitivity, precision/positive predictive value (PPV), and F-score were calculated (Table 2). The two sets of thresholds with the highest PPV and F-scores were for mutant read counts of ten or more and a minimum of 5% VAF. We observed that all of the 16 frozen samples achieved adequate exome coverage and depth. However, two of the 16 FFPE samples (samples 178 and 260) did not achieve the minimum median depth threshold of $50\times$. The ages of the two FFPE specimens that failed were 5 years and 10 years, respectively (the range for this cohort was 4–10 years). Whilst the initial starting quantities of DNA and following fragmentation were adequate, the total amount of post-adapter-ligation DNA was lower than expected (less than 400 ng), indicating inferior DNA quality. These samples failed the quality control criteria and were excluded from further analyses.

Table 2. Sensitivity, precision/positive predictive value (PPV), and F-Score for selected variant allele frequency (VAF) and tumour depth thresholds.

VAF (%)	Tumour Depth (X)	Combined Sensitivity	Combined Precision PPV	Combined F Score
2	5	0.775700935	0.83	0.801932367
5	5	0.775700935	0.83	0.801932367
10	5	0.76076555	0.81122449	0.785185185
15	5	0.712643678	0.765432099	0.738095238
20	5	0.732283465	0.801724138	0.765432099
2	10	0.778301887	0.829145729	0.802919708
5	10	0.778301887	0.829145729	0.802919708
10	10	0.763285024	0.81025641	0.786069652
15	10	0.715116279	0.763975155	0.738738739
20	10	0.744	0.801724138	0.771784232
2	15	0.773584906	0.83248731	0.80195599
5	15	0.773584906	0.83248731	0.80195599
10	15	0.758454106	0.813471503	0.785
15	15	0.709302326	0.767295597	0.737160121
20	15	0.736	0.807017544	0.769874477
2	20	0.763033175	0.829896907	0.795061728
5	20	0.763033175	0.829896907	0.795061728
10	20	0.747572815533981	0.810526316	0.777777778
15	20	0.695906433	0.762820513	0.727828746
20	20	0.717741935	0.801801802	0.757446809
2	25	0.759615385	0.822916667	0.79
5	25	0.759615385	0.822916667	0.79
10	25	0.748768473	0.808510638	0.777493606
15	25	0.704142012	0.767741935	0.734567901
20	25	0.729508197	0.809090909	0.767241379
2	30	0.747572816	0.814814815	0.779746835
5	30	0.747572816	0.814814815	0.779746835
10	30	0.736318408	0.8	0.766839378
15	30	0.694610778	0.753246753	0.722741433
20	30	0.716666667	0.788990826	0.751091703

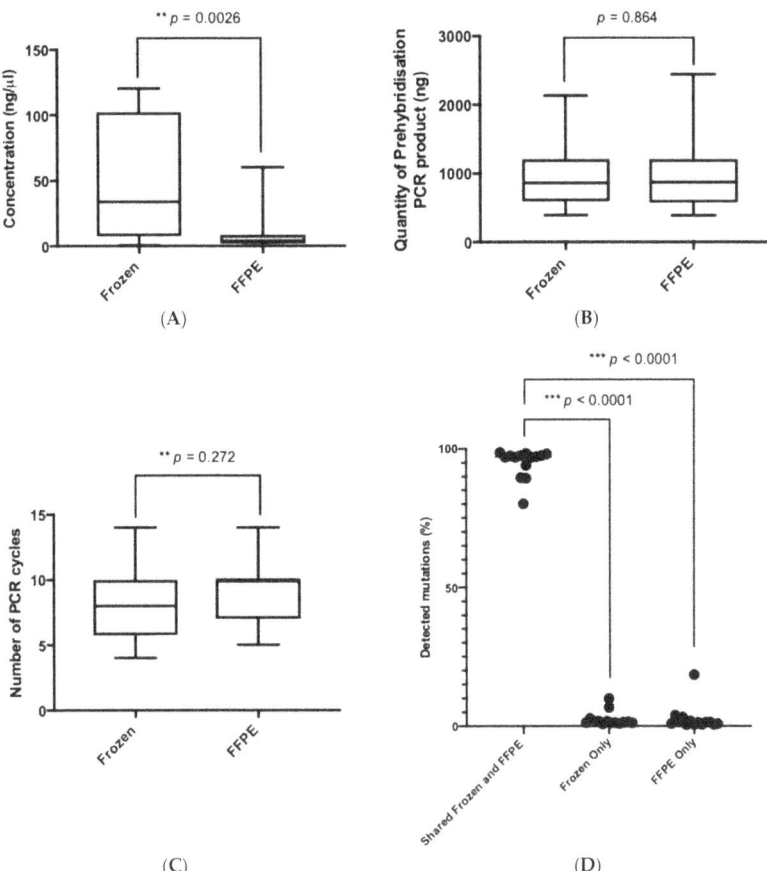

Figure 1. Mutational concordance between frozen and formalin-fixed paraffin-embedded (FFPE) gastro-oesophageal tumour samples. Box and whiskers plots showing the distribution of (**A**). The concentration of double-stranded DNA (nanograms per microlitre) extracted from FFPE and frozen gastro-oesophageal tumours. An increased double-stranded DNA yield was extracted from frozen tumour tissues compared with FFPE tissue ($p = 0.0026$,) (**B**). Prehybridisation PCR product (nanograms) (**C**). The number of PCR cycles required to generate the pre-hybridisation library from FFPE and frozen gastro-oesophageal tumour samples. No difference between FFPE and frozen samples was observed in terms of the overall quantity of pre-hybridisation PCR product generated, nor in terms of the number of PCR cycles required to generate the pre-hybridisation library prior to sequencing (**D**). Bar graph showing a high mutational concordance (range 80.1% to 98.68%) in terms of the percentage of shared mutations detected (in both frozen and FFPE samples) compared with mutations unique to frozen samples and FFPE samples.

3.3. Mutational Concordance between Frozen and FFPE Oesophageal Tumour Samples

To assess the mutational concordance between matched frozen and FFPE-derived gastro-oesophageal tumour DNA in the 14 matched samples that passed quality control criteria ($N = 28$), we cross-referenced mutations detected from exome sequencing. We observed that there was a high median mutational concordance of 97.07% (range 80.1% to 98.68%) between fresh-frozen and FFPE gastro-oesophageal tumour samples (Figure 1D, Table 3). There was no difference overall in the percentage of unique mutations found in DNA derived from FFPE compared with frozen tumour tissue ($p = 0.41$, Mann–Whitney U test). Given that 93% (90/96) of randomly selected mutations have previously been validated with Sanger sequencing, and that 95% (1791/1883) of mutations were recognised by both exome sequencing and the Ion Proton platform from our previous study [14], our current results demonstrate the feasibility of exome sequencing of FFPE-derived DNA samples from gastro-oesophageal tumours that have passed the described quality control criteria.

Table 3. The of percentage mutational concordance of matched fresh frozen and formalin-fixed paraffin-embedded (FFPE) gastro-oesophageal tumour samples.

Patient	Sample	Mutations Unique to Sample	% Unique to Sample
169	Frozen	1955	6.72
	FFPE	1129	3.88
	Shared	25,997	89.40
170	Frozen	456	1.65
	FFPE	250	0.90
	Shared	26,958	97.45
172	Frozen	471	1.73
	FFPE	361	1.32
	Shared	26,424	96.95
176	Frozen	853	2.72
	FFPE	1017	3.24
	Shared	29,508	94.04
177	Frozen	476	1.42
	FFPE	6205	18.48
	Shared	26,896	80.10
187	Frozen	3056	9.91
	FFPE	146	0.47
	Shared	27,630	89.61
195	Frozen	204	0.72
	FFPE	168	0.60
	Shared	27,790	98.68
203	Frozen	428	1.56
	FFPE	233	0.85
	Shared	26,811	97.59
218	Frozen	311	1.14
	FFPE	154	0.57
	Shared	26,738	98.29
220	Frozen	317	1.18
	FFPE	493	1.84
	Shared	25,978	96.98
249	Frozen	257	0.92
	FFPE	408	1.47
	Shared	27,119	97.61
254	Frozen	327	1.23
	FFPE	159	0.60
	Shared	26,076	98.17
259	Frozen	325	1.20
	FFPE	441	1.63
	Shared	26,234	97.16
267	Frozen	468	1.61
	FFPE	413	1.42
	Shared	28,209	96.97

3.4. Detection of Mutations within Cancer-Related Genes

To identify coding mutations in genes from exome sequencing that have also been implicated in other cancers, we correlated genes harbouring frameshift, non-synonymous, splice site, and stop-gained mutations with genes in the Cancer Genome Census (CGC) [20]. Overall, this comparison identified 120 cancer-related genes in the gastro-oesophageal samples from this study, with an average of 12 potentially deleterious CGC mutations (range 7–50) present in each sample (Figure 2). These mutations were further analysed to determine the dysregulation of cancer-associated pathways. Using this approach, we observed coding mutations in tumour-suppressor genes usually required for normal chromatin remodelling, including *ARID1A* (AT-rich interaction domain 1A gene), *BRD3* (Bromodomain-containing protein 3 gene), and *SMARCA4* (SWI/SNF-Related Matrix-Associated Actin-Dependent Regulator of Chromatin Subfamily A, Member 4 gene). In addition, 8 out of 16 tumours harboured mutations in well-established DNA repair-related tumour-suppressor genes, including *FANCE* (Fanconi Anemia Complementation Group E gene), *FANCF* (Fanconi Anaemia Complementation Group F gene), *MSH6* (MutS Homolog 6 gene), *PMS1* (PMS1 Homolog1, Mismatch Repair System Component gene), *PMS2* (PMS1 Homolog 2, Mismatch Repair System Component gene), *ERCC2* (ERCC Excision Repair 2, TFIIH Core Complex Helicase Subunit gene), or *SETD2* (SET Domain Containing 2 gene), suggestive of disrupted DNA repair pathway signalling in these tumours. Coding mutations in genes involved in Wnt signalling were detected, including mutations in *BCL9* (B-Cell CLL/Lymphoma 9 gene) and *AXIN1* (Axin 1 gene). Coding mutations in *TP53* were detected in 4 out of 16 tumours from exome sequencing. We also identified mutations in genes involved in RAS/RAF signalling, including *KRAS* (Kirsten ras oncogene) and *BRAF* (B-Raf Proto-Oncogene, Serine/Threonine Kinase gene). Mutations in therapeutically relevant genes were also observed, including those in *MET* (MET Proto-Oncogene, Receptor Tyrosine Kinase gene) and *FGFR1* (Fibroblast Growth Factor Receptor 1 gene).

3.5. Intratumoural Genetic Heterogeneity

Gastro-oesophageal tumours are known to be heterogeneous cancers [14,21]. Intratumoural heterogeneity with respect to actionable mutations has clinical implications for how targeted therapies might work [22,23]. Genomically distinct subpopulations of cells lead to differences among mutated loci in terms of the fraction of sequence reads displaying a mutant allele. A heterogeneous tumour will likely have a wider distribution of mutant-allele fractions among loci centred at a lower fraction, compared with a homogeneous tumour [24]. Taking this into consideration, we analysed exome sequencing results for each of the frozen and FFPE tumours. Moreover, we calculated the mutant-allele heterogeneity (MATH) score as the ratio of the width to the centre of its distribution of mutant-allele fractions among tumour-specific mutated loci (Supplementary Figure S1). We observed that the median MATH score for the frozen tumours was 32.95 (range 17.4 to 96.6), indicating notable differences in inter-tumoural heterogeneity in this set of gastro-oesophageal samples. The majority of the FFPE tumours (11 out of 14 samples) had higher MATH scores when compared with the corresponding frozen tumours ($p < 0.001$ Wilcoxon rank test, Figure 3A), suggesting that this analysis is likely to over-represent tumour heterogeneity in FFPE samples. In addition, the number of clonal clusters calculated by MATH was discordant in 9 out of 14 matched samples (Figure 3B). Although the median mutational concordance between fresh-frozen and FFPE gastro-oesophageal tumour samples was high (median 97%, range 80.1–98.68%), MATH analysis to assess tumour heterogeneity was not found to be reliable in FFPE samples.

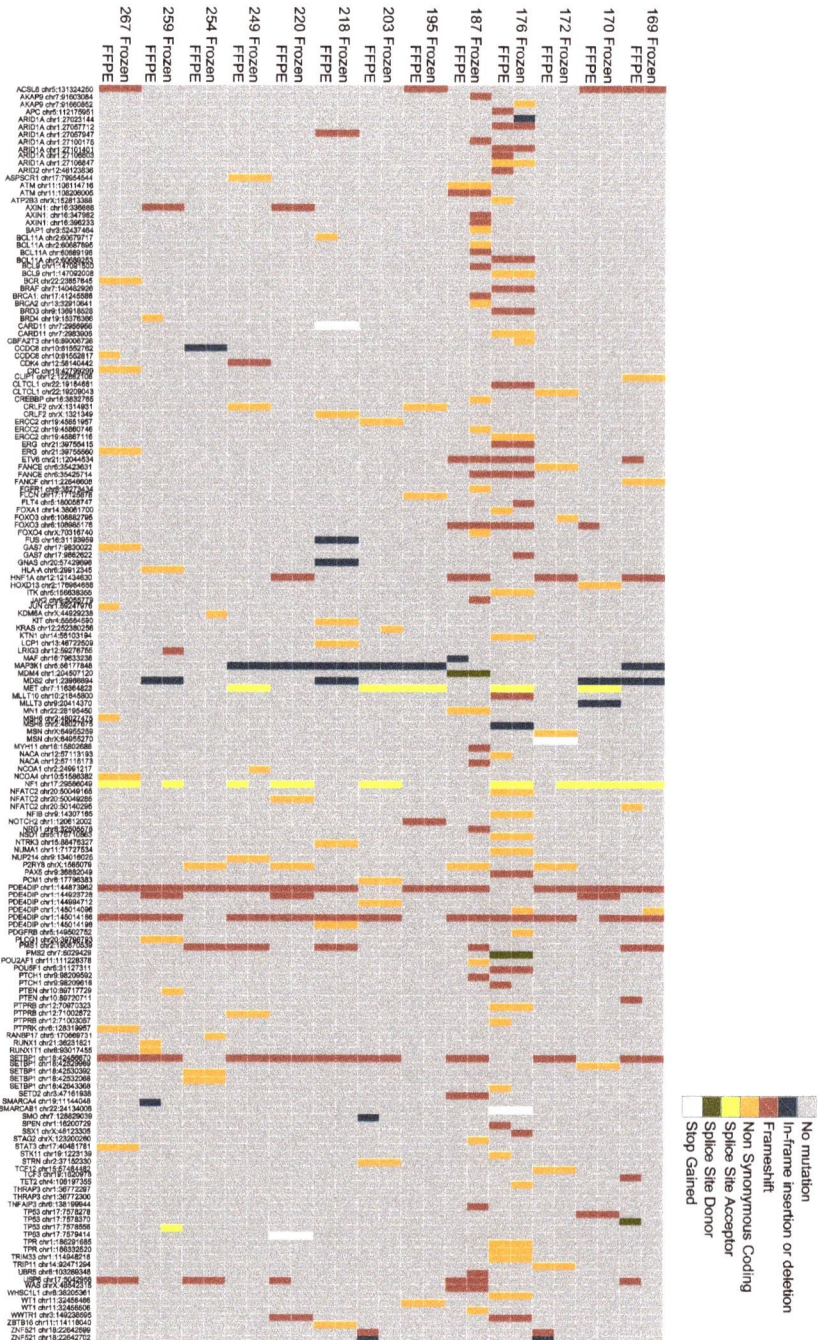

Figure 2. Detection of cancer-related genes from exome sequencing of gastro-oesophageal tumour DNA. Commutation plot showing the presence of mutations in genes from the Cancer Genome Census from exome sequencing of DNA extracted from frozen and formalin-fixed paraffin-embedded (FFPE) oesophageal tumours.

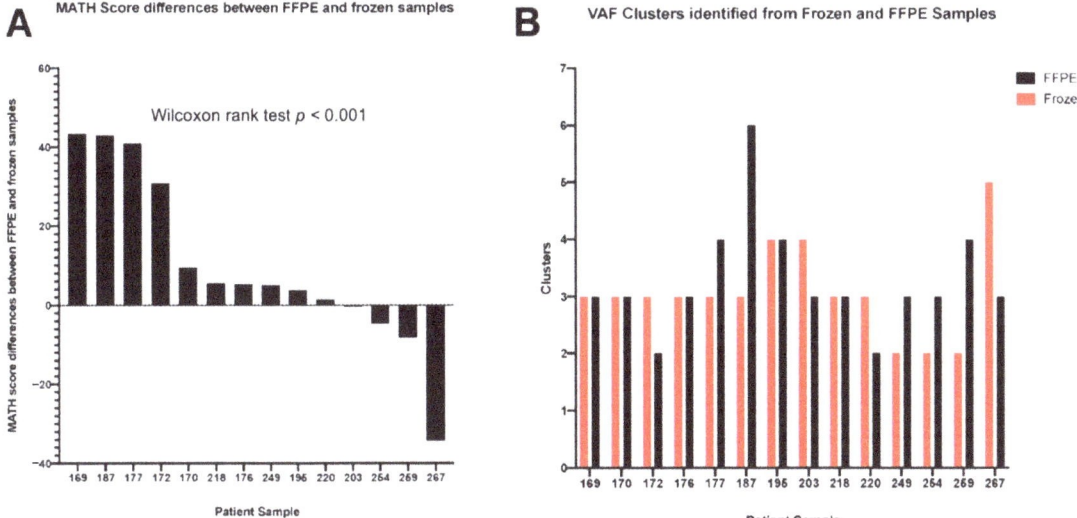

Figure 3. Differences in mutant-allele heterogeneity (MATH) scores and variant allele frequency (VAF) clusters identified from matched formalin-fixed paraffin-embedded (FFPE) and frozen gastro-oesophageal tumours. Histogram illustrating (**A**) differences in MATH scores between FFPE and frozen tumour samples—11 out of 14 FFPE tumours had higher MATH scores when compared with the corresponding frozen tumours ($p < 0.001$ Wilcoxon rank test); and (**B**) VAF clusters identified from FFPE and frozen samples.

4. Discussion

Considering the potential clinical impact of dissecting molecular mechanisms of treatment response and resistance within prospective clinical trials where only FFPE samples are available for analysis [25], the main purpose of this study was to assess the feasibility of using DNA extracted from FFPE gastro-oesophageal tumour for massively parallel sequencing. It is acknowledged that DNA cross-linking, degradation, and fragmentation occurring during the FFPE process has the potential to influence the reliability of mutational sequencing data [26–29]. Taking matched FFPE and frozen melanoma specimens as examples, a comparison of whole-exome sequencing data from 10 tumours revealed a very low overall mutational concordance (average 43.2%). However, the most clinically actionable mutations for this tumour type (*BRAF* and *NRAS*) were found to be concordant [30]. The authors from this study concluded that specialised library construction to account for low quality DNA is necessary before this approach could be used for routine clinical decision making. In contrast, studies relating to other tumour types and utilizing different massively parallel sequencing techniques have yielded more promising results; the concordance rate was found to be up to 96.8% in a lung cancer study comparing the variants of 27 cancer-related genes in 16 matched FFPE and frozen samples [31]. Mutational comparisons have also been undertaken in colorectal cancer (CRC) specimens; the detected concordance rate was up to 81.9% in a study of 33 matched metastatic CRC samples [32]. In a cohort of 10 paired metastatic liver CRC specimens, a high mutational concordance was observed when 212 amplicon regions in 48 cancer-related genes were sequenced, revealing 21 identical mutation calls and only two differing mutations [33]. Furthermore, Gao et al. conducted an extensive study using a 22-gene panel detecting 103 hotspot mutations in paired FFPE and fresh-frozen primary CRC tissues from 118 patients [34]. The investigators identified a concordance rate ranging from 73.8% to 100% and highlighted that important differences exist between the two tissue types.

We approached this problem by assessing DNA integrity prior to sequencing and analysing whole-exome sequencing data to define the mutational concordance of matched fresh-frozen and FFPE gastro-oesophageal tumours. As expected, DNA degradation was more pronounced in the FFPE biospecimens compared with the matched frozen samples. However, there was no significant differences in either the total quantity of pre-hybridisation PCR product generated or the number of PCR cycles required to generate the pre-hybridisation library prior to exome sequencing. Only two out of 16 FFPE samples failed quality control criteria with the inability to achieve the minimum median depth threshold of $50\times$. In the absence of normal/germline samples, we considered all variants likely to include many germline variants. Based on these variants, the subsequent calculation of PPV and F-scores, allowing for the calculation of true-positive, false-positive, and false-negative rates, using frozen tumour samples as a gold standard, identified the optimal filtering threshold as mutant read counts of 10 or more and a minimum of 5% VAF. Using this threshold, we observed a high median mutational concordance of 97% between DNA derived from fresh frozen and FFPE gastro-oesophageal tumours. Consistent with the literature, we also identified frequent mutations in genes responsible for chromatin remodelling, Wnt/β-catenin, and Receptor Tyrosine Kinase signalling [13]. Finally, we assessed intratumoural heterogeneity by calculating the MATH score, and the ratio of the width to the centre of its distribution of mutant-allele fractions among tumour-specific mutated loci, for each sample. We found that most FFPE gastro-oesophageal tumours in this study had higher MATH scores compared with the corresponding frozen tumours. FFPE samples are likely to over-estimate tumour heterogeneity due to the presence of artefactual substitutions in FFPE samples [35]. This result may lead to a more significant variation in observed VAFs, resulting in a higher MATH score.

Focusing on the two FFPE specimens that failed sequencing quality control, we have scrutinised the clinicopathological characteristics of patients included in this study, as well as the raw data generated after DNA extraction and before massively parallel sequencing, to evaluate whether, at any stage, sequencing failure could have been predicted. We found that none of the clinical characteristics were responsible. In particular, the age of the two FFPE specimens that failed were five years and ten years, respectively (the range for this cohort was 4–10 years). Furthermore, we confirmed that the initial quantities of DNA and following fragmentation were indeed adequate. However, the total amount of post-adapter-ligation DNA was lower than expected (less than 400 ng), which is an indication of inferior DNA quality. Whilst this finding could serve as a warning for investigators, we cannot definitively conclude that this factor alone should preclude the commencement of exome sequencing in future studies.

Our findings support the validity of massively parallel sequencing of FFPE gastro-oesophageal tissues as a discovery tool, recognising that only archival tumour blocks are available in the majority of completed phase III studies. Through rigorous assessment of DNA integrity and application of an optimal filtering threshold, a high level of mutational concordance between FFPE and frozen tissues can be achieved. However, subsequent orthogonal validation of actionable mutations is of utmost importance. In contrast, the assessment of intratumoural heterogeneity using the distribution of mutant allele fractions in FFPE gastro-oesophageal samples is much less reliable.

Supplementary Materials: The following are available online at https://www.mdpi.com/2077-0383/10/2/215/s1, Figure S1: MATH Profiles of intra-tumoural heterogeneity in matched grozen and FFPE gastro-oesophageal tumours.

Author Contributions: Conceptualization, I.Y.C., D.C., N.S., D.W., I.C., and S.R.; methodology, I.Y.C., L.A., A.C., S.K., K.F., I.A., N.M., A.W., and M.T.; software, S.H., J.A., A.R., and R.C.; validation, L.A. and M.L.-C.; formal analysis, I.Y.C., A.R., R.C., J.A., and S.H.; data curation, L.A., M.L.-C., R.B.; writing—original draft preparation, I.Y.C.; writing—review and editing, all authors. All authors have read and agreed to the published version of the manuscript.

Funding: We thank the following for financially supporting this work: the Thornton Foundation and the Royal Marsden Cancer Charity (funding to I.Y.C.), the Medical Research Council (I.Y.C. and D.C.), Cancer Research UK as part of Programme Funding (C.J.L.), Breast Cancer Now, working in partnership with Walk the Walk (S.H.). This work represents independent research supported by the National Institute for Health Research (NIHR) Biomedical Research Centre at The Royal Marsden NHS Foundation Trust and the Institute of Cancer Research, London. The views expressed are those of the authors and not necessarily those of the NIHR or the Department of Health and Social Care.

Institutional Review Board Statement: The study was conducted according to the guidelines of the Declaration of Helsinki, and approved by the Royal Marsden Hospital Ethics (CCR 2110).

Informed Consent Statement: Informed consent was obtained from all subjects involved in the study.

Data Availability Statement: The raw data supporting the conclusions of this article are available on request to the corresponding author.

Conflicts of Interest: The authors declare no conflict of interest.

References

1. Siegel, R.L.; Miller, K.D.; Jemal, A. Cancer statistics. *CA A Cancer J. Clin.* **2017**, *67*, 7–30. [CrossRef] [PubMed]
2. Rustgi, A.K.; El-Serag, H.B. Esophageal Carcinoma. *N. Engl. J. Med.* **2014**, *371*, 2499–2509. [CrossRef] [PubMed]
3. Siegel, R.L.; Miller, K.D.; Jemal, A. Cancer statistics. *CA Cancer J. Clin.* **2019**, *69*, 7–34. [CrossRef] [PubMed]
4. Bang, Y.-J.; Van Cutsem, E.; Feyereislova, A.; Chung, H.C.; Shen, L.; Sawaki, A.; Lordick, F.; Ohtsu, A.; Omuro, Y.; Satoh, T.; et al. Trastuzumab in combination with chemotherapy versus chemotherapy alone for treatment of HER2-positive advanced gastric or gastro-oesophageal junction cancer (ToGA): A phase 3, open-label, randomised controlled trial. *Lancet* **2010**, *376*, 687–697. [CrossRef]
5. Dutton, S.J.; Ferry, D.R.; Blazeby, J.M.; Abbas, H.; Dahle-Smith, A.; Mansoor, W.; Thompson, J.; Harrison, M.; Chatterjee, A.; Falk, S.; et al. Gefitinib for oesophageal cancer progressing after chemotherapy (COG): A phase 3, multicentre, double-blind, placebo-controlled randomised trial. *Lancet Oncol.* **2014**, *15*, 894–904. [CrossRef]
6. Waddell, T.; Chau, I.; Cunningham, D.; Gonzalez, D.; Okines, A.F.C.; Wotherspoon, A.; Saffery, C.; Middleton, G.; Wadsley, J.; Ferry, D.; et al. Epirubicin, oxaliplatin, and capecitabine with or without panitumumab for patients with previously untreated advanced oesophagogastric cancer (REAL3): A randomised, open-label phase 3 trial. *Lancet Oncol.* **2013**, *14*, 481–489. [CrossRef]
7. Ohtsu, A.; Shah, M.A.; Van Cutsem, E.; Rha, S.Y.; Sawaki, A.; Park, S.R.; Lim, H.Y.; Yamada, Y.; Wu, J.; Langer, B.; et al. Bevacizumab in Combination with Chemotherapy as First-Line Therapy in Advanced Gastric Cancer: A Randomized, Double-Blind, Placebo-Controlled Phase III Study. *J. Clin. Oncol.* **2011**, *29*, 3968–3976. [CrossRef]
8. Fuchs, C.S.; Tomasek, J.; Yong, C.J.; Dumitru, F.; Passalacqua, R.; Goswami, C.; Safran, H.; Dos Santos, L.V.; Aprile, G.; Ferry, D.R.; et al. Ramucirumab monotherapy for previously treated advanced gastric or gastro-oesophageal junction adenocarcinoma (REGARD): An international, randomised, multicentre, placebo-controlled, phase 3 trial. *Lancet* **2014**, *383*, 31–39. [CrossRef]
9. Wilke, H.; Muro, K.; Van Cutsem, E.; Oh, S.-C.; Bodoky, G.; Shimada, Y.; Hironaka, S.; Sugimoto, N.; Lipatov, O.; Kim, T.-Y.; et al. Ramucirumab plus paclitaxel versus placebo plus paclitaxel in patients with previously treated advanced gastric or gastro-oesophageal junction adenocarcinoma (RAINBOW): A double-blind, randomised phase 3 trial. *Lancet Oncol.* **2014**, *15*, 1224–1235. [CrossRef]
10. Bang, Y.-J.; Xu, R.-H.; Chin, K.; Lee, K.-W.; Park, S.H.; Rha, S.Y.; Shen, L.; Qin, S.; Xu, N.; Im, S.-A.; et al. Olaparib in combination with paclitaxel in patients with advanced gastric cancer who have progressed following first-line therapy (GOLD): A double-blind, randomised, placebo-controlled, phase 3 trial. *Lancet Oncol.* **2017**, *18*, 1637–1651. [CrossRef]
11. Ross-Innes, C.S.; Wheatley, T.; Weaver, J.M.; Lynch, A.G.; Kingsbury, Z.; Ross, M.T.; Humphray, S.; Bentley, D.; Fitzgerald, R.C.; Becq, J.; et al. Whole-genome sequencing provides new insights into the clonal architecture of Barrett's esophagus and esophageal adenocarcinoma. *Nat. Genet.* **2015**, *47*, 1038–1046. [CrossRef] [PubMed]
12. Stachler, M.D.; Taylor-Weiner, A.; Peng, S.; McKenna, A.; Agoston, A.T.; Odze, R.D.; Davison, J.M.; Nason, K.S.; Loda, M.; Leshchiner, I.; et al. Paired exome analysis of Barrett's esophagus and adenocarcinoma. *Nat. Genet.* **2015**, *47*, 1047–1055. [CrossRef] [PubMed]
13. Dulak, A.M.; Stojanov, P.; Peng, S.; Lawrence, M.S.; Fox, C.; Stewart, C.; Bandla, S.; Imamura, Y.; Schumacher, S.E.; Shefler, E.; et al. Exome and whole-genome sequencing of esophageal adenocarcinoma identifies recurrent driver events and mutational complexity. *Nat. Genet.* **2013**, *45*, 478–486. [CrossRef] [PubMed]
14. Chong, I.Y.; Cunningham, D.; Barber, L.J.; Campbell, J.; Chen, L.; Kozarewa, I.; Fenwick, K.; Assiotis, I.; Guettler, S.; Garcia-Murillas, I.; et al. The genomic landscape of oesophagogastric junctional adenocarcinoma. *J. Pathol.* **2013**, *231*, 301–310. [CrossRef] [PubMed]
15. The Cancer Genome Atlas Research Network Integrated genomic characterization of oesophageal carcinoma. *Nat. Cell Biol.* **2017**, *541*, 169–175. [CrossRef]

16. Yakovleva, A.; Plieskatt, J.L.; Jensen, S.; Humeida, R.; Lang, J.; Li, G.; Bracci, P.; Silver, S.; Bethony, J.M. Fit for genomic and proteomic purposes: Sampling the fitness of nucleic acid and protein derivatives from formalin fixed paraffin embedded tissue. *PLoS ONE* **2017**, *12*, e0181756. [CrossRef]
17. Li, H.; Durbin, R. Fast and accurate short read alignment with Burrows-Wheeler transform. *Bioinformatics* **2009**, *25*, 1754–1760. [CrossRef]
18. McKenna, A.; Hanna, M.; Banks, E.; Sivachenko, A.; Cibulskis, K.; Kernytsky, A.; Garimella, K.; Altshuler, D.; Gabriel, S.B.; Daly, M.J.; et al. The Genome Analysis Toolkit: A MapReduce framework for analyzing next-generation DNA sequencing data. *Genome Res.* **2010**, *20*, 1297–1303. [CrossRef]
19. Greytak, S.R.; Engel, K.B.; Bass, B.P.; Moore, H.M. Accuracy of Molecular Data Generated with FFPE Biospecimens: Lessons from the Literature. *Cancer Res.* **2015**, *75*, 1541–1547. [CrossRef]
20. Futreal, P.A.; Coin, L.; Marshall, M.; Down, T.A.; Hubbard, T.; Wooster, R.; Rahman, N.; Stratton, M.R. A census of human cancer genes. *Nat. Rev. Cancer* **2004**, *4*, 177–183. [CrossRef]
21. Marusyk, A.; Almendro, V.; Polyak, K. Intra-tumour heterogeneity: A looking glass for cancer? *Nat. Rev. Cancer* **2012**, *12*, 323–334. [CrossRef] [PubMed]
22. Stahl, P.; Seeschaaf, C.; Lebok, P.; Kutup, A.; Bockhorn, M.; Izbicki, J.R.; Bokemeyer, C.; Simon, R.; Sauter, G.; Marx, A.H. Heterogeneity of amplification of HER2, EGFR, CCND1 and MYC in gastric cancer. *BMC Gastroenterol.* **2015**, *15*, 1–13. [CrossRef] [PubMed]
23. Wakatsuki, T.; Yamamoto, N.; Sano, T.; Chin, K.; Kawachi, H.; Takahari, D.; Ogura, M.; Ichimura, T.; Nakayama, I.; Osumi, H.; et al. Clinical impact of intratumoral HER2 heterogeneity on trastuzumab efficacy in patients with HER2-positive gastric cancer. *J. Gastroenterol.* **2018**, *53*, 1186–1195. [CrossRef] [PubMed]
24. Mroz, E.A.; Rocco, J.W. MATH, a novel measure of intratumor genetic heterogeneity, is high in poor-outcome classes of head and neck squamous cell carcinoma. *Oral Oncol.* **2013**, *49*, 211–215. [CrossRef] [PubMed]
25. Normanno, N.; Rachiglio, A.M.; Roma, C.; Fenizia, F.; Esposito, C.; Pasquale, R.; La Porta, M.L.; Iannaccone, A.; Micheli, F.; Santangelo, M.; et al. Molecular diagnostics and personalized medicine in oncology: Challenges and opportunities. *J. Cell. Biochem.* **2013**, *114*, 514–524. [CrossRef]
26. Esteve-Codina, A.; Arpí, O.; Martinez-García, M.; Pineda, E.; Mallo, M.; Gut, M.; Carrato, C.; Rovira, A.; López, R.; Tortosa, A.; et al. A Comparison of RNA-Seq Results from Paired Formalin-Fixed Paraffin-Embedded and Fresh-Frozen Glioblastoma Tissue Samples. *PLoS ONE* **2017**, *12*, e0170632. [CrossRef]
27. Suciu, B.A.; Pap, Z.; Dénes, L.; Brînzaniuc, K.; Copotoiu, C.; Pávai, Z. Allele-specific PCR method for identification of EGFR mutations in non-small cell lung cancer: Formalin-fixed paraffin-embedded tissue versus fresh tissue. *Romanian J. Morphol. Embryol. Rev. Roum. Morphol. Embryol.* **2016**, *57*, 495–500.
28. Lehmann, U.; Kreipe, H. Real-Time PCR Analysis of DNA and RNA Extracted from Formalin-Fixed and Paraffin-Embedded Biopsies. *Methods* **2001**, *25*, 409–418. [CrossRef]
29. Grünberg, J.; Verocay, M.C.; Rébori, A.; Pouso, J. Comparison of chronic peritoneal dialysis outcomes in children with and without spina bifida. *Pediatr. Nephrol.* **2007**, *22*, 573–577. [CrossRef]
30. De Paoli-Iseppi, R.; Johansson, P.A.; Menzies, A.M.; Dias, K.-R.; Pupo, G.M.; Kakavand, H.; Wilmott, J.S.; Mann, G.J.; Hayward, N.K.; Dinger, M.E.; et al. Comparison of whole-exome sequencing of matched fresh and formalin fixed paraffin embedded melanoma tumours: Implications for clinical decision making. *Pathology* **2016**, *48*, 261–266. [CrossRef]
31. Spencer, D.H.; Sehn, J.K.; Abel, H.J.; Watson, M.A.; Pfeifer, J.D.; Duncavage, E.J. Comparison of Clinical Targeted Next-Generation Sequence Data from Formalin-Fixed and Fresh-Frozen Tissue Specimens. *J. Mol. Diagn.* **2013**, *15*, 623–633. [CrossRef] [PubMed]
32. Solassol, J.; Ramos, J.; Lopez-Crapez, E.; Saifi, M.; Mangé, A.; Vianès, E.; Lamy, P.; Costes, V.; Maudelonde, T. KRAS Mutation Detection in Paired Frozen and Formalin-Fixed Paraffin-Embedded (FFPE) Colorectal Cancer Tissues. *Int. J. Mol. Sci.* **2011**, *12*, 3191–3204. [CrossRef] [PubMed]
33. Betge, J.; Kerr, G.; Miersch, T.; Leible, S.; Erdmann, G.; Galata, C.L.; Zhan, T.; Gaiser, T.; Post, S.; Ebert, M.P.; et al. Amplicon Sequencing of Colorectal Cancer: Variant Calling in Frozen and Formalin-Fixed Samples. *PLoS ONE* **2015**, *10*, e0127146. [CrossRef] [PubMed]
34. Gao, X.H.; Li, J.; Gong, H.F.; Yu, G.Y.; Liu, P.; Hao, L.Q.; Liu, L.J.; Bai, C.G.; Zhang, W. Comparison of Fresh Frozen Tissue with Formalin-Fixed Paraffin-Embedded Tissue for Mutation Analysis Using a Multi-Gene Panel in Patients With Colorectal Cancer. *Front. Oncol.* **2020**, *10*, 310. [CrossRef]
35. Do, H.; Dobrovic, A. Sequence Artifacts in DNA from Formalin-Fixed Tissues: Causes and Strategies for Minimization. *Clin. Chem.* **2015**, *61*, 64–71. [CrossRef]

Article

The Prognostic Role of Early Skeletal Muscle Mass Depletion in Multimodality Management of Patients with Advanced Gastric Cancer Treated with First Line Chemotherapy: A Pilot Experience from Modena Cancer Center

Margherita Rimini [1], Annarita Pecchi [2], Francesco Prampolini [2], Chiara Bussei [3], Massimiliano Salati [1], Daniela Forni [2], Francesca Martelli [2], Filippo Valoriani [3], Fabio Canino [1], Alessandro Bocconi [1], Fabio Gelsomino [1], Linda Reverberi [3], Stefania Benatti [1], Federico Piacentini [1], Renata Menozzi [3], Massimo Dominici [1], Gabriele Luppi [1] and Andrea Spallanzani [1,*]

1. Division of Oncology, Department of Oncology and Hematology, University Hospital of Modena, 41122 Modena, Italy; margherita.rimini@gmail.com (M.R.); massisalati@gmail.com (M.S.); fabiocanino05@gmail.com (F.C.); alessandro.bocconi@gmail.com (A.B.); fabiogelsomino83@yahoo.it (F.G.); stefania.benatti@unimore.it (S.B.); federico.piacentini@unimore.it (F.P.); massimo.dominici@unimore.it (M.D.); luppi.gabriele@aou.mo.it (G.L.)
2. Department of Radiology, University Hospital of Modena, 41122 Modena, Italy; pecchi.annarita@aou.mo.it (A.P.); prampolini.francesco@aou.mo.it (F.P.); danielaforni92@gmail.com (D.F.); francesca.martelli1992@gmail.com (F.M.)
3. Division of Metabolic Disease and Clinical Nutrition, University Hospital of Modena, 41122 Modena, Italy; bussei.chiara@aou.mo.it (C.B.); valorianifilippo@gmail.com (F.V.); reverberi.linda@policlinico.mo.it (L.R.); menozzi.renata@aou.mo.it (R.M.)
* Correspondence: andrea.spallanzani@gmail.com; Tel.: +39-05-9422-3310

Abstract: Background: Few data about the link between nutritional status and survival are available in the metastatic gastric cancer (GC) setting. The aim of this work was to evaluate the prognostic role of tissue modifications during treatment and the benefit of a scheduled nutritional assessment in this setting. Methods: Clinical and laboratory variables of 40 metastatic GC patients treated at Modena Cancer Center were retrieved: 20 received a nutritional assessment on the oncology's discretion, the other 20 received a scheduled nutritional assessment at baseline and every 2–4 weeks. Anthropometric parameters were calculated on Computed Tomography (CT) images at the baseline and after 3 months of chemotherapy. Results: A correlation between baseline Eastern Cooperative Oncology Group Performance Status (ECOG PS), Lymphocyte to Monocyte Ratio (LMR), C-reactive protein (PCR), Prognostic Nutritional Index (PNI) and Overall survival (OS) was highlighted. Among the anthropometric parameters, early skeletal muscle mass depletion (ESMMD) >10% in the first months of treatment significantly impacted on mOS ($p = 0.0023$). A link between ESMMD and baseline LDH > 460 U/L, baseline CRP > 2.2 mg/dL and weight decrease during treatment emerged. Patients evaluated with a nutritional scheduled support experienced a mean gain in subcutaneous and visceral fat of 11.4% and 10.21%, respectively. Conclusion: We confirm the prognostic impact of ESMMD > 10% during chemotherapy in metastatic GC. The prognostic role of a scheduled nutritional assessment deserves further confirmation in large prospective trials.

Keywords: gastric cancer; sarcopenia; nutritional status

1. Introduction

The prognosis of patients with advanced gastric cancer is still poor due to the absence of potentially curative options [1]. Palliative chemotherapy improves survival and quality of life (QoL) compared to best supportive care both in first and second line setting [2]. In recent years, the development of new drugs alone or in combination with chemotherapy, helped to raise the bar of median overall survival over 12 months at the expense of increased treatment related toxicities [3,4]. The introduction of anti-HER2 treatment in first such as the development of ramucirumab alone or in combination with chemotherapy in second line provided nearly 14–16 months of median overall survival in patients with new diagnosis of metastatic gastric cancer [5–7]. In fact, alongside progress in the pharmacological field, the target has moved to an adequate patient selection. The research of clinic-pathological prognostic and predictive factors is one of the main objectives of prospective studies and retrospective analysis [8,9].

Some prognostic scores have been developed combining inflammation-related and nutrition-related markers, such as the neutrophil-to-lymphocyte ratio (NLR) platelets to Lymphocyte ratio (PLR), lymphocyte to monocyte ratio (LMR) and prognostic nutritional index (PNI): the prognostic role of these parameters and other factors such as performance status and neoplastic markers (CEA and CA 19.9) is well known in patients with advanced gastric cancer [10,11].

Almost two decades ago it was identified the close link between malnutrition and survival and the impact of sarcopenia on tolerance to chemotherapy, longer hospitalization, quality of life and mortality, but to date, many malnourished cancer patients still receive inadequate nutritional support, mainly due to the poor awareness of the problem and inefficient collaboration between oncologists and clinical nutritionists [12].

An adequate evaluation of patients' nutritional status in metastatic setting cannot ignore the assessment of skeletal muscle mass and skeletal muscle density using computed tomography scan. Previous studies in various types of cancer highlighted the strong association between survival, treatment toxicities and the amount of muscle and adipose tissue at diagnosis such as its modification during chemotherapy [13–16].

A recent metanalysis focused on the effects of dietary interventions on nutritional status of gastric cancer patients undergoing gastrectomy, but few data are available in patients with metastatic gastric cancer treated with palliative chemotherapy [17].

The aim of our work is to evaluate the incidence of sarcopenia such as the prognostic and predictive role of muscle and visceral tissue modifications during the first 3 months of chemotherapy in patients with metastatic gastric cancer. In a subsequent pivotal analysis, we matched two different group of patients to evaluate the role of an adequate nutritional support during palliative chemotherapy.

2. Materials and Methods

Patients with recurrent or metastatic gastric cancer who received fluoropyrimidines and platinum based first-line chemotherapy in Modena Cancer Center from November 2015 through December 2019 were retrospectively studied. All patients had histologically proven adenocarcinoma of stomach with at least one metastatic lesion as confirmed by diagnostic imaging. Computed Tomography (CT) scan was performed every 2–4 months in most patients to evaluate treatment efficacy. The study was approved by local Ethic Committee (n° 427/2019/OSS/AOUMO). All alive patients provided written informed consent.

Clinical and laboratory data were reported from the hospital electronic medical database at diagnosis and first CT re-evaluation including the following variables: age, gender, performance status (ECOG), height, weight, Body-Mass Index (BMI), blood count, neutrophil/lymphocyte ratio (NLR), platelets/lymphocyte ratio (PLR), lymphocyte/monocyte ratio (LMR), systemic inflammatory index (SII) lactate dehydrogenase (LDH), C-reactive protein (CRP), albumin, Sodium (Na^+), Potassium (K^+), CEA, CA 19.9 and prognostic nutritional index (PNI).

In the second part of the work, we searched for differences in terms of clinical, anthropometric and survival outcomes between the first group of patients which received a nutritional evaluation at oncology's discretion and the second group of patients which received a standardized nutritional evaluation at the baseline and then every 2–4 weeks during treatment.

The nutritional evaluation was defined as an individualized counselling aimed to collecting data about the dietary intake, usual dietary pattern, intolerances or food aversions, digestive difficulties, patients' psychological status, autonomy and need for help in the act of eating. In addition, a symptom assessment was included in the nutritional evaluation. Each nutritional assessment resulted in dietary advice and, if necessary, in prescription of oral implementations.

2.1. Body Composition Parameter Measurements

All patients included in the study underwent CT scan at the time of diagnosis and after 2–4 months, as part of the diagnostic and therapeutic path planned by the cancer center.

CT exams were performed at our hospital using a 64-slice CT scanner (Lightspeed VCT, GE Healthcare, Milwaukee, WI, USA).

Baseline and follow-up CT examinations were loaded on an Advantage Workstation (VolumeShare 7, GE Healthcare, Milwaukee, WI, USA) and non-contrast images at the level of the third lumbar vertebra (L3) were used for reconstructions and measurements of quantitative and qualitative body composition parameters.

According to literature, skeletal muscle cross-sectional areas including the psoas, paraspinal muscles and abdominal muscles were identified and quantified using the preestablished HU thresholds for muscle (HU-30 to 150), whereas subcutaneous and visceral adipose cross-sectional areas were quantified using HU thresholds for fat tissue (HU-150 to-30) (Figure 1).

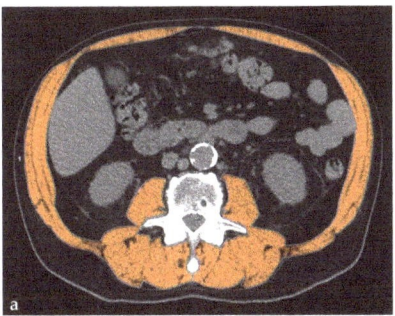

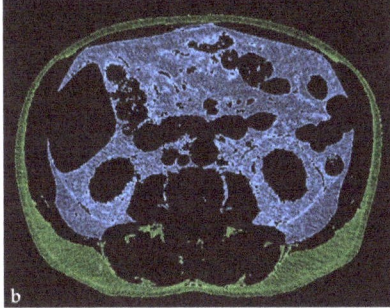

Figure 1. Measurement of body composition parameters with cross-sectional computed tomography (CT) images at the level of third lumbar vertebra. (**a**) Skeletal muscle area (**b**) Subcutaneous and Visceral fat areas.

The skeletal muscle mass index (SMI, cm^2/m^2) was calculated by dividing these skeletal muscle areas by height squared and similarly visceral fat index (VFI, cm^2/m^2) and subcutaneous fat index (SFI, cm^2/m^2) were calculated by normalizing each fat area for height.

Total adipose index (TAI) was calculated by adding SFI + VFI.

Relative changes of body composition occurred in the period between baseline and follow-up CT scans were also quantified for each patient by calculating delta (Δ) parameters: ΔSMI (defined also as ESMMD), ΔSFI, ΔVFI, ΔTAI. SMI reduction between baseline and first evaluation was classified as early skeletal muscle mass depletion (ESMMD).

In addition, the quality of skeletal muscle at the time of the diagnosis was examined by calculating the mean attenuation (MA) of skeletal muscle and the intramuscular adipose tissue content (IMAC) of paraspinal muscles.

Therefore, only for baseline CT scans, MA, i.e., density of the skeletal muscle tissue was measured in HU and IMAC was calculated according to literature by dividing CT density of the multifidus muscles (HU) with CT density of subcutaneous fat (HU).

Higher IMAC indicates a greater content of adipose tissue in muscle and, consequently, suggests a lower skeletal muscle quality [18,19].

We used specific cut-off values for SMI, MA, SFI and VFI. We used these cut-off values in accordance with their prognostic role highlighted in two large cohorts reported by Martin et al. and Ebady et al. [14,19]. Sarcopenia was defined as SMI < 43 cm^2/m^2 in male patients with BMI < 25 kg/m^2 and SMI < 53 cm^2/m^2 if BMI > 25 kg/m^2; in female patients, sarcopenia was set at SMI < 41 kg/m^2 irrespective of BMI. Cut-off values for MA were <41 HU in non-overweight patients (BMI < 25 kg/m^2) and <33 HU if BMI > 25 kg/m^2 for both sexes. Sarcopenic obesity was defined as sarcopenia combined with overweight or obesity (BMI > 25 kg/m^2). The cut off values for VFI, SFI and TAI were 52.9 cm^2/m^2 in males and 51.5 cm^2/m^2 in females, 50 cm^2/m^2 in males and 42 cm^2/m^2 in females and 107.7 cm^2/m^2 in males and 102.2 cm^2/m^2 in females, respectively [14,20].

2.2. Statistical Analysis

Data on baseline characteristics and body composition are shown as mean and SD. The median overall survival (OS) and progression free survival (PFS) were determined using the Kaplan–Meier method. Differences in demographic and clinical data between groups were evaluated using the Fisher exact test for categorical variables and independent *t*-test for continuous variables. The best cut-off for laboratory values were defined by ROC curve distribution.

Cox proportional hazards regression model was used to determine the relationship of explanatory variables to survival as hazard ratios (HR) and 95% confidence intervals (CI). Logistic regression was used to describe and explain the relationship between dependent binary variables and independent variables. Odds ratio (OR) together with 95% confidence interval (CI) were provided for logistic regression analyses. Independent variable statistically significant in the univariate analyses were used to build the multivariate analysis. All tests were 2-sided and $p < 0.05$ was considered statistically significant.

MedCalc package (MedCalc1 version 16.8.4) was used for all statistical analyses.

3. Results
3.1. Patients Characteristics

The present study included 40 patients with a confirmed diagnosis of advanced gastric adenocarcinoma treated with first-line chemotherapy between November 2015 to December 2019 in Modena Cancer Center. The main characteristics of patients enrolled in the study are summarized in Table 1. Overall, 82.5% of patients were younger than 70 years and the 60% of patients were male. The ECOG performance status was 0–1 in the 87.5% of patients at baseline. Since we considered patients with advanced disease, in our sample, only six patients (15%) were submitted to a previous gastrectomy. The first line regimens were mainly doublet chemotherapy with fluoropirimidin and platinum-derivative: 26 patients performed folfox (5-fluorouracil + oxaliplatin), four patients the TOGA regimen (cisplatin + 5-fluorouracil + trastuzumab), four patients a triplete regimen with EOX (epirubicin + oxaliplatin + capecitabine), three patients Xelox (capecitabine + oxaliplatin), and three patients monotherapy with 5-fluorouracil as De Gramont regimen.

Table 1. Patients' characteristics.

Variable	N(%)
Age	
<70 years	33 (82.5%)
≥70 years	7 (17.5%)
Gender	
Male	24 (60.0%)
Female	16 (40.0%)
Site of primary tumor	
Gastroesophageal junction	5 (12.5%)
Fundus	3 (7.5%)
Body	12 (30.0%)
Fundus and body	4 (10.0%)
GE junction, fundus and body	1 (2.5%)
Antrum	7 (17.5%)
Body and antrum	6 (15.0%)
Diffuse/linitis	2 (5.0%)
Previous gastrectomy	
Yes	6 (15.0%)
No	34 (85%)
Eastern Cooperative Oncology Group Performance Status (ECOG PS) at 1^line chemotherapy start	
0–1	35 (87.5%)
≥2	5 (12.5%)
N° of metastatic sites at 1^line chemotherapy start	
1	12 (30.0%)
≥2	27 (67.5%)
Unknown	1 (2.5%)
Metastatic site at 1^line chemotherapy start	
Liver	5 (12.5%)
Nodes	11 (27.5%)
Peritoneum	24 (60.0%)
Lung	4 (10.0%)
Bone	11 (27.5%)
Others	5 (12.5%)
Body mass index—BMI (kg/m^2)	
<25	28 (70.0%)
≥25	12 (30.0%)
Prognostic nutritional index—PNI	
<38.6	8 (20.0%)
≥38.6	18 (45.0%)
Unknown	14 (35.0%)
Type of first line treatment	
Single agent	2 (5.0%)
Combination	38 (95.0%)
Laboratory parameter at first-line chemotherapy start	
Neutrophil-lymphocyte Ratio—NLR (Mean ± standard deviation)	5.1 ± 3.5
<4.8	17 (42.5%)
≥4.8	11 (27.5%)
Unknown	12 (30.0%)
Platelet-lymphocyte ratio—PLR (Mean ± standard deviation)	260.8 ± 127.1
<217	12 (30.0%)
≥217	16 (40.0%)
Unknown	12 (30.0%)

Table 1. Cont.

Variable	N(%)
Lymphocyte-monocyte ratio—LMR (Mean ± standard deviation)	3.0 ± 1.4
≤2.1	7 (17.5%)
>2.1	21 (52.5%)
Unknown	12 (30.0%)
Systemic Immune-Inflammation Index (SII) (Mean ± standard deviation) ($\times 10^3$ cells/µL)	1465 ± 1041
≤1110	20 (30.0%)
>1110	16 (40.0%)
Unknown	12 (30.0%)
Albumine (Mean ± standard deviation) (g/dL)	3.6 ± 0.5
≤3.5	19 (47.5%)
>3.5	17 (42.5%)
Unknown	4 (10.0%)
C reactive Protein—PCR (Mean ± standard deviation) (mg/dL)	3,2 ± 4,6
<2.2	13 (32.5%)
≥2.2	8 (20.0%)
Unknown	19 (47.5%)
Carcinoembryonic antigen—CEA (Mean ± standard deviation) (ng/mL)	201.6 ± 683.2
≤5	23 (57.5%)
>5	14 (35.0%)
Unknown	3 (7.5%)
Carbohydrate antigen 19.9—Ca 19.9 (Mean ± standard deviation) (U/mL)	622 ± 1856
≤37	20 (50.0%)
>37	17 (42.5%)
Unknown	3 (7.5%)

The median duration of first line chemotherapy was 6 months (range 1.68–16.38 months); in 7 of 40 (17%) patients an early discontinuation of the treatment was required due to toxicities or worsening of patient clinical conditions.

The mainly reported toxicity was blood count alteration with neutropenia and anemia in 11 patients (27%); afterward, gastrointestinal alterations (mainly nausea and vomit) and peripheral neuropathy in 8 patients (19%). The grade of these adverse events was not reported in our clinical records but none of these was a grade 4. Overall, 20 patients (50%) were reported to receive a second line therapy, consisting prevalently in the association ramucirumab and paclitaxel accordi2ng to the guidelines. In particular, 8/20 (40%) patients in the first group and 12/20 (60%) patients in second group were treated with a second line therapy.

Concerning the anthropometric characteristics, median BMI of the entire sample was 23.59 kg/m². The prevalence of baseline sarcopenia and sarcopenic obesity were 42.5% (17/40) and 7% (3/40), respectively.

3.2. Prognostic Factors

The first part of our analysis was addressed to research clinical and anthropometric prognostic parameters and the correlation between these variables and clinical benefit in the whole sample.

Overall, after a median follow-up of 16.4 months, mOS was 12.07 months, whereas mPFS was 6.18 months.

All covariates retrieved were tested within a univariate model.

We evaluated the prognostic impact of baseline clinical, laboratory and anthropometric measures finding a significant interaction between ECOG (ECOG 2 vs. ECOG 0/1. HR

12.74; 95% C.I. 0.66 to 243.85, $p < 0.001$), LMR (LMR > 2.1 vs. LMR < 2.1. HR 3.47; 95% C.I. 1.35 to 8.91, p 0.0095), PCR (PCR > 2.2 vs. PCR < 2.2. HR 3.71; 95% C.I. 1.38 to 9.93, p 0.009), PNI (PNI > 38.6 vs. PNI < 38.6. HR 3.58; 95% C.I. 1.36 to 9.42, p 0.009) and overall survival. Concerning the anthropometric parameters, only ESMMD > 10% from baseline to the first radiological revaluation significantly impact on mOS (HR 2.57, 95% CI 1.13–5.82, $p = 0.0023$) (Table 2).

Following adjustment for significantly prognostic covariates at univariate analysis, a multivariate analysis was performed, which confirmed ECOG PS (0–1 vs. 2 HR 49.32, 95% CI 7.32–331.95, $p = 0.0001$) and ESMMD > 10% (HR 2.47 95% CI 1.05–7.09, $p = 0.0375$) as the only independent prognostic factors in terms of OS and PFS (Figure 2).

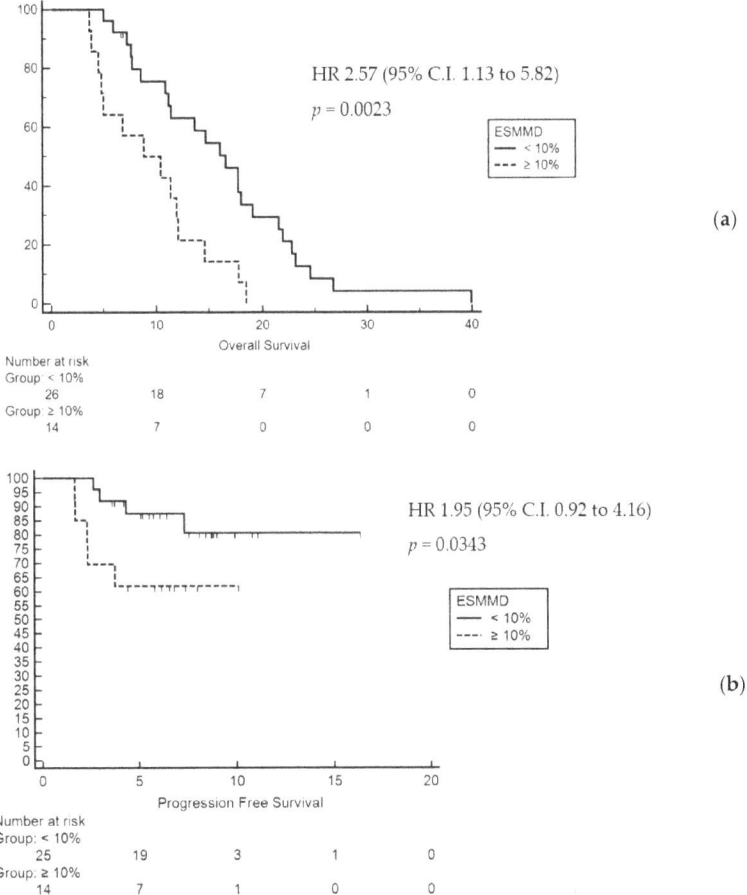

Figure 2. Kaplan–Meier curves for overall survival (a) and progression free survival (b) according to early skeletal muscle mass depletion (ESMMD). HR: Hazard Ration; CI: Confidence Interval.

Moreover, by performing a logistic regression analysis, ECOG PS was highlighted to be the only clinical parameter correlated with clinical benefit (defined as stable disease and/or partial response vs. progression disease) (OR 7.25, 95% C.I. 0.9876 to 53.2239, $p = 0.0004$).

Overall, no correlation has been highlighted between anthropometric parameters and toxicities from treatment.

On the other hand, a relationship has been reported between several clinical and bio-humoral variables and radiological assessment of early variation of SMI. In particular, our analysis confirmed a strong link between ESMMD and baseline LDH > 460 U/l (OR 7.91; 95% CI 1.31–47.51, p = 0.0046), baseline CRP > 2.2 mg/dL (OR 20.0; 95% CI 1.65–241.73, p = 0.006) and weight decrease during treatment (OR 0.82; 95% C.I. 0.71 to 0.94, p = 0.0009).

Table 2. Uni and multivariate analysis for overall survival.

	Univariate		Multivariate
	HR (95% CI)	p	
Age (≥65 vs. <65 years)	1.08 (0.57–2.07)	0.8110	
ECOG PS (2 vs. 0–1)	12.75 (0.67–243.86)	<0.0001	0.0001
Site of M (>1 vs. 1)	1.92 (0.90–4.11)	0.058	
NLR (≥4.8 vs. <4.8)	2.00 (0.84–4.75)	0.0711	
LMR (<2.1 vs. ≥2.1)	3.03 (0.88–10.46)	0.0060	
PCR (≥2.2 vs. <2.2 mg/dL)	3.1 (0.98–9.78)	0.0055	
CEA (≥5 vs. <5 ng/mL)	0.67 (0.33 to 1.36)	0.2763	
PNI (≥38.6 vs. <38.6)	0.34 (0.11–1.06)	0.0058	
SII (≥1110 vs. <1110 (×10³ cells/µL)	0.95 (0.44–2.07)	0.9104	
BMI (<25 vs. ≥25 kg/m²)	0.79 (0–37–1.70)	0.5215	
IMAC (≤−0.33 vs. >−0.33)	0.67 (0.34–1.32)	0.2233	
VFI (≥52.9 cm²/m² in males and 51.5 cm²/m² in females vs. <52.9 cm²/m² in males and 51.5 cm²/m² in females)	1.24 (0.66–2.36)	0.5010	
SFI (≤50 cm²/m² in males and 42 cm²/m² in females vs. >50 cm²/m² in males and 42 cm²/m² in females)	0.76 (0.40–1.43)	0.3921	
Sarcopenia sec. Martin (Yes vs. No)	1.40 (0.72–2.73)	0.3058	
Sarcopenia at revaluation sec. Martin (Yes vs. No)	2.24 (1.07–4.69	0.0117	
ESMMD (≥10% vs. <10%)	2.57 (1.13–5.83)	0.0036	0.0375

3.3. Role of Nutritional Assessment

The second part of our analysis was focused on the role of an early and scheduled nutritional evaluation. We searched for differences in terms of clinical, anthropometric and survival outcomes between the first group of patients which received a nutritional evaluation at oncology's discretion and the second group of patients which received a standardized nutritional evaluation at the baseline and then every 2–4 weeks during treatment. Overall, 20 patients were included in the first group of patients and 20 patients were included in the second group of patients.

Clinical characteristics were well balanced between the two groups of patients as shown in Table 3.

No significant differences in terms of OS and PFS were reported between the two groups of patients; in return, significative differences in adipose tissue modification during treatment have been highlighted. In particular, our analysis showed that patients reserved to a nutritional scheduled support experienced a mean gain in subcutaneous fat (SFI) of 11.4% at the first radiological evaluation vs. baseline; contrarily, patients reserved to an occasional nutritional support experienced a mean lost in SFI of 3.97% at the first radiological evaluation vs. baseline. Consistently, we demonstrated in patients submitted to a scheduled nutritional support a mean gain in visceral fat of 8.55% at the first radiological evaluation vs. baseline, whereas in patients without a scheduled nutritional evaluation, we found a mean loss of visceral fat of 10.21% at the first revaluation vs. baseline. No significant differences in median ESMMD (−7.52% vs.−2.94%) or median ΔBMI (−3.7% vs.−1.7%) were reported in the two groups of patients.

Table 3. Patients categorized according to the nutritional approach.

	Occasional Nutritional Evaluation (n = 20)	Systematic Nutritional Evaluation (n = 20)	p
	Age		
<70 years	16 (80%)	17 (85%)	1.00
≥70 years	4 (20%)	3 (15%)	
	Gender		
Male	13 (65%)	11 (55%)	0.54
Female	7 (35%)	9 (45%)	
	Site of primary tumor		
Gastroesophageal junction	4 (20%)	1 (5%)	0.2334
Fundus	3 (15%)	0	
Body	4 (20%)	8 (40%)	
Fundus and body	2 (10%)	2 (10%)	
GE junction, fundus and body	1 (5%)	0	
Antrum	3 (15%)	4 (20%)	
Body and antrum	3 (15%)	3 (15%)	
Diffuse/linitis	0	2 (10%)	
	Previous gastrectomy		
Yes	3 (15%)	3 (15%)	
No	17 (85%)	17 (85%)	
	ECOG PS at 1ˆline chemotherapy start		
0–1	19 (95%)	16 (80%)	0.3416
≥2	1 (5%)	4 (20%)	
	N° of metastatic sites at 1ˆline chemotherapy start		
1	7 (35%)	5 (25%)	0.7311
≥2	13 (65%)	14 (70%)	
Unknown	0	1 (5%)	
	Metastatic site at 1ˆline chemotherapy start		
Liver	1 (5%)	4 (20%)	0.1173
Nodes	8 (40%)	3 (15%)	
Peritoneum	11 (55%)	13 (65%)	
Lung	1 (5%)	3 (15%)	
Bone	8 (40%)	3 (15%)	
Others	4 (20%)	1 (5%)	
	Body mass index—BMI (kg/m^2)		
<25	14 (70%)	14 (70%)	1.00
≥25	6 (30%)	6 (30%)	
	Prognostic nutritional index—PNI		
<38.6	2 (10%)	6 (30%)	0.2077
≥38.6	9 (45%)	9 (45%)	
Unknown	9 (45%)	5 (25%)	
	Type of first line treatment		
Single agent	1 (5%)	1 (5%)	1.00
Combination	19 (95%)	19 (95%)	
	Laboratory parameter at first-line chemotherapy start		
Neutrophil-lymphocyte Ratio—NLR (Mean ± standard deviation)	4.6 ± 1.9	5.5 ± 4.2	
<4.8	7 (35%)	10 (50%)	0.3765
≥4.8	5 (25%)	6 (30%)	
Unknown	8 (40%)	4 (20%)	

Table 3. Cont.

	Occasional Nutritional Evaluation (n = 20)	Systematic Nutritional Evaluation (n = 20)	p
Platelet-lymphocyte ratio—PLR (Mean ± standard deviation)	240.4 ± 81.9	276.1 ± 150.6	
<217	5 (25%)	7 (35%)	0.3835
≥217	7 (35%)	9 (45%)	
Unknown	8 (40%)	4 (20%)	
Lymphocyte-monocyte ratio—LMR (Mean ± standard deviation)	2.8 ± 1.4	3.1 ± 1.5	
≤2.1	3 (15%)	4 (20%)	0.3858
>2.1	9 (45%)	12 (60%)	
Unknown	8 (40%)	4 (20%)	
Lactate dehydrogenase—LDH (Mean ± standard deviation) (U/L)	631 ± 460	505 ± 661	
≤460	8 (40%)	15 (75%)	0.0769
>460	6 (30%)	2 (10%)	
Unknown	6 (30%)	3 (15%)	
Albumine (Mean ± standard deviation) (g/dL)	3,7 ± 0,5	3,4 ± 0,5	
≤ 3.5	8 (40%)	11 (55%)	0.6056
> 3.5	10 (50%)	7 (35%)	
Unknown	2 (10%)	2 (10%)	
C reactive Protein—PCR (Mean ± standard deviation) (mg/dL)	3.7 ± 5.2	3.0 ± 4.2	
<2.2	4 (20%)	9 (45%)	0.0820
≥2.2	3 (15%)	5 (25%)	
Unknown	13 (65%)	6 (30%)	
Carcinoembryonic antigen—CEA (Mean ± standard deviation) (ng/mL)	178.5 ± 537.3	216.2 ± 744.4	
≤5	11 (55%)	12 (60%)	0.8283
>5	7 (35%)	7 (35%)	
Unknown	2 (10%)	1 (5%)	
Carbohydrate antigen 19.9—Ca 19.9 (Mean ± standard deviation) (U/mL)	646.7 ± 1013.6	604.9 ± 2217.4	
≤37	9 (45%)	11 (55%)	0.529
>37	9 (45%)	8 (40%)	
Unknown	2 (10%)	1 (5%)	

4. Discussion

Recently, the role of sarcopenia in gastric cancer has been focused among perioperative setting. Preoperative muscle mass quality and malnutrition are strictly related to higher surgical risk and delayed and prematurely interrupted adjuvant treatment [21]. Few data are available on the prognostic role of malnutrition in mGC patients [22,23].

In this study, we evaluated a small cohort of 40 advanced GC patients treated with first line palliative chemotherapy in Modena Cancer Center between 2016 and 2019. We evaluated the prognostic impact of baseline clinical, laboratory and anthropometric measures finding a significant interaction between ECOG (ECOG 0/1 vs. ECOG 2, $p < 0.001$), LMR (LMR > 2.1 vs. LMR < 2.1, p 0.0095), PCR (PCR > 2.2 vs. PCR < 2.2, p 0.009), PNI (PNI > 38.6 vs. PNI < 38.6, p 0.009) and overall survival.

In our group of patients, the prevalence of baseline sarcopenia and sarcopenic obesity were 42.5% (17/40) and 7% (3/40) but neither baseline sarcopenia nor BMI at diagnosis significantly affected survival. Conversely, ESMMD > 10% (reported in 14/40 patients) and sarcopenia at first re-evaluation (reported in 18/40 patients) during palliative chemotherapy were associated with shorter mPFS and mOS. In multivariate analysis, in addition to ECOG performance status, only early SMI reduction >10% was statistically relevant and associated with both worse PFS and OS (median PFS 7.3 months vs. 4.4 months, p 0.038; median OS

16.5 months vs. 8.5 months, *p* 0.0375). The relevant role of ECOG performance status was highlighted also for its significant impact on clinical benefit at first evaluation (OR 7.25; 95% C.I. 0.9876 to 53.2239; *p* 0.049).

The prevailing role of ESMMD over baseline sarcopenia in metastatic setting has been previously reported not only for gastric cancer patients [20] but also in patients with different gastrointestinal cancers [24–27]. In the IMPACT trial, in particular, in patients with metastatic pancreatic cancer, ESMMD $\geq$ 10% was significantly associated with worse OS (HR: 2.16; 95% CI 1.23–3.78; *p* = 0.007) and PFS (HR: 2.31; 95% CI 1.30–4.09; *p* = 0.004) [27].

Beside the role of SMI depletion, another point of our study was the evaluation of the prognostic impact of muscle tissue quality (IMAC and MA) as well as early changes in subcutaneous and visceral adipose tissue during chemotherapy, but none of these parameters were clinically relevant maybe due to the small sample size of the study. The prognostic role of muscle quality at baseline is reported in other setting [19,27–31] but in a recent Dutch series enrolled 88 mGC patients treated with capecitabine and oxaliplatin as first line chemotherapy, no correlation between muscle attenuation and survival was confirmed [24].

Several studies confirmed a well-known association between muscle mass depletion and systemic inflammation [21,32,33]. Systemic inflammation has been reported as a strong prognostic factor in cancer progression. In patients with cancer, pro-inflammatory mediators cause an energetic imbalance between catabolic and anabolic pathways. IL-6, IL-2, IL-10, epidermal growth factor (EGF) and IFN exert their effect by activating the signal transducer and activator of transcription 3 (STAT3) producing loss of muscle mass. The levels of IL-6, TNFa and CRP have been reported to be significantly up-regulated in sarcopenia patients. The activation of a pro-inflammatory status can also lead to insulin resistance and muscle depletion through the activation of the ubiquitin-proteasome proteolytic pathway [34]. In our series, we confirmed the strong link between early muscle mass loss and systemic inflammatory indexes because we noted that baseline LDH > 460, CRP > 2.2 and weight decrease during treatment significantly predicted ESMMD.

The second part of our work was an exploratory analysis on the role of a scheduled nutritional evaluation.

As we know, the nutritional support should be considered as an integrated treatment in patients receiving palliative anti-cancer treatment. Patients identified by screening for unintentional weight loss in last 3–6 years or decreased oral intake, should receive adequate nutritional counselling and support but few studies reported a significative benefit of nutritional support in advanced cancer patients [12,17,35,36].

In our center from 2018, all patients with mGC were evaluated through MUST screening test and then taking charge from a nutritional perspective. They performed a nutritional evaluation every 2–4 weeks alongside the scheduled oncological examination. Before 2018, the nutritional path was at the discretion of oncologists and often the first nutritional evaluation was delayed.

Twenty patients were diagnosed in 2016–2017 and subjected to an occasional involvement of the nutritional team; conversely, the other group of patients were evaluated at diagnosis and then every 2 or 4 weeks with scheduled nutritional visit. No significant difference in OS and PFS were reported but relevant difference in adipose tissue modification has been found.

About subcutaneous fat, a mean gain of 15.38% of SFI vs. baseline SFI was reported between patients with nutritional scheduled support (+11.4% at 3 months vs. baseline) vs. patients with occasional nutritional evaluation (−3.97% at 3 months vs. baseline). Concurrently, a relevant mean gain of 18.76% was reported about the visceral fat between patients in the first group (+8.55% vs. baseline) vs. patients in the latter one (−10.21% vs. baseline).

No relevant difference in median ESMMD (−7.52% vs. −2.94%) or median ΔBMI (−3.7% vs. −1.7%) were reported between the 2 groups.

The prognostic role of adipose tissue in gastrointestinal cancers is still debating [37]. In patients with pancreatic and biliary carcinoma underwent resection, high VSR (visceral to subcutaneous ratio) was reported as a negative prognostic factor in a single Japanese series [38,39]. In a classic trial, enrolled patients underwent gastrectomy followed by adjuvant chemotherapy, a marked loss of visceral or subcutaneous fat significantly predicted shorter DFS and OS [40].

In a large series of 1473 gastrointestinal and respiratory metastatic cancer patients, low TAI (total adipose index) was associated with increased mortality (mOS 19.8 months vs. 14.0 months) [19]. In metastatic colorectal cancer, higher VFI has been associated with shorter OS in patients treated with chemotherapy and anti-VEGF antibody but not in those treated with chemotherapy alone [41]. In a post hoc analysis of two non-randomized phase II trials in the same setting, low SFI (HR 1.63; 1.23–2.17) and low VFI (HR 1.48; 1.09–2.02) were associated with an increased risk of dying confirming the protective role of obesity [42].

In addition, in our series, this protective role was confirmed although not statistically significative maybe due to the small sample size: patients with a higher baseline SFI (>50 cm^2/m^2 in males and > 42 cm^2/m^2 in females) experienced an increased median overall survival (13.65 vs. 11.94 months), such as patients with a higher VFI (>52.9 cm^2/m^2 in males and >51.5 cm^2/m^2 in females; mOS 13.65 vs. 11.34 months). Moreover, patients with VFI gain during chemotherapy experienced an increased median overall survival (16.02 months vs. 11.18 months), such as patients with SFI gain (14.64 months vs. 11.18 months) and patients with TAI gain (13.65 months vs. 11.35 months).

Our analysis has several limitations: firstly, the limited number of patients and the retrospective design of the trial. Secondly, we reported a number of patients treated with a consequent second line therapy, which could have influenced the survival outcomes of the two groups of patients considered. Thirdly, patients without available CT scans or lost at follow up were excluded from this trial leading to a possible selection bias. Moreover, we could not have a comprehensive report of the relation between body composition parameters and chemotherapy toxicities or quality of life due to few medical records about these items and the retrospective nature of the study.

5. Conclusions

In conclusion, as reported in other metastatic setting, we confirm the prognostic impact of ESMMD > 10% during the first 3 months of first line chemotherapy in metastatic gastric cancer. The impact of ESMMD > 10% is independent from weight loss and could be predicted by some immune-inflammatory markers such as CRP and LDH at baseline.

The prognostic role of a scheduled nutritional assessment could not be highlighted, perhaps due to the sample size of this series, but a relevant gain in adipose tissue (SFI, VFI, TAI) is reported in this group of patients, suggesting clinical benefit due to the protective role of obesity in metastatic gastrointestinal cancers; therefore, a scheduled nutritional assessment and intervention should be evaluated in metastatic gastric cancer patients. However, the role of this approach deserves further confirmation in large prospective trials.

Author Contributions: Conception and design: A.S., M.S., A.P., F.P. (Francesco Prampolini), C.B., F.V.; Acquisition of data (acquired and managed patients): All authors; Analysis and interpretation of data: A.S., F.P. (Francesco Prampolini); Writing, review and/or revision of the manuscript: A.S., M.R., F.C., F.P. (Francesco Prampolini); Final approval of manuscript: All authors. All authors have read and agreed to the published version of the manuscript.

Funding: This research received no external funding.

Institutional Review Board Statement: The Ethical Review Board of each Institutional Hospital approved the present study. This study was performed in line with the principles of the Declaration of Helsinki.

Informed Consent Statement: Informed consent was obtained from all subjects involved in the study.

Data Availability Statement: Data available on request from the authors.

Conflicts of Interest: The authors declare no conflict of interest.

References

1. Salati, M.; Di Emidio, K.; Tarantino, V.; Cascinu, S. Second-line treatments: Moving towards an opportunity to improve survival in advanced gastric cancer? *ESMO Open* **2017**, *2*, e000206. [CrossRef]
2. Wagner, A.D.; Syn, N.L.X.; Moehler, M.; Grothe, W.; Yong, W.P.; Tai, B.-C.C.; Ho, J.; Unverzagt, S.; Wagner, D.A.; Syn, L.X.N.; et al. Chemotherapy for advanced gastric cancer Systematic Review. *Cochrane Database Syst. Rev.* **2017**, *2017*, 8. [CrossRef]
3. Shitara, K.; Bang, Y.-J.; Iwasa, S.; Sugimoto, N.; Ryu, M.-H.; Sakai, D.; Chung, H.-C.; Kawakami, H.; Yabusaki, H.; Lee, J.; et al. Trastuzumab Deruxtecan in Previously Treated HER2-Positive Gastric Cancer. *N. Engl. J. Med.* **2020**, *382*, 2419–2430. [CrossRef]
4. Shitara, K.; Van Cutsem, E.; Bang, Y.J.; Fuchs, C.; Wyrwicz, L.; Lee, K.W.; Kudaba, I.; Garrido, M.; Chung, H.C.; Lee, J.; et al. Efficacy and Safety of Pembrolizumab or Pembrolizumab Plus Chemotherapy vs Chemotherapy Alone for Patients with First-line, Advanced Gastric Cancer: The KEYNOTE-062 Phase 3 Randomized Clinical Trial. *JAMA Oncol.* **2020**, *6*, 1571–1580. [CrossRef] [PubMed]
5. Wilke, H.; Muro, K.; Van Cutsem, E.; Oh, S.C.; Bodoky, G.; Shimada, Y.; Hironaka, S.; Sugimoto, N.; Lipatov, O.; Kim, T.Y.; et al. Ramucirumab plus paclitaxel versus placebo plus paclitaxel in patients with previously treated advanced gastric or gastro-oesophageal junction adenocarcinoma (RAINBOW): A double-blind, randomised phase 3 trial. *Lancet Oncol.* **2014**, *15*, 1224–1235. [CrossRef]
6. Fuchs, C.S.; Tomasek, J.; Yong, C.J.; Dumitru, F.; Passalacqua, R.; Goswami, C.; Safran, H.; dos Santos, L.V.; Aprile, G.; Ferry, D.R.; et al. Ramucirumab monotherapy for previously treated advanced gastric or gastro-oesophageal junction adenocarcinoma (REGARD): An international, randomised, multicentre, placebo-controlled, phase 3 trial. *Lancet* **2014**, *383*, 31–39. [CrossRef]
7. Bang, Y.-J.; Van Cutsem, E.; Feyereislova, A.; Chung, H.C.; Shen, L.; Sawaki, A.; Lordick, F.; Ohtsu, A.; Omuro, Y.; Satoh, T.; et al. Trastuzumab in combination with chemotherapy versus chemotherapy alone for treatment of HER2-positive advanced gastric or gastro-oesophageal junction cancer (ToGA): A phase 3, open-label, randomised controlled trial. *Lancet* **2010**, *376*, 687–697. [CrossRef]
8. Demirelli, B.; Babacan, N.A.; Ercelep, Ö.; Öztürk, M.A.; Kaya, S.; Tanrıkulu, E.; Khalil, S.; Hasanov, R.; Alan, Ö.; Telli, T.A.; et al. Modified Glasgow Prognostic Score, Prognostic Nutritional Index and ECOG Performance Score Predicts Survival Better than Sarcopenia, Cachexia and Some Inflammatory Indices in Metastatic Gastric Cancer. *Nutr. Cancer* **2021**, *73*, 230–238. [CrossRef]
9. Ter Veer, E.; van Kleef, J.J.; Schokker, S.; van der Woude, S.O.; Laarman, M.; Mohammad, N.H.; Sprangers, M.A.; van Oijen, M.G.; van Laarhoven, H.W. Prognostic and predictive factors for overall survival in metastatic oesophagogastric cancer: A systematic review and meta-analysis. *Eur. J. Cancer* **2018**, *103*, 214–226. [CrossRef]
10. Casadei-Gardini, A.; Scarpi, E.; Ulivi, P.; Palladino, M.A.; Accettura, C.; Bernardini, I.; Spallanzani, A.; Gelsomino, F.; Corbelli, J.; Marisi, G.; et al. Prognostic role of a new inflammatory index with neutrophil-to-lymphocyte ratio and lactate dehydrogenase (CII: Colon Inflammatory Index) in patients with metastatic colorectal cancer: Results from the randomized Italian Trial in Advanced Colorectal Cancer. *Cancer Manag. Res.* **2019**, *11*, 4357–4369. [CrossRef]
11. Grenader, T.; Waddell, T.; Peckitt, C.; Oates, J.; Starling, N.; Cunningham, D.; Bridgewater, J. Prognostic value of neutrophil-to-lymphocyte ratio in advanced oesophago-gastric cancer: Exploratory analysis of the REAL-2 trial. *Ann. Oncol.* **2016**, *27*, 687–692. [CrossRef]
12. Arends, J.; Bachmann, P.; Baracos, V.; Barthelemy, N.; Bertz, H.; Bozzetti, F.; Fearon, K.; Hütterer, E.; Isenring, E.; Kaasa, S.; et al. ESPEN guidelines on nutrition in cancer patients. *Clin. Nutr.* **2017**, *36*, 11–48. [CrossRef]
13. Cushen, S.J.; Power, D.G.; Murphy, K.P.; McDermott, R.; Griffin, B.T.; Lim, M.; Daly, L.; MacEneaney, P.; O'Sullivan, K.; Prado, C.M.; et al. Impact of body composition parameters on clinical outcomes in patients with metastatic castrate-resistant prostate cancer treated with docetaxel. *Clin. Nutr. ESPEN* **2016**, *13*, e39–e45. [CrossRef]
14. Martin, L.; Birdsell, L.; MacDonald, N.; Reiman, T.; Clandinin, M.T.; McCargar, L.J.; Murphy, R.; Ghosh, S.; Sawyer, M.B.; Baracos, V.E. Cancer Cachexia in the Age of Obesity: Skeletal Muscle Depletion Is a Powerful Prognostic Factor, Independent of Body Mass Index. *J. Clin. Oncol.* **2013**, *31*, 1539–1547. [CrossRef]
15. Ryan, A.M.; Prado, C.M.; Sullivan, E.S.; Power, D.G.; Daly, L.E. Effects of weight loss and sarcopenia on response to chemotherapy, quality of life, and survival. *Nutrition* **2019**, *67–68*, 110539. [CrossRef]
16. Omarini, C.; Palumbo, P.; Pecchi, A.; Draisci, S.; Balduzzi, S.; Nasso, C.; Barbolini, M.; Isca, C.; Bocconi, A.; Moscetti, L.; et al. Predictive Role of Body Composition Parameters in Operable Breast Cancer Patients Treated with Neoadjuvant Chemotherapy. *Cancer Manag. Res.* **2019**, *11*, 9563–9569, PMCID:PMC6859164. [CrossRef] [PubMed]
17. Rinninella, E.; Cintoni, M.; Raoul, P.; Pozzo, C.; Strippoli, A.; Bria, E.; Tortora, G.; Gasbarrini, A.; Mele, M.C. Effects of nutritional interventions on nutritional status in patients with gastric cancer: A systematic review and meta-analysis of randomized controlled trials. *Clin. Nutr. ESPEN* **2020**, *38*, 28–42. [CrossRef]
18. Hamaguchi, Y.; Kaido, T.; Okumura, S.; Kobayashi, A.; Shirai, H.; Yagi, S.; Kamo, N.; Okajima, H.; Uemoto, S. Impact of Skeletal Muscle Mass Index, Intramuscular Adipose Tissue Content, and Visceral to Subcutaneous Adipose Tissue Area Ratio on Early Mortality of Living Donor Liver Transplantation. *Transplantation* **2017**, *101*, 565–574. [CrossRef] [PubMed]

19. Waki, Y.; Irino, T.; Makuuchi, R.; Notsu, A.; Kamiya, S.; Tanizawa, Y.; Bando, E.; Kawamura, T.; Terashima, M. Impact of Preoperative Skeletal Muscle Quality Measurement on Long-Term Survival After Curative Gastrectomy for Locally Advanced Gastric Cancer. *World J. Surg.* 2019, *43*, 3083–3093. [CrossRef]
20. Ebadi, M.; Martin, L.; Ghosh, S.; Field, C.J.; Lehner, R.; Baracos, E.V.; Mazurak, V.C. Subcutaneous adiposity is an independent predictor of mortality in cancer patients. *Br. J. Cancer* 2017, *117*, 148–155. [CrossRef] [PubMed]
21. Lin, J.X.; Lin, J.P.; Xie, J.; Wang, J.; Lu, J.; Chen, Q.; Cao, L.; Lin, M.; Tu, R.; Zheng, C.; et al. Prognostic Value and Association of Sarcopenia and Systemic Inflammation for Patients with Gastric Cancer Following Radical Gastrectomy. *Oncologist* 2019, *24*. [CrossRef] [PubMed]
22. Sugiyama, K.; Narita, Y.; Mitani, S.; Honda, K.; Masuishi, T.; Taniguchi, H.; Kadowaki, S.; Ura, T.; Ando, M.; Tajika, M.; et al. Baseline Sarcopenia and Skeletal Muscle Loss During Chemotherapy Affect Survival Outcomes in Metastatic Gastric Cancer. *Anticancer. Res.* 2018, *38*, 5859–5866. [CrossRef] [PubMed]
23. Rinninella, E.; Cintoni, M.; Raoul, P.; Pozzo, C.; Strippoli, A.; Bria, E.; Tortora, G.; Gasbarrini, A.; Mele, M.C. Muscle mass, assessed at diagnosis by L3-CT scan as a prognostic marker of clinical outcomes in patients with gastric cancer: A systematic review and meta-analysis. *Clin. Nutr.* 2020, *39*, 2045–2054. [CrossRef]
24. Dijksterhuis, W.P.M.; Pruijt, M.J.; Van Der Woude, S.O.; Klaassen, R.; Kurk, S.A.; Van Oijen, M.G.H.; Van Laarhoven, H.W.M. Association between body composition, survival, and toxicity in advanced esophagogastric cancer patients receiving palliative chemotherapy. *J. Cachex Sarcopenia Muscle* 2019, *10*, 199–206. [CrossRef]
25. Choi, Y.; Oh, D.-Y.; Kim, T.-Y.; Lee, K.-H.; Han, S.-W.; Im, S.-A.; Bang, Y.-J. Skeletal Muscle Depletion Predicts the Prognosis of Patients with Advanced Pancreatic Cancer Undergoing Palliative Chemotherapy, Independent of Body Mass Index. *PLoS ONE* 2015, *10*, e0139749. [CrossRef]
26. Blauwhoff-Buskermolen, S.; Versteeg, K.S.; De Van Der Schueren, M.A.E.; Braver, N.R.D.; Berkhof, J.; Langius, J.A.E.; Verheul, H.M.W. Loss of Muscle Mass During Chemotherapy Is Predictive for Poor Survival of Patients with Metastatic Colorectal Cancer. *J. Clin. Oncol.* 2016, *34*, 1339–1344. [CrossRef]
27. Basile, D.; Parnofiello, A.; Vitale, M.G.; Cortiula, F.; Gerratana, L.; Fanotto, V.; Lisanti, C.; Pelizzari, G.; Ongaro, E.; Bartoletti, M.; et al. The IMPACT study: Early loss of skeletal muscle mass in advanced pancreatic cancer patients. *J. Cachex. Sarcopenia Muscle* 2019, *10*, 368–377. [CrossRef] [PubMed]
28. Rier, H.N.; Jager, A.; Sleijfer, S.; van Rosmalen, J.; Kock, M.C.; Levin, M.-D. Low muscle attenuation is a prognostic factor for survival in metastatic breast cancer patients treated with first line palliative chemotherapy. *Breast* 2017, *31*, 9–15. [CrossRef] [PubMed]
29. Antoun, S.; Lanoy, E.; Iacovelli, R.; Albiges-Sauvin, L.; Loriot, Y.; Merad-Taoufik, M.; Fizazi, K.; Di Palma, M.; Baracos, V.E.; Escudier, B. Skeletal muscle density predicts prognosis in patients with metastatic renal cell carcinoma treated with targeted therapies. *Cancer* 2013, *119*, 3377–3384. [CrossRef] [PubMed]
30. Ataseven, B.; Luengo, T.G.; Du Bois, A.; Waltering, K.-U.; Traut, A.; Heitz, F.; Alesina, P.F.; Prader, S.; Meier, B.; Schneider, S.; et al. Skeletal Muscle Attenuation (Sarcopenia) Predicts Reduced Overall Survival in Patients with Advanced Epithelial Ovarian Cancer Undergoing Primary Debulking Surgery. *Ann. Surg. Oncol.* 2018, *25*, 3372–3379. [CrossRef]
31. Van Dijk, D.; Bakens, M.; Coolsen, M.; Rensen, S.; Van Dam, R.; Bours, M.; Weijenberg, M.; De Jong, C.; Damink, S.O. Reduced survival in pancreatic cancer patients with low muscle attenuation index. *HPB* 2016, *18*, e756. [CrossRef]
32. Feliciano, E.M.C.; Kroenke, C.H.; Meyerhardt, J.A.; Prado, C.M.; Bradshaw, P.T.; Kwan, M.L.; Xiao, J.; Alexeeff, S.; Corley, D.; Weltzien, E.; et al. Association of Systemic Inflammation and Sarcopenia with Survival in Nonmetastatic Colorectal Cancer: Results From the C SCANS Study. *JAMA Oncol.* 2017, *3*, e172319. [CrossRef] [PubMed]
33. Kim, E.Y.; Kim, Y.S.; Seo, J.-Y.; Park, I.; Ahn, H.K.; Jeong, Y.M.; Kim, J.H.; Kim, N. The Relationship between Sarcopenia and Systemic Inflammatory Response for Cancer Cachexia in Small Cell Lung Cancer. *PLoS ONE* 2016, *11*, e0161125. [CrossRef] [PubMed]
34. Da Fonseca, G.W.P.; Farkas, J.; Dora, E.; Von Haehling, S.; Lainscak, M. Cancer Cachexia and Related Metabolic Dysfunction. *Int. J. Mol. Sci.* 2020, *21*, 2321. [CrossRef] [PubMed]
35. Caccialanza, R.; Cereda, E.; Caraccia, M.; Klersy, C.; Nardi, M.; Cappello, S.; Borioli, V.; Turri, A.; Imarisio, I.; Lasagna, A.; et al. Early 7-day supplemental parenteral nutrition improves body composition and muscle strength in hypophagic cancer patients at nutritional risk. *Clin. Nutr.* 2018, *37*, S14. [CrossRef]
36. De Waele, E.; Mattens, S.; Honoré, P.M.; Spapen, H.; De Grève, J.; Pen, J.J. Nutrition therapy in cachectic cancer patients. The Tight Caloric Control (TiCaCo) pilot trial. *Appetite* 2015, *91*, 298–301. [CrossRef]
37. Kapoor, N.D.; Twining, P.K.; Groot, O.Q.; Pielkenrood, B.J.; Bongers, M.E.R.; Newman, E.T.; Verlaan, J.J.; Schwab, J.H. Adipose tissue density on CT as a prognostic factor in patients with cancer: A systematic review. *Acta Oncol.* 2020, *59*, 1488–1495. [CrossRef]
38. Okumura, S.; Kaido, T.; Hamaguchi, Y.; Kobayashi, A.; Shirai, H.; Yao, S.; Yagi, S.; Kamo, N.; Hatano, E.; Okajima, H.; et al. Visceral Adiposity and Sarcopenic Visceral Obesity are Associated with Poor Prognosis After Resection of Pancreatic Cancer. *Ann. Surg. Oncol.* 2017, *24*, 3732–3740. [CrossRef]
39. Okumura, S.; Kaido, T.; Hamaguchi, Y.; Kobayashi, A.; Shirai, H.; Fujimoto, Y.; Iida, T.; Yagi, S.; Taura, K.; Hatano, E.; et al. Impact of Skeletal Muscle Mass, Muscle Quality, and Visceral Adiposity on Outcomes Following Resection of Intrahepatic Cholangiocarcinoma. *Ann. Surg. Oncol.* 2016, *24*, 1037–1045. [CrossRef]

40. Park, H.S.; Kim, H.S.; Beom, S.H.; Rha, S.Y.; Chung, H.C.; Kim, J.H.; Chun, Y.J.; Lee, S.W.; Choe, E.-A.; Heo, S.J.; et al. Marked Loss of Muscle, Visceral Fat, or Subcutaneous Fat After Gastrectomy Predicts Poor Survival in Advanced Gastric Cancer: Single-Center Study from the CLASSIC Trial. *Ann. Surg. Oncol.* **2018**, *25*, 3222–3230. [CrossRef]
41. Guiu, B.; Petit, J.M.; Bonnetain, F.; Ladoire, S.; Guiu, S.; Cercueil, J.-P.; Krausé, D.; Hillon, P.; Borg, C.; Chauffert, B.; et al. Visceral fat area is an independent predictive biomarker of outcome after first-line bevacizumab-based treatment in metastatic colorectal cancer. *Gut* **2009**, *59*, 341–347. [CrossRef] [PubMed]
42. Brandl, A. Prognostischer Einfluss von Fettgewebsdichte und Muskelmasse beim fortgeschrittenen kolorektalen Karzinom. Prognostic value of adipose tissue and muscle mass in advanced colorectal cancer. *Coloproctology* **2019**, *41*, 218–219. [CrossRef]

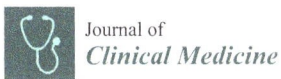

Journal of Clinical Medicine

Article

Role of Baseline Computed-Tomography-Evaluated Body Composition in Predicting Outcome and Toxicity from First-Line Therapy in Advanced Gastric Cancer Patients

Silvia Catanese [1,†], Giacomo Aringhieri [2,3,†], Caterina Vivaldi [1,2,*], Francesca Salani [1], Saverio Vitali [3], Irene Pecora [4], Valentina Massa [1], Monica Lencioni [1], Enrico Vasile [1], Rachele Tintori [2], Francesco Balducci [2], Alfredo Falcone [1,2], Carla Cappelli [3] and Lorenzo Fornaro [1]

1. Unit of Medical Oncology, Azienda Ospedaliero-Universitaria Pisana, Via Roma 67, 56126 Pisa, Italy; catanesesilvia@gmail.com (S.C.); f.salani1@gmail.com (F.S.); valentinamassa22@gmail.com (V.M.); monicalencioni65@gmail.com (M.L.); envasile@gmail.com (E.V.); alfredo.falcone@med.unipi.it (A.F.); lorenzo.fornaro@gmail.com (L.F.)
2. Department of Translational Research and New Surgical and Medical Technologies, University of Pisa, Via Savi 6, 56126 Pisa, Italy; giacomo.aringhieri@unipi.it (G.A.); racheletintori@hotmail.com (R.T.); francescocbalducci@gmail.com (F.B.)
3. Diagnostic and Interventional Radiology, Azienda Ospedaliero-Universitaria Pisana, Via Roma 67, 56126 Pisa, Italy; vitalisaverio@gmail.com (S.V.); carlacappelli1@gmail.com (C.C.)
4. Unit of Medical Oncology, Ospedale della Misericordia di Grosseto, Azienda Usl Sud Est, Via Senese 161, 58100 Grosseto, Italy; irene.pecora@gmail.com
* Correspondence: caterinavivaldi@gmail.com; Tel.: +39-050-992466
† Equally contributed to this paper.

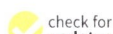

Citation: Catanese, S.; Aringhieri, G.; Vivaldi, C.; Salani, F.; Vitali, S.; Pecora, I.; Massa, V.; Lencioni, M.; Vasile, E.; Tintori, R.; et al. Role of Baseline Computed-Tomography-Evaluated Body Composition in Predicting Outcome and Toxicity from First-Line Therapy in Advanced Gastric Cancer Patients. *J. Clin. Med.* **2021**, *10*, 1079. https://doi.org/10.3390/jcm10051079

Academic Editor: Angelica Petrillo

Received: 1 February 2021
Accepted: 26 February 2021
Published: 5 March 2021

Publisher's Note: MDPI stays neutral with regard to jurisdictional claims in published maps and institutional affiliations.

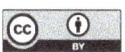

Copyright: © 2021 by the authors. Licensee MDPI, Basel, Switzerland. This article is an open access article distributed under the terms and conditions of the Creative Commons Attribution (CC BY) license (https://creativecommons.org/licenses/by/4.0/).

Abstract: Sarcopenia is recognised as a predictor of toxicity and survival in localised and locally advanced gastric cancer (GC). Its prognostication power in advanced unresectable or metastatic GC (aGC) is debated. The survival impact of visceral and subcutaneous fat distribution (visceral fat area (VFA)/subcutaneous fat area (SFA)) is ambiguous. Our aim was to determine the influence of body composition parameters (BCp) on toxicity and survival in aGC patients undergoing palliative treatment. BCp were retrospectively assessed by baseline computed tomography for 78 aGC patients who received first-line chemotherapy from March 2010 to January 2017. Correlations between BCp and toxicity and survival were calculated by χ^2-test and by log-rank-test and Cox-model, respectively. Sarcopenia fails to show association with progression-free survival (PFS) ($p = 0.44$) and overall survival (OS) ($p = 0.88$). However, sarcopenia influences the development of high-grade neutropenia ($p = 0.048$) and mucositis ($p = 0.054$). VFA/SFA (high vs. all the rest) results as a strong predictor of objective response ($p = 0.02$) and outcome (PFS, $p = 0.001$; OS, $p = 0.02$). At multivariate analysis for PFS, prognostic factors are VFA/SFA ($p = 0.03$) and a neutrophil–lymphocyte ratio >3. The same factors remain significant for OS (each $p = 0.03$) along with Eastern Cooperative Oncology Group (ECOG) performance status ($p = 0.008$) and number of metastatic sites ≥ 2 ($p < 0.001$). In our cohort of aGC, VFA/SFA exhibit a robust impact on survival, with a higher sensitivity than sarcopenia.

Keywords: gastric cancer; metastatic; body composition; sarcopenia; visceral fat area; subcutaneous fat area; outcome; toxicity

1. Introduction

Gastric cancer (GC) is the fifth most common malignancy and the third leading cause of cancer death worldwide [1]. Sixty percent of cases are inoperable or advanced at diagnosis (aGC), requiring palliative chemotherapy treatment [2]. Body weight changes are common in patients with aGC, even though they do not strictly correlate with body composition changes. The body of literature investigating the prognostic role of body composition has progressively increased in recent years [3]. The actual gold standard to evaluate skeletal muscle mass and adipose tissue distribution variations is the analysis of a computed tomography (CT) scan at the level of the third lumbar vertebra (L3) [4,5]. The depletion of skeletal muscle mass (sarcopenia) has been recognised as a poor outcome predictor in many solid tumours and in localised and locally aGC [6–11]. Moreover, after gastrectomy, baseline preoperative sarcopenia constitutes an independent risk factor for postoperative surgical complications and infections [9–11]. Despite this evidence, in the case of advanced disease, the impact of sarcopenia remains controversial [12–16]. The association with treatment-related toxicity has been mainly investigated in the perioperative setting: in two retrospective series, a trend toward a moderately positive correlation with treatment reduction, postponement or discontinuation was observed [17,18]. Though data are not conspicuous, sarcopenia was not confirmed as a predictor of toxicity in the metastatic setting [12,15]. The alteration of adipose tissue distribution among the visceral and the subcutaneous compartment is a known metabolic disruption occurring during the progression of neoplastic disease [19]. The ratio between visceral fat area (VFA) and subcutaneous fat area (SFA) has shown a negative prognostic impact in many retrospective series in gastrointestinal cancers, despite the fact that the majority were in the preoperative or perioperative setting [20–24].

Considering the poor prognosis of aGC, a further exploration of these parameters appeared necessary to clarify their role as outcome and toxicity predictors and improve our quality care. The aim of our work was to define which body composition parameter better correlates with outcome and chemotherapy-derived toxicity in a homogeneous cohort of Caucasian aGC patients treated with first-line palliative chemotherapy.

2. Materials and Methods

2.1. Study Population

We retrospectively evaluated the medical records of consecutive patients diagnosed with advanced esophagogastric junction carcinoma or aGC, who received at least one cycle of first-line doublet chemotherapy at our Azienda Ospedaliero-Universitaria Pisana from March 2010 to January 2017. All selected cases had a histologically proven diagnosis of adenocarcinoma. Patients whose CT scans lacked images of the third lumbar vertebra within 30 days prior to treatment initiation or patients who had palliative systemic therapy before CT evaluation were excluded (study inclusion flow-chart, Figure A1). Collected clinicopathological data included: age, sex, height, weight, Eastern Cooperative Oncology Group (ECOG) performance status (PS), primary tumour and metastatic sites, previous treatment history, human epidermal growth factor receptor 2 (HER2) status, baseline laboratory values (complete blood count with differential count and serum chemistry), chemotherapy regimen and administration, radiological response, survival status and last follow-up. Neutrophils–lymphocytes ratio (NLR) and platelets–lymphocytes ratio (PLR) were also collected at baseline (before cycle one administration) and dichotomised according to literature data cut-offs for metastatic gastric cancer patients: NLR > vs. $\leq$ 3 and PLR > vs. $\leq$ 200 [25,26].

All patients signed institutionally approved written informed consent before treatment administration.

2.2. Treatment

Only patients who received standard first-line palliative systemic therapy were included. Treatments consisted of the combination of fluoropyrimidine and platinum compound according to modified FOLFOX-6 regimen (mFOLFOX6) (5-FU 400 mg/m^2 bolus on day 1 and 2400 mg/m^2 continuous infusion from day 1 to 3 plus oxaliplatin 85 mg/m^2 on day 1, in a two-weekly cycle) and CapOX regimen (capecitabine 1000 mg/m^2, taken orally two times a day on days 1 to 14 plus oxaliplatin 130 mg/m^2 on day 1, in a three-weekly cycle). 5-FU was preferred over capecitabine in the case of dysphagia or contraindication to oral fluoropyrimidine (such as concomitant treatment with oral anticoagulants), while capecitabine was preferred in case of a patient's request for an oral treatment. In case of

HER2-positive disease, trastuzumab was added to the chemotherapy backbone. Treatment was discontinued in case of disease progression, unacceptable toxicity, or on patient's request. Toxicity was assessed using the Common Terminology Criteria for Adverse Events (version 4.03) by recording the highest grade of each adverse event throughout all administered cycles [27]. In the case of the development of neurotoxicity of high grade (G3–G4), according to CTCAE oxaliplatin administration was discontinued and maintenance with fluoropyrimidine monotherapy was provided.

2.3. Efficacy and Outcome

Response evaluation was performed according to Response Evaluation Criteria in Solid Tumours version 1.1 (RECIST 1.1), using radiological follow-up assessments obtained every 8 to 12 weeks during treatment [28]. Progression-free survival (PFS) and overall survival (OS) were defined as the time from first-line chemotherapy initiation to the date of radiological/clinical progression or death from any cause and to the date of death or last follow-up, respectively.

2.4. Body Composition Parameters Assessment

Slice thickness of included CT exams ranged from 2.5 to 3 mm. To evaluate the quantitative assessment of skeletal muscle mass, visceral and subcutaneous fat tissue for each patient, portal phase CT images, performed prior to the initiation of therapy, were analysed by a trained radiologist who was blinded to clinical data on GE advantage workstation (software version 4.7, G.E. Healthcare, Milwaukee, WI, USA).

Measurements of the total muscle areas were made on transverse images at the third lumbar vertebra (L3) level, with the transverse processes fully visible. First, visceral and subcutaneous fat was segmented, and VFA and SFA were separately calculated. Then, after visceral and subcutaneous fat removal, the skeletal muscle area was measured using automatic tissue-specific Hounsfield unit (HU) thresholds, according to literature values (-50 to 140 HU).

The VFA/SFA ratio was calculated for each patient. Since no specific thresholds are known to define normal VFA/SFA values, we divided the study population into quartiles, as previously performed by other groups in oesophageal cancers [23]. Quartiles (Q) were defined as follows: Q1 the lowest, Q4 the highest. In addition, the VFA/SFA variable was treated as dichotomous with Q4 being defined as the "high ratio" and Q1–3 as "all the rest ratio".

Sarcopenia was categorized according to the Martin cut-off values for Skeletal Muscle Index (SMI, defined as Skeletal Muscle Area (SMA) measured at L3 vertebra normalized for height squared), considering sex and body mass index (BMI), which demonstrated a strong correlation with poor outcome in a large cohort of patients affected by gastrointestinal and respiratory tract tumours. In detail, sarcopenia was defined in male patients as SMI < 43 cm^2/m^2 if BMI < 25 kg/m^2 and SMI < 53 cm^2/m^2 if BMI ≥ 25 kg/m^2, and in female patients as SMI < 41 kg/m^2 irrespective of BMI [6].

2.5. Statistical Analysis

Descriptive statistics were provided as the proportion or medians with standard deviations and ranges for continuous variables. The association of sarcopenia, and different VFA/SFA ratio cut-offs with clinicopathological parameters, efficacy and toxicity were performed using the Pearson's χ^2 test or Fisher's exact test for categorical variables. Continuous variables were analysed with the Mann–Whitney U test. PFS and OS were estimated applying the Kaplan–Meyer method and compared by the mean of the log-rank test. A multivariable Cox proportional hazard model was built to identify prognostic predictors of outcome: only factors with a two-sided p-value < 0.05 by the log-rank test were included. The analysis was performed using the statistical software Medcalc version 14.8.1 (Medcalc, Ostend, Belgium).

3. Results

3.1. Patient Characteristics and Body Composition Parameters Distribution

Characteristics of the 78 patients included and the correlations with body composition variables are depicted in Table 1. Median age was 67 years (range 35–80). Most of the patients (72%) were male and presented more than two metastatic sites (62%) of which lymph nodes and peritoneum had the highest frequency. Sixteen patients (24%) were HER2 positive. At baseline, 47% of patients were of normal weight, only 6% were obese, according to BMI categories.

Table 1. Patient characteristics according to loss of muscle mass and abdominal fat distribution.

Characteristics	All Patients	Sarcopenia		p-Value	VFA/SFA		p-Value
	(n = 78) N (%)	Yes (n = 34) N (%)	No (n = 44) N (%)		All the Rest (n = 43) N (%)	High (n = 14) N (%)	
Age, years Median, (range)	67, (35–80)	70, (35–80)	66, (37–79)	0.29	66, (35–80)	65, (55–78)	0.87
Sex Female/male	22 (18)/56 (72)	12 (35)/22 (65)	10 (23)/34 (77)	0.33	13 (30)/30 (70)	2 (14)/12 (86)	0.40
ECOG PS 0 vs. 1–2	34 (44)/44 (56)	12 (35)/22 (65)	22 (50)/22 (50)	0.28	23 (54)/20 (46)	4 (29)/10 (71)	0.19
Primary tumour site EGJ/PGC/DGC	32 (41)/26 (33)/20 (27)	13 (38)/10 (30)/11 (32)	19 (43)/16 (36)/9 (20)	0.48	12 (28)/21 (49)/10 (23)	8 (58)/3 (21)/3 (21)	0.10
Primary tumour surgery Yes/no	22 (28)/56 (72)	31 (91)/3 (9)	41 (93)/3 (7)	0.95	15 (35)/28 (65)	3 (21)/11 (79)	0.62
N° metastatic sites 1 vs. ≥2	30 (38)/48 (62)	12 (35)/22 (65)	18 (41)/26 (59)	0.78	20 (46)/23 (54)	1 (7)/13 (93)	0.02
Metastatic sites							
Liver	30 (38)	11 (32)	19 (43)	0.46	20 (47)	5 (36)	0.69
Lung	6 (7)	4 (12)	2 (5)	0.45	2 (5)	3 (22)	0.16
Lymph nodes	52 (66)	24 (71)	28 (64)	0.68	24 (56)	13 (93)	0.02
Peritoneum	39 (50)	17 (50)	22 (50)	0.81	22 (51)	6 (43)	0.81
Bone	7 (9)	6 (18)	1 (2)	0.05	2 (5)	3 (21)	0.16
HER2 * Yes/no	16 (24)/51 (76)	7 (25)/21 (75)	9 (23)/30 (77)	0.91	10 (25)/30 (75)	2 (25)/6 (75)	0.65
NLR>3 Yes/no/na	39 (50)/38 (49,9)/1 (0,1)	18 (53)/15 (44)/1 (3)	21 (48)/23 (52)/–	0.71	21 (49)/22 (51)	8 (62)/5 (38)	0.62
PLR >200 Yes/no/na	36 (46)/40 (51,8)/2 (0,2)	13 (38)/20 (59)/1 (3)	23 (52)/20 (45)/1 (3)	0.32	24 (57)/18 (43)	4 (31)/9 (69)	0.18

Table 1. Cont.

Characteristics	All Patients	Sarcopenia	p-Value	VFA/SFA	p-Value
BMI ≤20/20–24.9/25–30/≥30	17 (23)/37 (47)/19 (24)/5 (6)	–	–	–	–
SMI, median (range; SD) Female	40.65 (25.48–61.94; 8.55)	–	–	–	–
Male	48.51 (32.73–68.70; 8.50)	–	–	–	–
VFA [§], median (Range; SD)	89.10 (3.56–407.77; 88.57)	–	–	–	–
SFA [§], median (Range; SD)	108.99 (0.88–355.97; 80.55)	–	–	–	–

VFA/SFA, visceral fat area/subcutaneous fat area; ECOG PS, Eastern Cooperative Oncology Group (ECOG) performance status; EGJ, esophago–gastric junction cancer; PGC, proximal gastric cancer; DGC, distal gastric cancer; HER2, epidermal growth factor receptor 2; NLR, neutrophil–lymphocyte ratio; PLR, platelet–lymphocyte ratio; BMI, body mass index (kg/m^2); SMI, skeletal muscle index (cm^2/m^2); VFA, visceral fat area (cm^2); SFA, subcutaneous fat area (cm^2) * Data available for 67 patients (pts); [§] Data available for 57 pts.

3.1.1. Skeletal Muscle

The mean L3 SMI was 40.65 cm^2/m^2 (range: 25.48–61.94) for females and 48.51 cm^2/m^2 (range: 32.73–68.70) for males. As per Martin's cut-off values, 34% of patients were judged to be sarcopenic. No significant associations were observed between sarcopenia and clinico–pathological characteristics, except for a higher prevalence of bone metastasis in patients with a loss of muscle mass ($p = 0.05$).

3.1.2. Adipose Tissue

Regarding fat distribution parameters, assessable in 57 patients, the median VFA was 89.10 cm^2 (range: 3.56–407.77), the median SFA was 108.99 cm^2 (range: 0.88–355.97) and the median VFA/SFA ratio was 1.09 (range: 0.17–4.05). According to quartiles of the VFA/SFA ratio, patients were classified as follows: first quartile cases (Q1: ≤0.58); second quartile cases (Q2: 0.59–1.09): third quartile cases (Q3: 1.10–1.53); and fourth quartile cases (Q4: ≥1.54). Due to the findings of efficacy and survival for each Q group (see Section 3.2.1, Figure A3a,b and Table A1), we defined a dichotomous VFA/SFA ratio: group Q4 as the "high VFA/SFA" and groups Q1–3 as the "all the rest VFA/SFA". Only fourteen patients presented a high VFA/SFA ratio. All clinicopathological characteristics were stratified and analysed in the aforementioned groups. Significant differences in terms of the presence of ≥2 metastatic sites and especially lymph nodes metastasis among the high VFA/SFA ratio group was noticed ($p = 0.02$).

3.2. Body Composition Parameters and Outcome

3.2.1. Efficacy

At a median follow-up of 52.2 months (range: 31.25–87.66), 74 patients (95%) had progressed, and 70 (90%) had died: median PFS (mPFS) was 5.9 months (95% CI: 4.8–7.2) and median OS (mOS) was 10.8 months (95% CI: 9.5–12.9).

Neither PFS (hazard ratio (HR): 0.83, 95% CI: 0.53–1.32; $p = 0.44$) nor OS (HR: 0.97, 95% CI: 0.60–1.55; $p = 0.88$) differed between sarcopenic and non-sarcopenic patients (Figure A2).

As shown in Figure A3a,b, Kaplan–Meyer curves were calculated for each Q group of the VFA/SFA ratio. A statistically significant worsening of PFS (p = 0.01) and a trend toward worse OS (p = 0.08) were observed for Q4 compared to any other group in a univariate Cox proportional hazards model (Table A1). Therefore, we proceed to analyse the VFA/SFA ratio as dichotomous groups: Q1–3 as "all the rest VFA/SFA ratio" and Q4 as the "high VFA/SFA ratio". Looking at Q1–3 vs. Q4 survival comparison, patients in the high VFA/SFA group experienced a statistically significant worse PFS (HR: 2.49, 95% CI: 1.11–5.61; p = 0.001) and OS (HR: 2.02, 95% CI: 0.93–4.41; p = 0.02) compared to those in the all the rest of the VFA/SFA group (Figure 1a,b).

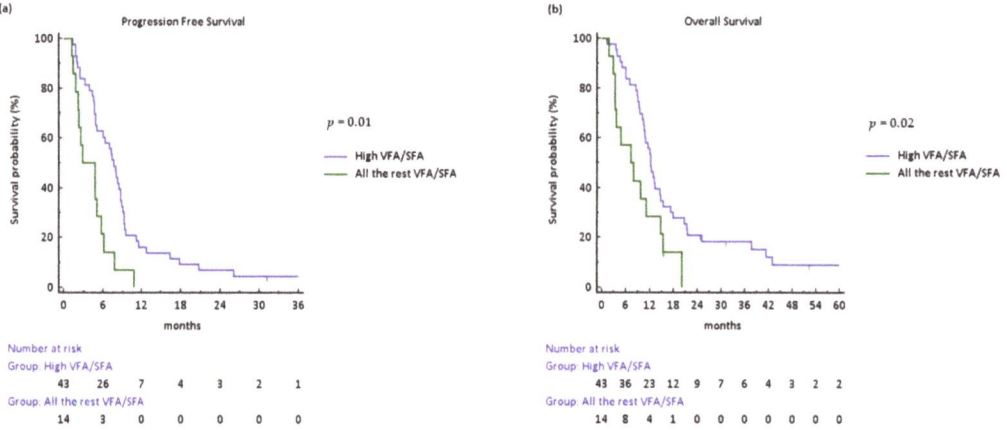

Figure 1. Kaplan–Meyer curves according to VFA/SFA ratio: (**a,b**) progression-free and overall survival stratified by high vs. all the rest, respectively. Abbreviations: VFA/SFA, visceral fat area/subcutaneous fat area.

3.2.2. Activity

Partial response (PR) was achieved in 28 patients (no complete responses were observed; response rate, RR: 35.9%), and disease control was achieved in 55 patients (disease control rate, DCR: 70.5%).

The presence of sarcopenia did not affect activity (PR vs. stable disease (SD) vs. progressive disease (PD): p = 0.55) or DCR (p = 0.44).

Conversely, a significant difference in treatment activity was noticed among the 57 patients belonging to different VFA/SFA quartiles ratio, with no PD observed in Q1 group in contrast to PD probability of 50% in the Q4 group (p = 0.02). The statistically significant difference was retained also when responses were compared as presence vs. absence of DCR (p = 0.03) (Figure 2).

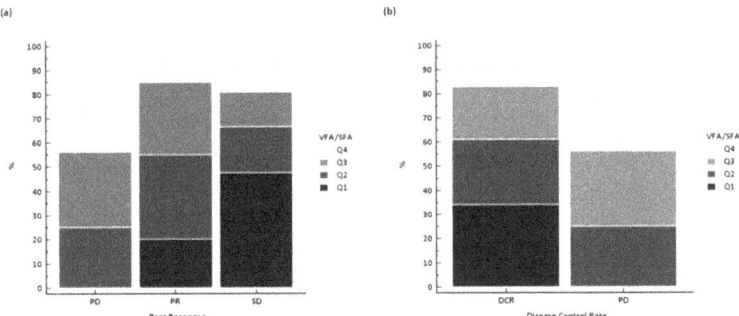

Figure 2. Response according to the VFA/SFA ratio, stratified by quartiles: (**a**) best response; and (**b**) disease control rate. Abbreviations: VFA/SFA, visceral fat area/subcutaneous fat area; Q, quartile; PD, progressive disease; PR, partial response; SD, stable disease; DCR, disease control rate.

3.3. Cox Proportional Hazards Model for Survival of Body Composition and Clinical Parameters

3.3.1. Univariate Analysis

As previously discussed, at univariate analysis, sarcopenia showed no prognostic impact, while the VFA/SFA ratio as a dichotomous variable was strongly prognostic for both PFS and OS. ECOG PS was highly prognostic in the log-rank test both for PFS ($p = 0.02$) and OS ($p = 0.03$). The presence of bone lesions represented the strongest clinical predictor of OS ($p < 0.001$). Systemic inflammatory parameters such as NLR and PLR confirmed their prognostic impact on OS ($p = 0.007$ and $p = 0.04$, respectively), with NLR also being associated with PFS ($p = 0.008$) (Table 2).

Table 2. Univariate analyses for progression-free survival and overall survival.

Variables	Progression-Free Survival		Overall Survival	
	HR (95% CI)	*p*-Value	HR (95% CI)	*p*-Value
Age ≥ vs. < 67 years	0.85 (0.54–1.35)	0.47	0.73 (0.46–1.18)	0.18
ECOG PS 0 vs. 1–2	0.58 (0.37–0.92)	0.02	0.59 (0.37–0.95)	0.03
Primary tumour surgery Yes vs. no	0.70 (0.43–1.13)	0.16	0.69 (0.42–1.13)	0.16
N° metastatic sites 1 vs. ≥2	0.64 (0.41–1.01)	0.06	0.63 (0.39–1.01)	0.06
Metastatic sites				
Liver	0.91 (0.57–1.44)	0.68	0.67 (0.42–1.07)	0.09
Lung	1.56 (0.57–4.30)	0.29	1.27 (0.46–3.47)	0.61
Lymph nodes	1.21 (0.75–1.75)	0.43	1.31 (0.81–2.12)	0.29
Peritoneum	1.07 (0.67–1.68)	0.77	1.40 (0.87–2.24)	0.16
Bone	2.10 (0.72–6.15)	0.05	4.35 (0.97–19.57)	<0.001
NLR > 3 Yes vs. no	1.81 (1.13–2.90)	0.008	1.88 (1.16–3.05)	0.007
PLR > 200 Yes vs. no	1.44 (0.90–2.30)	0.11	1.63 (1.00–2.65)	0.04
SMI Yes vs. no	0.83 (0.53–1.32)	0.44	0.96 (0.60–1.55)	0.88
VFA/SFA All the rest vs. high	0.40 (0.18–0.90)	0.002	0.49 (0.23–1.10)	0.02

Abbreviations: HR, hazard ratio; ECOG PS, ECOG performance status; NLR, neutrophil–lymphocyte ratio; PLR, platelet–lymphocyte ratio; SMI, skeletal muscle index; VFA/SFA, visceral fat area/subcutaneous fat area.

3.3.2. Multivariate Analysis

At multivariate analysis, the VFA/SFA ratio retained its prognostic role for PFS ($p = 0.03$) and OS ($p = 0.02$), as did NLR for both survival parameters (each $p = 0.03$). ECOG PS (0 vs. 1–2) and the presence of bone metastases maintained their independent value for OS ($p = 0.008$ and $p < 0.001$, respectively) (Table 3).

Table 3. Multivariate analysis for progression-free and overall survival.

Variables	Progression-Free Survival		Overall Survival	
	HR (95% CI)	p-Value	HR (95% CI)	p-Value
ECOG PS 0 vs. 1–2	1.59 (0.90–2.81)	0.11	2.36 (1.25–4.44)	0.008
N° metastatic sites 1 vs. ≥2	0.99 (0.52–1.87)	0.97	1.35 (0.67–2.63)	0.41
Metastatic sites Bone	2.32 (0.86–6.26)	0.09	9.63 (3.16–29.37)	<0.001
NLR>3 Yes vs. no	2.00 (1.08–3.69)	0.03	2.19 (1.08–4.45)	0.03
PLR >200 Yes vs. no	–	–	1.59 (0.80–3.19)	0.18
VFA/SFA All the rest vs. high	2.23 (1.08–4.59)	0.03	2.42 (1.44–5.13)	0.02

Abbreviations: HR, hazard ratio; ECOG PS, ECOG Performance Status; NLR, neutrophil to lymphocyte ratio; PLR, platelet to lymphocyte ratio; VFA/SFA, visceral fat area/subcutaneous fat area.

3.4. Body Composition Parameters as Toxicity Predictors

3.4.1. Treatment Exposure

Thirty percent of patients received at least six cycles of chemotherapy, 8 being the median number (range 1–12). In 36 patients (46.2%), the doses of fluoropyrimidine and/or oxaliplatin were reduced or treatment administration was postponed due to toxicity. Treatment was discontinued due to adverse events in six patients (7.7%).

Chemotherapy administration was not significantly influenced by the presence of sarcopenia ($p = 0.29$) or visceral/subcutaneous adipose tissue distribution alterations ($p = 0.95$).

3.4.2. Adverse Events

A grade 3–4 hematologic adverse event was reported in 27 patients (35%). Grade 3–4 non-hematologic adverse events affected only nine patients (12%).

Sarcopenia seemed to be significantly associated with grade 3–4 neutropenia ($p = 0.048$): among patients who suffered from grade 3–4 neutropenia, 61.9% were sarcopenic compared to 18.2% who did not present muscle mass reduction. The development of mucositis of any grade was also significantly associated with sarcopenia (55.9 vs. 44.1%, $p = 0.054$). VFA/SFA ratios did not show any correlation with toxicity.

4. Discussion

In our study, sarcopenia was observed in nearly half of the enrolled population and did not affect the response and survival of aGC patients treated with first-line doublet chemotherapy. Indeed, sarcopenia had an impact on the development of grade 3–4 hematologic toxicity and any grade mucositis. Of note, a higher proportion of visceral fat over subcutaneous fat was convincingly associated with an unfavourable prognosis, without showing the influence on treatment tolerance.

The impact of sarcopenia on toxicity has been to date scarcely investigated in first-line aGC: almost no association was found in the literature, except for a correlation between baseline sarcopenic obesity and grade 2–4 neurotoxicity [12,13]. The body of evidence in the perioperative setting suggests a significant association between sarcopenia and dose-limiting toxicity and early treatment termination [17,18]; in contrast, we did not find a negative impact of sarcopenia on treatment compliance and exposure. The correlation we identified with high-grade neutropenia in sarcopenic patients could possibly be explained by the known association with lean and muscle mass with pharmacokinetics parameters such as drug distribution, metabolism and the clearance of chemotherapeutic agents, especially for hydrophilic ones such as fluoropyrimidines [8,29].

Although several studies reported an association between the loss of skeletal muscle mass and OS [6,7,9,12,14], we did not observe such a correlation. This was possibly due to the reduced power of the study and the relatively small number of obese patients (6%, Table 1), considering that the survival prediction of Martin's cutoffs was greater in overweight and obese patients [6]. In line with our data, two recent studies in the same setting and in a Caucasian population achieved comparable negative results in terms of OS. Dijksterhuis et al. observed no association between skeletal muscle and survival in advanced esophagogastric cancer patients receiving palliative chemotherapy. In an extensive retrospective analysis of baseline CT scans from the phase 3 EXPAND trial, sarcopenia was identified as a predictor only for PFS [15,16].

Rather than skeletal muscle quantity, the quality of skeletal muscle mass appears to be relevant for survival. Of uttermost importance, this can be studied on CT scan: the skeletal muscle density (SMD) and the mean muscle attenuation (MA) are both parameters of skeletal muscle infarction by adipose tissue, which compromises muscle properties. This issue has been primarily investigated by a Japanese retrospective study on aGC that showed lower SMD as independent predictor of survival in association with more than two metastatic sites [13]. Interestingly, Hacker et al., in the analysis of 761 radiological and clinical data from advanced esophagogastric cancer patients treated with first-line chemotherapy achieved similar conclusions: MA constituted the only powerful body composition parameter with a prognostic value for OS, although large differences in MA were translated into only moderate differences in an expected cohort [16].

Considering that reduced SMD and/or MA, whose prognostic impact has been extensively discussed, are consequences of higher cytoplasmatic depots of intramyocellular lipid droplets as well as intermuscular adipocytes [30], we might infer that the impact on outcome observed for VFA/SFA in our work should be inscribed in the same context.

The role of baseline visceral and subcutaneous fat amount and distribution has been explored in the operable setting in localised colorectal cancer patients undergoing surgery, and in locally advanced rectal cancer planned to receive neoadjuvant chemoradiotherapy: a correlation of higher VFA/SFA ratio with poorer disease-free survival (DFS) was demonstrated [20,21]. The same results concerning these fat parameters were obtained in patients affected by squamous oesophageal cancer after esophagectomy [23]. In a single centre study cohort from the phase 3 CLASSIC (Capecitabine and Oxaliplatin Adjuvant Study in Stomach Cancer) trial, the marked loss of VFA and SFA, analysed as indexes normalized by height squared (VFI and SFI, respectively), appeared as a poor prognostic factor for DFS both in the group receiving adjuvant chemotherapy, and in the surgery-only group; the negative correlation with OS was demonstrated only in the interventional arm [24]. This last evidence was in line with a retrospective evaluation of preoperative body composition parameters in 507 upper gastrointestinal cancer patients: in this study, low visceral fat cases experienced a higher overall mortality rate [22]. However, the results of these two works should not be considered to be conflicting with the other literature evidence and our findings. In fact, adipose tissue parameters were investigated as single entities, instead of a proportion of visceral and subcutaneous fat components.

Chronic insulin resistance is a known metabolic disruption occurring in malignant tumours in early stages prior to the development of weight loss and cachexia, actively contributing to its pathogenesis [19]. Body composition parameters and especially visceral adipose tissue have been shown to significantly correlate with insulin signalling [31]. The adipose tissue is an endocrine organ, secreting adipocytokines like adiponectin and leptin and cytokines (IL-1, IL-6, TNF-α), which regulates appetite, inflammation, insulin sensitivity and fat metabolism itself. Excess of adipose tissue, particularly the visceral component, metabolically more active than the subcutaneous one, is strongly associated with inflammatory cytokines production, the upregulation of nuclear factor-kB leading to increased nitric oxide and reactive oxygen species, which further propagate inflammation. Thus, visceral adipose tissue activity along with insulin resistance, and systemic inflammation would promote and perpetuate a pro-tumorigenic environment [19]. In this context, our findings appear convincing and we should highlight the point that VFA/SFA is independently associated with response, PFS and OS. Moreover, at multivariate analysis, the only other factor that retained significance for PFS was the inflammation parameter NLR. Lastly, along with known prognostic factors for OS like ECOG PS and a higher number of metastatic sites, VFA/SFA and NLR maintained their prognostic role in the multivariate model. Due to the mentioned evidence, we suggest that the VFA/SFA ratio is the best factor that depicts the metabolic changes occurring during cancer initiation and progression.

We are aware of the limitations of our study represented by its retrospective design, the single centre recruitment, and the small sample size of enrolled patients. Nevertheless, it represents a homogeneous aGC population of Caucasian patients treated with the actual standard of care in first-line doublet chemotherapy.

5. Conclusions

Our study confirms the absence of a prognostic role for sarcopenia in the advanced setting and shows the VFA/SFA ratio, readily assessable during routine radiological exams, as a potential game changer in the natural history of aGC. Further investigation on this putative prognostic biomarker is warranted, along with the exploration of new nutritional, hormonal and/or anti-inflammatory interventions (for example adiponectin replacement) to better clarify its possible role as a therapeutic target.

Author Contributions: Conceptualization, S.C., G.A., C.V., F.S., I.P., C.C. and L.F.; methodology S.C. and G.A.; software S.C. and G.A.; validation, S.C., G.A., C.V., F.S., I.P., C.C. and L.F.; formal analysis, S.C. and G.A.; investigation, S.C., G.A., C.V., F.S., S.V., I.P., V.M., M.L., E.V., R.T., F.B., A.F., A.F., C.C., L.F.; resources, S.C., G.A., C.V., F.S., S.V., I.P., V.M., M.L., E.V., R.T., F.B., A.F., A.F., C.C., L.F.; data curation, S.C., G.A., C.V., F.S., S.V., I.P., V.M., M.L., E.V., R.T., F.B., A.F., A.F., C.C., L.F.; writing—original draft preparation, S.C., G.A., C.V. and L.F.; writing—review and editing, S.C., G.A., C.V., F.S., S.V., I.P., V.M., M.L., E.V., R.T., F.B., A.F., A.F., C.C., L.F.; visualization, S.C., G.A., C.V., F.S., S.V., I.P., V.M., M.L., E.V., R.T., F.B., A.F., A.F., C.C., L.F.; supervision, C.V., C.C. and L.F.; project administration, S.C., G.A. and L.F.; funding acquisition, not applicable. All authors have read and agreed to the published version of the manuscript.

Funding: This research received no external funding.

Institutional Review Board Statement: The study was conducted according to the guidelines of the Declaration of Helsinki. No formal protocol approval by the local IRB was required due to the nature of the study.

Informed Consent Statement: Informed consent for treatment administration and data collection was obtained from all subjects involved in the study.

Data Availability Statement: All data are already presented in the manuscript.

Conflicts of Interest: The authors declare no conflict of interest.

Appendix A

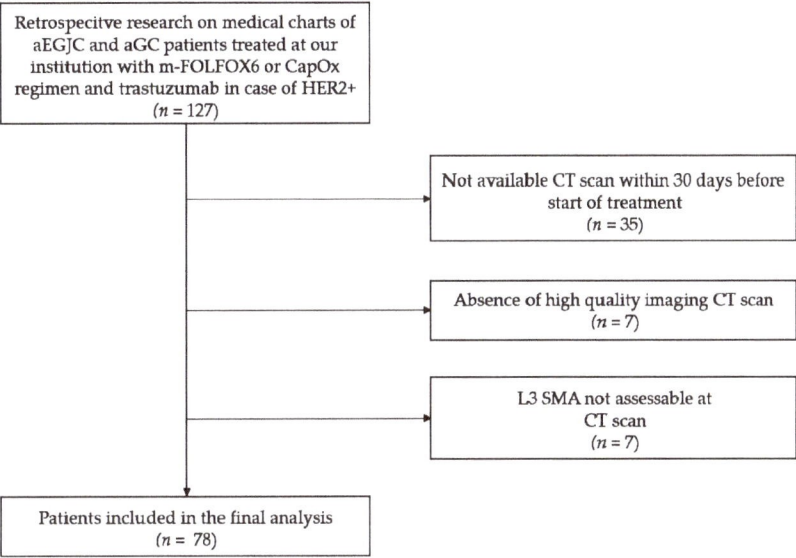

Figure A1. Patient's selection flow-chart. Abbreviations: aEGJC, advanced oesophagogastric junction cancer; aGC, advanced gastric cancer; HER2, epidermal growth factor receptor 2; CT, computed tomography; L3 SMA, third lumbar vertebra skeletal muscle area.

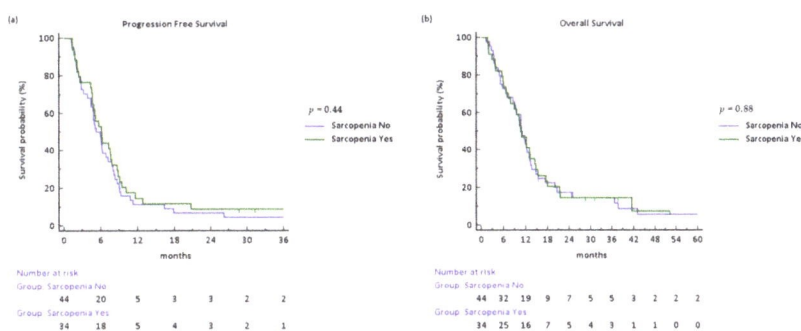

Figure A2. Kaplan–Meyer curves according to presence or absence of sarcopenia: (**a**) progression-free survival; and (**b**) overall survival.

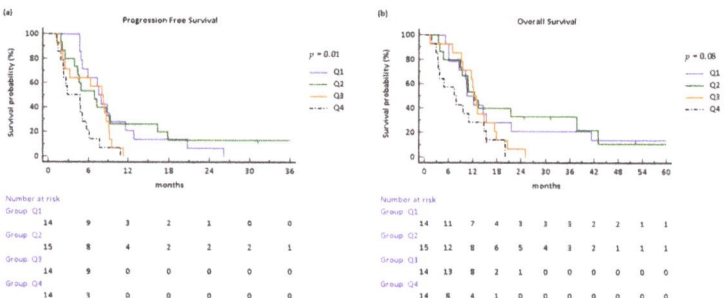

Figure A3. Kaplan–Meyer curves according to the VFA/SFA ratio: (**a**,**b**) progression-free and overall survival stratified by quartiles, respectively.

Table A1. Univariate analysis for progression-free and overall survival according to VFA/SFA ratio stratified by quartiles.

VFA/SFA Quartile	N°	Progression-Free Survival		Overall Survival	
		HR (95% CI)	p-Value	HR (95% CI)	p-Value
Q4 (≥1.54)	14	1 (Reference Value)	0.01	1 (Reference Value)	0.08
Q3 (1.10–1.53)	14	1.89 (0.74–4.84)	–	1.56 (0.63–3.88)	–
Q2 (0.59–1.09)	15	2.85 (1.16–6.97)	–	2.42 (1.02–5.78)	–
Q1 (≤0.58)	14	2.76 (1.14–6.71)	–	2.16 (0.89–5.21)	–

Abbreviations: VFA/SFA, visceral fat area/subcutaneous fat area; N°, number of cases; HR, hazard ratio; Q, quartile.

References

1. Siegel, R.L.; Miller, K.D.; Jemal, A. Cancer statistics, 2020. *CA Cancer J. Clin.* **2020**, *70*, 7–30. [CrossRef]
2. Glimelius, B.; Ekström, K.; Hoffman, K.; Graf, W.; Sjödén, P.-O.; Haglund, U.; Svensson, C.; Enander, L.-K.; Linné, T.; Sellsröm, H.; et al. Randomized comparison between chemotherapy plus best supportive care with best supportive care in advanced gastric cancer. *Ann. Oncol.* **1997**, *8*, 163–168. [CrossRef]
3. Brown, J.C.; Feliciano, E.M.C.; Caan, B.J. The evolution of body composition in oncology-epidemiology, clinical trials, and the future of patient care: Facts and numbers. *J. Cachex Sarcopenia Muscle* **2018**, *9*, 1200–1208. [CrossRef] [PubMed]
4. Mourtzakis, M.; Prado, C.M.M.; Lieffers, J.R.; Reiman, T.; McCargar, L.J.; Baracos, V.E. A practical and precise approach to quantification of body composition in cancer patients using computed tomography images acquired during routine care. *Appl. Physiol. Nutr. Metab.* **2008**, *33*, 997–1006. [CrossRef]
5. Maurovichhorvat, P.; Massaro, J.M.; Fox, C.S.; Moselewski, F.; Odonnell, C.J.; Hoffmann, U. Comparison of anthropometric, area- and volume-based assessment of abdominal subcutaneous and visceral adipose tissue volumes using multi-detector computed tomography. *Int. J. Obes.* **2006**, *31*, 500–506. [CrossRef]
6. Martin, L.; Birdsell, L.; Macdonald, N.; Reiman, T.; Clandinin, M.T.; McCargar, L.J.; Murphy, R.; Ghosh, S.; Sawyer, M.B.; Baracos, V.E. Cancer Cachexia in the Age of Obesity: Skeletal Muscle Depletion Is a Powerful Prognostic Factor, Independent of Body Mass Index. *J. Clin. Oncol.* **2013**, *31*, 1539–1547. [CrossRef]
7. Prado, C.M.; Lieffers, J.R.; McCargar, L.J.; Reiman, T.; Sawyer, M.B.; Martin, L.; E Baracos, V. Prevalence and clinical implications of sarcopenic obesity in patients with solid tumours of the respiratory and gastrointestinal tracts: A population-based study. *Lancet Oncol.* **2008**, *9*, 629–635. [CrossRef]
8. Prado, C.M.; Baracos, V.E.; McCargar, L.J.; Reiman, T.; Mourtzakis, M.; Tonkin, K.; Mackey, J.R.; Koski, S.; Pituskin, E.; Sawyer, M.B. Sarcopenia as a Determinant of Chemotherapy Toxicity and Time to Tumor Progression in Metastatic Breast Cancer Patients Receiving Capecitabine Treatment. *Clin. Cancer Res.* **2009**, *15*, 2920–2926. [CrossRef] [PubMed]
9. Rinninella, E.; Cintoni, M.; Raoul, P.; Pozzo, C.; Strippoli, A.; Bria, E.; Tortora, G.; Gasbarrini, A.; Mele, M.C. Muscle mass, assessed at diagnosis by L3-CT scan as a prognostic marker of clinical outcomes in patients with gastric cancer: A systematic review and meta-analysis. *Clin. Nutr.* **2020**, *39*, 2045–2054. [CrossRef]

10. Zhuang, C.-L.; Huang, D.-D.; Pang, W.-Y.; Zhou, C.-J.; Wang, S.-L.; Lou, N.; Ma, L.-L.; Yu, Z.; Shen, X. Sarcopenia is an Independent Predictor of Severe Postoperative Complications and Long-Term Survival After Radical Gastrectomy for Gastric Cancer: Analysis from a Large-Scale Cohort. *Medicine* **2016**, *95*, e3164. [CrossRef]
11. Levolger, S.; van Vugt, J.L.A.; de Bruin, R.W.F.; Ijzermans, J.N.M. Systematic review of sarcopenia in patients operated on for gastrointestinal and hepatopancreatobiliary malignancies. *BJS* **2015**, *102*, 1448–1458. [CrossRef]
12. Sugiyama, K.; Narita, Y.; Mitani, S.; Honda, K.; Masuishi, T.; Taniguchi, H.; Kadowaki, S.; Ura, T.; Ando, M.; Tajika, M.; et al. Baseline Sarcopenia and Skeletal Muscle Loss During Chemotherapy Affect Survival Outcomes in Metastatic Gastric Cancer. *Anticancer. Res.* **2018**, *38*, 5859–5866. [CrossRef]
13. Hayashi, N.; Ando, Y.; Gyawali, B.; Shimokata, T.; Maeda, O.; Fukaya, M.; Goto, H.; Nagino, M.; Kodera, Y. Low skeletal muscle density is associated with poor survival in patients who receive chemotherapy for metastatic gastric cancer. *Oncol. Rep.* **2015**, *35*, 1727–1731. [CrossRef] [PubMed]
14. Lee, J.S.; Kim, Y.S.; Kim, E.Y.; Jin, W. Prognostic significance of CT-determined sarcopenia in patients with advanced gastric cancer. *PLoS ONE* **2018**, *13*, e0202700. [CrossRef]
15. Dijksterhuis, W.P.; Pruijt, M.J.; Van Der Woude, S.O.; Klaassen, R.; Kurk, S.A.; Van Oijen, M.G.; Van Laarhoven, H.W. Association between body composition, survival, and toxicity in advanced esophagogastric cancer patients receiving palliative chemotherapy. *J. Cachex Sarcopenia Muscle* **2019**, *10*, 199–206. [CrossRef] [PubMed]
16. Hacker, U.T.; Hasenclever, D.; Linder, N.; Stocker, G.; Chung, H.; Kang, Y.; Moehler, M.; Busse, H.; Lordick, F. Prognostic role of body composition parameters in gastric/gastroesophageal junction cancer patients from the EXPAND trial. *J. Cachex Sarcopenia Muscle* **2019**, *11*, 135–144. [CrossRef]
17. Tan, B.; Brammer, K.; Randhawa, N.; Welch, N.; Parsons, S.; James, E.; Catton, J. Sarcopenia is associated with toxicity in patients undergoing neo-adjuvant chemotherapy for oesophago-gastric cancer. *Eur. J. Surg. Oncol.* **2015**, *41*, 333–338. [CrossRef]
18. Palmela, C.; Velho, S.; Agostinho, L.; Branco, F.; Santos, M.; Santos, M.P.C.; Oliveira, M.H.; Strecht, J.; Maio, R.; Cravo, M.; et al. Body Composition as a Prognostic Factor of Neoadjuvant Chemotherapy Toxicity and Outcome in Patients with Locally Advanced Gastric Cancer. *J. Gastric Cancer* **2017**, *17*, 74–87. [CrossRef]
19. Dev, R.; Bruera, E.; Dalal, S. Insulin resistance and body composition in cancer patients. *Ann. Oncol.* **2018**, *29*, ii18–ii26. [CrossRef] [PubMed]
20. Moon, H.-G.; Ju, Y.-T.; Jeong, C.-Y.; Jung, E.-J.; Lee, Y.-J.; Hong, S.-C.; Ha, W.-S.; Park, S.-T.; Choi, S.-K. Visceral Obesity May Affect Oncologic Outcome in Patients with Colorectal Cancer. *Ann. Surg. Oncol.* **2008**, *15*, 1918–1922. [CrossRef]
21. Clark, W.; Siegel, E.M.; Chen, Y.A.; Zhao, X.; Parsons, C.M.; Hernandez, J.M.; Weber, J.; Thareja, S.; Choi, J.; Shibata, D. Quantitative Measures of Visceral Adiposity and Body Mass Index in Predicting Rectal Cancer Outcomes after Neoadjuvant Chemoradiation. *J. Am. Coll. Surg.* **2013**, *216*, 1070–1081. [CrossRef]
22. Harada, K.; Baba, Y.; Ishimoto, T.; Kosumi, K.; Tokunaga, R.; Izumi, D.; Ida, S.; Imamura, Y.; Iwagami, S.; Miyamoto, Y.; et al. Low Visceral Fat Content is Associated with Poor Prognosis in a Database of 507 Upper Gastrointestinal Cancers. *Ann. Surg. Oncol.* **2015**, *22*, 3946–3953. [CrossRef]
23. Okamura, A.; Watanabe, M.; Mine, S.; Nishida, K.; Imamura, Y.; Kurogochi, T.; Kitagawa, Y.; Sano, T. Clinical Impact of Abdominal Fat Distribution on Prognosis After Esophagectomy for Esophageal Squamous Cell Carcinoma. *Ann. Surg. Oncol.* **2015**, *23*, 1387–1394. [CrossRef]
24. Park, H.S.; Kim, H.S.; Beom, S.H.; Rha, S.Y.; Chung, H.C.; Kim, J.H.; Chun, Y.J.; Lee, S.W.; Choe, E.-A.; Heo, S.J.; et al. Marked Loss of Muscle, Visceral Fat, or Subcutaneous Fat After Gastrectomy Predicts Poor Survival in Advanced Gastric Cancer: Single-Center Study from the CLASSIC Trial. *Ann. Surg. Oncol.* **2018**, *25*, 3222–3230. [CrossRef]
25. Kim, H.; Ro, S.M.; Yang, J.H.; Jeong, J.W.; Lee, J.E.; Roh, S.Y.; Kim, I.-H. The neutrophil-to-lymphocyte ratio prechemotherapy and postchemotherapy as a prognostic marker in metastatic gastric cancer. *Korean J. Intern. Med.* **2018**, *33*, 990–999. [CrossRef] [PubMed]
26. Wang, J.; Qu, J.; Li, Z.; Che, X.; Liu, J.; Teng, Y.; Jin, B.; Zhao, M.; Liu, Y.; Qu, X. Pretreatment platelet-to-lymphocyte ratio is associated with the response to first-line chemotherapy and survival in patients with metastatic gastric cancer. *J. Clin. Lab. Anal.* **2017**, *32*, e22185. [CrossRef]
27. Common Terminology Criteria for Adverse Events (CTCAE) Protocol Development CTEP. Available online: https://ctep.cancer.gov/protocoldevelopment/electronic_applications/ctc.htm (accessed on 29 January 2021).
28. Schwartz, L.H.; Litière, S.; De Vries, E.; Ford, R.; Gwyther, S.; Mandrekar, S.; Shankar, L.; Bogaerts, J.; Chen, A.; Dancey, J.; et al. RECIST 1.1—Update and clarification: From the RECIST committee. *Eur. J. Cancer* **2016**, *62*, 132–137. [CrossRef]
29. Prado, C.M.; Baracos, V.E.; McCargar, L.J.; Mourtzakis, M.; Mulder, K.E.; Reiman, T.; Butts, C.A.; Scarfe, A.G.; Sawyer, M.B. Body Composition as an Independent Determinant of 5-Fluorouracil–Based Chemotherapy Toxicity. *Clin. Cancer Res.* **2007**, *13*, 3264–3268. [CrossRef] [PubMed]
30. Aubrey, J.; Esfandiari, N.; Baracos, V.E.; Buteau, F.A.; Frenette, J.; Putman, C.T.; Mazurak, V.C. Measurement of skeletal muscle radiation attenuation and basis of its biological variation. *Acta Physiol.* **2014**, *210*, 489–497. [CrossRef] [PubMed]
31. Doyle, S.L.; Donohoe, C.L.; Lysaght, J.; Reynolds, J.V. Visceral obesity, metabolic syndrome, insulin resistance and cancer. *Proc. Nutr. Soc. USA* **2012**, *71*, 181–189. [CrossRef]

MDPI
St. Alban-Anlage 66
4052 Basel
Switzerland
Tel. +41 61 683 77 34
Fax +41 61 302 89 18
www.mdpi.com

Journal of Clinical Medicine Editorial Office
E-mail: jcm@mdpi.com
www.mdpi.com/journal/jcm